MASTER THE BOARDS

Internal Medicine

SECOND EDITION

OTHER EDUCATIONAL TOOLS BY CONRAD FISCHER, MD

Books

Master the Boards USMLE® Step 2 CK

Master the Boards USMLE® Step 3

Master the Wards Internal Medicine Clerkship:
Survive Clerkship & Ace the Shelf

Internal Medicine Question Book

Master the Boards USMLE® Medical Ethics

Flashcards

USMLE® Diagnostic Test Flashcards:
The 200 Questions You Need to Know for the Exam for Steps 2 & 3

USMLE® Examination Flashcards:
The 200 "Most Likely Diagnosis" Questions You Will See on the Exam for Steps 2 & 3

USMLE® Pharmacology and Treatment Flashcards:
The 200 Questions You're Most Likely to See on Steps 1, 2 & 3

USMLE® Physical Findings Flashcards:
The 200 Questions You're Most Likely to See on the Exam

Online

Dr. Conrad Fischer's USMLE® Disease Deck Revised! (*app*)

Dr. Conrad Fischer's Comprehensive Cases

Updated USMLE® Step 3 Qbank

MASTER THE BOARDS

Internal Medicine

THE HIGHEST-YIELD REVIEW FOR THE ABIM® EXAM

SECOND EDITION

Conrad Fischer, MD

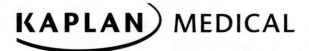

© 2013, 2011 by Conrad Fischer, MD

The authors of the following sections have granted Conrad Fischer, MD, and Kaplan Publishing exclusive use of their work:

Niket Sonpal, MD—Chapter 6: Gastroenterology

Published by Kaplan Publishing, a division of Kaplan, Inc.
395 Hudson Street, 4th Floor
New York, NY 10014

Printed in the United States of America

10 9 8 7 6 5 4 3 2 1

ISBN-13: 978-1-60978-880-3

Kaplan Publishing books are available at special quantity discounts to use for sales promotions, employee premiums, or educational purposes. For more information or to purchase books, please call the Simon & Schuster special sales department at 866-506-1949.

DEDICATION

This book is dedicated to:

Conrad Fischer, MD

Conrad is an amazing educator with tremendous passion and commitment. The author wishes to recognize himself for the months of backbreaking work it took to stay up night after night to create this book.

ACKNOWLEDGMENTS

The author wishes to acknowledge dear Debbie C., who patiently waited for another book to be born. Thank you for being so kind and warm.

Dr. Sonpal would like to acknowledge and dedicate his chapter to his mom. Thank you for supporting me in all my dreams.

About the Author

Conrad Fischer, MD, is director of educational development for the Department of Medicine at Jamaica Hospital Medical Center in New York City. Jamaica Hospital is a robust window on the world of medicine. Dr. Fischer is also chairman of medicine for Kaplan Medical, teaching USMLE Steps 1, 2, and 3, Internal Medicine Board Review and Attending Recertification, and USMLE Step 1 Physiology. Dr. Fischer is associate professor of physiology, pharmacology, and medicine at Touro College of Osteopathic Medicine in New York City.

Niket Sonpal, MD, author of the Gastroenterology chapter, is chief resident at Lenox Hill Hospital and assistant clinical professor at Touro College of Osteopathic Medicine in New York City. He is also co-author of *Master the Boards USMLE Step 2 CK* and a member of the faculty on Kaplan Medical's Step 2 High-Yield course.

SECTION EDITORS

All of the section editors are faculty members in the Department of Medicine at Jamaica Hospital Medical Center. The author expresses his appreciation to each of the following individuals for ensuring the accuracy of the following chapters:

Cardiology: Beppy Edasery, MD; Sudheer Chauhan, MD

Dermatology: Farshad Bagheri, MD

Endocrinology: Richard Pinsker, MD; Narinder Kukar, MD

Gastroenterology: Asit Mehta, MD; Avani Patel, MD

General Internal Medicine: Sudheer Chauhan, MD; Ratilal T. Patel, MD; Naveen Pathak, MD

Geriatrics: Kaushik Doshi, MD; Surendra Mahadevia, MD

Hematology: Jose Cervantes, MD; Kunal Patel, MD

Infectious Diseases: Farshad Bagheri, MD

Nephrology: Sudheer Chauhan, MD

Neurology: Hasit Thakur, MD

Oncology: Jose Cervantes, MD; Kunal Patel, MD

Pulmonary: Craig Thurm, MD; Mohammad Babury, MD; Mahendra C. Patel, MD; Artur Shalonov, MD; Samir Sarkar, MD

Rheumatology: Jebun Nahar, MD; Katerina Teller, MD; Eduardo Andre, MD

Women's Health: Jebun Nahar, MD

TABLE OF CONTENTS

AUTHOR'S NOTE

It is my sincere hope that I have created a unique and useful book to prepare you for the American Board of Internal Medicine (ABIM) examination or for greater depth of study in internal medicine. Initially, the volume of information you must absorb will seem overwhelming. All I can tell you for sure is:

- While the knowledge you must eventually acquire seems infinite, it isn't.
- The amount you need for this standardized test is certainly finite.

The format this book follows is the pattern of the most frequently asked questions on the exam:

1. What is the most likely diagnosis?

2. What is the best initial test?

3. What is the most accurate test?

4. Which of the following physical findings is most likely to be found in this patient?

5. What is the best initial therapy?

In addition, we will show you the most likely results of EKGs, x-rays, and CT and MRI scans to be found on the test.

Studying a lot can feel hard and painful. It is an effort. I will share with you, then, the solvent for painful efforts in the area of medicine.

- Everything you are learning here is useful to help people.
- The "smartest" or most knowledgeable that most people ever are in medicine is the day they walk into their boards. This is, therefore, a high point or peak experience. Don't waste it.
- You can always rest later; you can't study for your boards later.

My suggestion on how to use this book is:

1. Study one subject as a time.

2. Read it in multiple (3 to 4) different sources.

3. Use a book of practice questions only after you have studied the subject. Don't start with practice questions.

If you study a small number of subjects repetitively, it will provide more depth and you will develop a greater sense of satisfaction. It may feel slower, but it is more focused and you become more confident.

What Do I Do if I Hate Certain Subspecialties?

Not to worry! Say you love pulmonary and hate hematology, or the other way around. You actually can pass the ABIM examination by picking your favorite subjects and studying them really, really well. Remember, on the ABIM exam, no one ever asks your ranking. A "pass" is as good as the 99th percentile in the eyes of the world. Therefore, for the less attentive person, it is better to…I am sorry, what was I saying?

Ah yes! For those with limited attention, it is better to study the things you like really well than to be superficial over every subject. I myself studied this way. Only later did I fully learn the other subjects.

Your "Calling"

I have spent just short of 30 years in the classroom. I taught my first class, physiology, by accident as a 19-year-old college junior. I spent another year teaching physics to college students. I was never sick and I had no sick relatives. How, then, did I know to go to medical school? Because it is a calling. A calling means you try to grasp where your great passion and the world's great need meet.

As a physician, you are different from the other healthcare providers. No other branch of caregivers needed a law to limit them to 80 hours a week of work. Anyone can do a job if it is easy. The reason we are "professional" is that we get the job done whether it is easy or not. At the end of the day, we are not done when our shift is done. We are done when the job is done. We are done when people are taken care of, not when the clock hits a certain hour. I was on rounds today, a Saturday morning on a 3-day holiday weekend. The resident had been up all night and was tired and hungry. He wanted to stop and to leave. But he did not. He took care of patients. He started to develop a nosebleed and had to sit down, and continued to present patients and do the right thing, despite bleeding.

We do not seek suffering for ourselves. We do not create pain or make the process needlessly difficult. When pain comes in the process of our mission, our goal, our duty, however, we do not avoid it. This is the process of our training that makes us, as physicians, better than the other professions.

In a homogenized world where everyone is supposed to be the same, we as doctors are simply not the same. We work harder, study longer, and stay past any arbitrary outside clock until our duty is fulfilled.

This book is the culmination and the result of decades of classroom experience and thousands of patients seen. I hope you will find it useful. If you use it correctly, you will "master the boards" as well as relieve suffering.

And that is a mighty fine thing to do in this lifetime!

IMPLICATIONS OF BOARD CERTIFICATION

Board certification in the past was considered a sign of excellence. Currently, however, when the pass rate has been averaging 80% to 90%, board certification has become simply a sign of competence. This has led to tremendous difficulties in employability for those not certified. The examination is not graded on a curve, so theoretically, everyone taking the examination in a certain year could pass.

IS MY RESIDENCY EXPERIENCE ENOUGH?

Let us say you went to a busy, well-run residency where you had enormous clinical exposure and great teaching. Is it enough to prepare for your boards?

ABSOLUTELY NOT!

It doesn't matter if you do a 300-year-long residency in a great program. It is not enough. There are simply too many subjects that you need to cover. There are too many diseases that you never see because they are never admitted to the hospital where the majority of teaching occurs. There are more than 7,000 primary test takers a year for the ABIM exam, and there are only a few hundred cases of Brugada syndrome in the history of the world's literature. Even if every case were seen by ten residents, it still would not be enough. Did you see Alport syndrome? Liddle syndrome? Is there a case of Churg-Strauss syndrome for every morning report for every hospital?

The answer is: You need to study for boards to supplement your experience because there are just too many unusual diseases you will not see for a long time. The good news is: There are many, many things you will study just for boards that you will later diagnose and recognize simply because you learned them for a test.

FAIRNESS

Is the test fair?

ABSOLUTELY!

No one designing the ABIM exam is trying to fool you or make you fail. There is a rigorous intellectual honesty to the test. Your efforts are not lost. If you follow the blueprint for the exam, all you need is honest study and rigorous effort for a short period of time. And you will succeed.

Dr. Conrad Fischer

2013, New York City

How to Use This Book

Master the Boards: Internal Medicine is not a textbook—it is a review book: a review of the information that you need to know for this exam.

The layout is primarily presented as an outline, mostly with the use of short phrases either in paragraph form or in bulleted or numbered lists. Comparative material is presented in tables, and there are images that represent some of the issues discussed in the text. In each chapter, the emphasis is on presentation, etiology, diagnostic tests, and treatment. In addition, key words in making a diagnosis; major associations with the disease; and choosing the best initial test, the most accurate test, the best initial therapy, and the most effective therapy are covered. Tips and sidebars direct you to targeted information and can help you complete a brief final review prior to taking your exam.

About the Internal Medicine Certification Exam

The Internal Medicine Certification Exam is given on several dates, usually in August each year, at Pearson VUE centers worldwide. The exam is taken in a single day over about 10 hours, which includes time for registration, three optional breaks, and an optional tutorial and survey. There are four 2-hour sessions of the exam, and a single session may have as many as 60 questions. This computer-based test consists of between 270 and 352 questions. Questions are single best answer (multiple-choice), and the majority (more than 75%) are based on patient presentations.

Normal laboratory values are provided to you and some questions require you to interpret a visual such as an electrocardiogram.

Breakdown of the ABIM by Subspecialty

The breakdown of the examination by subspecialty is:

Medical content category	Percentage
Cardiovascular Disease	14%
Pulmonary Disease	10%
Gastroenterology	9%
Infectious Disease	9%
Rheumatology/Orthopedics	8%
Endocrinology, Diabetes, and Metabolism	8%
Medical Oncology	7%
Hematology	6%
Nephrology/Urology	6%
Allergy/Immunology	3%
Psychiatry	4%
Neurology	4%
Dermatology	3%
Obstetrics/Gynecology	2%
Ophthalmology	2%
Otorhinolaryngology	2%
Miscellaneous	3%
Total	100%

Internal Medicine Certification Exam Eligibility Requirements

In order to sit for the exam, you must be a graduate of an accepted medical school (accredited by the Liaison Committee on Medical Education in the United States, the Committee for Accreditation of Canadian Medical Schools, or the American Osteopathic Association). Otherwise, you must have an Educational Commission for Foreign Medical Graduates certificate or comparable credentials from the Medical Council of Canada, or documented training if you used the Fifth Pathway (per the American Medical Association) to enter graduate medical education in the United States. In addition, you must have completed 36 calendar months of Accreditation Council for Graduate Medical Education–accredited graduate medical education before August 31 of the year you take the exam. You must also demonstrate competence in the care of patients in a clinical setting. Please refer to the ABIM website (www.abim.org) for complete details about your eligibility.

REGISTRATION

The registration period for the Internal Medicine Certification Exam is from December 1 through February 1. You must complete and submit an application form, which can be done online. When the form has been successfully transmitted to ABIM, you will receive a confirmation number. This number should be kept for your records. Once you have submitted your application, you will receive instructions on contacting a Pearson VUE test center to schedule your exam. If there are any changes to your name or contact information between registration and your test date, you must notify ABIM in writing online or by mail. At the time of publication, the registration fee is $1,280. For the most accurate, up-to-date information about registration and test day procedures, visit the ABIM website.

SCORING

Passing Score

This exam is pass-fail. Because this determination is based on your overall performance on the exam, it is important to answer as many questions as possible; unanswered questions are scored as incorrect. The passing score is determined by the examination committee and approved by ABIM's board of directors. A general rule, however, is that you must answer approximately two-thirds of the questions correctly in order to pass. In 2012, 81% of first-time test takers passed the Internal Medicine Certification Exam.

Score Reporting

Three months after the last date of the exam in your area, results are released and you will receive a score report in the mail. However, the ABIM website indicates when results are released, and you can find out whether you passed or failed by checking the exam history section of your ABIM account. Your actual score report is available only by mail.

ON THE DAY OF THE EXAM

1. Arrive at the test center at least 30 minutes before your scheduled testing time to allow for check-in. If you arrive late, you may not be permitted to take the exam.
2. You must bring your confirmation and two forms of ID. The first must be an acceptable, unexpired form of identification with a recent photograph. Acceptable forms of identification include a driver's license or a U.S. passport. Your secondary ID must include your signature, but not necessarily a photo. Examples include a valid credit or debit card or a Social

Security card. The names on both forms of ID must match the name with which you registered for the exam.

3. Be prepared to leave all personal items outside the testing area, including wallets or purses, cell phones, watches, pens, and paper.

About the ABIM Maintenance of Certification Exam

When you pass the ABIM Certification Exam, you are certified as a diplomate of ABIM. This certification is valid for only 10 years, after which time you must pass the ABIM Maintenance of Certification Exam. The exam is given twice per year, once in the spring and once in the fall.

Review Beyond the ABIM

Others besides those taking the Internal Medicine Certification Exam for the first time may find this book helpful. While the material goes beyond that needed for the USMLE, knowledge for that exam is presented (and reflective of the types of questions typically asked). Physicians who need to recertify in internal medicine may find that a reading of this book is a useful way to prepare. It may also be used as a quick office reference guide, although there are no specifics in terms of dosing of drugs or the use of precise treatment protocols.

So whatever your goal, you should find this review book useful in terms of strengthening your internal medicine knowledge. You might even learn something that you previously did not know. Study all parts thoroughly and never assume that because something is uncommon, you will not see a question on it. So study everything well, and good luck.

GENERAL INTERNAL MEDICINE

INTRODUCTION

General internal medicine, which includes all screening, is one of the most highly tested areas of the boards. Although this chapter is brief, nearly every fact is eligible to be tested. The American Board of Internal Medicine (ABIM) examination is meant to test the basic competence of the general internist. As such, the level of oncology tested, for example, always includes the current screening recommendations for cancer, whereas specific types of chemotherapy for a disease such as multiple myeloma may not be tested at all. You do not need to go to medical school to know that screening tests detect cancer, but you *do* have to go to medical school to know which ones will lower mortality.

> What screening tests lower mortality? Mammography, PAP smears, and colonoscopy.

▶ **TIP**

Do not walk into the exam without knowing the most current screening recommendations.

Whose Recommendations Are You Tested On?

ABIM and all board examinations predominantly use the recommendations of the United States Preventive Services Task Force (USPSTF), an independent panel that has no financial incentive for its recommendations.

For example, USPSTF states clearly that there is no definite recommendation to screen men for prostate cancer with prostate specific antigen (PSA). On the other hand, the American Urological Association recommends screening with PSA and a digital rectal examination starting at the age of 40. You are **not** tested on the recommendations of private organizations with a strong financial interest in the outcome of a test. The National Cancer Institute permissively recommends screening PSA starting at the age of 50. "Permissively" means they acknowledge the controversy and let you know Medicare will pay for the test at age 50.

> There is no definite mortality benefit with the use of PSA. PSA is not recommended as a general screening test.

This book will not engage in lengthy pro and con discussions; rather, it will give direct recommendations on what you should answer if the question comes up. Although the exam includes a number of challenging and complicated subjects, this book's purpose is to give you an answer with the minimum number of facts to memorize. This does not mean this book is superficial or incomplete; it simply means it will jump to the bottom-line answer.

How Do the Boards Handle Controversial or Unclear Areas of Medicine?

The boards are absolutely not the place where controversies will be worked out. If a question seems controversial or the answer unclear based on your understanding of the best current data, you may want to consider that a number of questions on your examination are experimental. This means they are being tested to see how many people get them right.

The boards have a simple solution to controversial issues: The right answer will be the one that is most broadly supported by current research.

For example:

Which of the following statements concerning prostate cancer is correct?

a. PSA should be offered routinely at age 40.
b. PSA should be offered routinely at age 50.
c. Digital rectal examination should be offered routinely at age 40.
d. Screening with PSA lowers mortality.
e. A rapidly rising level of PSA is associated with an increased risk of prostate cancer.

Answer: The correct answer is (e). This statement is correct. The question is intelligently put because it sidesteps the issue of whether you should be doing the test in favor of a statement that everyone can agree upon. Another correct statement could have been: "If a man fully understanding the risks and benefits of PSA testing is requesting the test, then the test should be performed."

▶ TIP

Every boards question appears as an experimental question at least once before it joins the scored portion of the exam.

How Do I Answer Questions Concerning Recommendations that Have Recently Changed?

Never try to "time" the exam in terms of answering based on what was correct when you think the question was written. Answer based on your understanding of the recommendation on the day of the test. For instance, on February 24, 2010, the recommendation for influenza vaccination was changed to include all adults, not just those over age 50. Do not answer based on whether you think that a new question could be written, edited, and incorporated into the ABIM examination given in August of the same year. Rather, answer based on the current recommendation at the time of your exam.

The reason it takes several weeks to get your grade after taking the test is that ABIM is reviewing the questions, partly to see how they are answered and partly to discard questions that may have become inaccurate since the time the exam was written. ABIM will discard questions whose answers have changed in light of new recommendations.

> You will not be penalized because your knowledge is more current than the content of the exam.

CANCER SCREENING

Breast Cancer

The strongest evidence shows that screening for breast cancer is most effective beginning at age 50. There is controversy surrounding screening between the ages of 40 and 50. However, the boards have never engaged in this controversy. The greatest benefit of screening with mammography has always been in those above the age of 50.

Which of the following is most likely to benefit a patient with breast cancer?

a. Screening with ultrasound
b. Screening with MRI
c. Tamoxifen in those with 2 first-degree relatives with breast cancer
d. Soy diet
e. Exercise
f. Low-fat diet
g. BRCA testing

Answer: The correct answer is (c). Estrogen inhibition is an underutilized therapy to prevent breast cancer. Tamoxifen and raloxifene are not routinely recommended in those with an average risk of cancer, but having relatives with breast cancer markedly increases the risk of cancer. Ultrasound helps distinguish cystic from solid lesions, particularly in younger women. MRI as a screening method is not yet of clear value. Although soy diets and exercise may have some benefit, it is not nearly as clear as that of antiestrogen therapy. In women with a strong family history suggestive of a mutation, BRCA testing will detect an increased risk of breast and other cancers, such as ovarian. However, it is not clear what the right therapeutic intervention in those with a positive test is.

BRCA Testing

BRCA is associated with an increased risk of cancer, especially with a family history of cancer.

- The **intervention** for a positive test is **not clear**.
- Prophylactic mastectomy (and oophorectomy) for a positive test is **not clearly recommended** for all who test positive.

> It is not enough just to detect an increased risk of cancer. To intervene, you must detect an increased risk of cancer that you can do something about.

- There is **no clear mortality benefit** to routine BRCA testing.
- **BRCA** is associated with an **increased risk of ovarian cancer, in addition to numerous other cancers, such as prostate and pancreas.**

First-degree relatives = siblings and parents

Tamoxifen and raloxifene will also treat osteoporosis in addition to decreasing the risk of breast cancer.

Prophylactic Tamoxifen and Raloxifene Prevent Breast Cancer

Tamoxifen and raloxifene reduce the risk of breast cancer by 50% to 70%. When a patient has multiple first-degree relatives with breast cancer, tamoxifen is FDA-approved for prevention of breast cancer in premenopausal women; in postmenopausal women, either tamoxifen or raloxifene should be used to prevent the development of breast cancer. The best age at which to start treatment is not precisely known. There is no clear benefit when starting before age 40. The greatest benefit is in those above age 50. Treatment should be continued for at least 5 years.

The most common adverse effects of tamoxifen are:

- Hot flashes
- Leg cramps
- **Endometrial cancer** (unusual)
- Deep vein **thrombosis**
- Cataracts

► **TIP**

Boards questions have to be clear. The boards will not provide a scenario in which the patient's age is equivocal or unclear.

The benefits of the prophylactic use of tamoxifen were clearly measurable even after 10 years of use. The adverse effects did not persist or occur after 5 years. In addition to markedly reducing the risk of breast cancer, there was a 30% reduction in the risk of osteoporotic fractures.

Lifetime Risk of Developing Breast Cancer in a Woman with No Children			
Age	No family history	One first-degree relative	Two first-degree relatives
40	10%	18%	29%
50	9%	16%	26%
60	6.5%	13%	21%

This table demonstrates the enormous increase in risk because of a family history of breast cancer.

If, for a 40-year-old woman with 2 relatives with cancer, we add in:

- Giving birth before age 20
- Menarche at age 11

The lifetime risk of breast cancer rises to 43%.

Colon Cancer

- Screening for colon cancer should begin by age 50.
- Colonoscopy is superior to all other modalities.
- Colonoscopy is performed every 10 years in the average risk population.
- Virtual (or CT) colonoscopy is never the right answer.
- Barium enema, fecal occult blood testing, and sigmoidoscopy are inferior to colonoscopy.

Special Circumstances for Colon Cancer Screening				
One family member with colon cancer	**Three family members, 2 generations, 1 premature (before age 50)**	**Familial adenomatous polyposis (FAP)**	**Inflammatory bowel disease (IBD)**	**Gardner syndrome, Juvenile polyposis, and Peutz-Jeghers syndrome**
Start at age 40 or 10 years earlier than the age the family member was diagnosed, whichever is **earlier**. Screen at regular intervals afterward.	Start at age 25 with colonoscopy every 10 years.	Screening sigmoidoscopy every 1–2 years starting at age 12.	Colonoscopy after 8–10 years of colonic involvement. Test every 1–2 years.	No additional screening.

Cervical Cancer

- Pap smears start at age 21, **irrespective** of the age of onset of **sexual activity**.
- No screening is necessary for those above age 65.
- There is no need for Pap smear in those who have had a hysterectomy.
- Pap every 3 years or every 5 years combined with HPV testing

Which of the following results in the greatest benefit?

a. Pap smear
b. Colonoscopy
c. Mammography
d. Annual chest x-ray in heavy smokers
e. PSA

> Chlamydia screening is routine for all sexually active women.

> Cervical screening: Pap and HPV testing every 5 years

Answer: The correct answer is (c). The changes in screening recommendations have not changed the answer to the most frequently asked cancer screening question. The mammogram has always been the most beneficial of all the cancer screening methods, and women above the age of 50 have always been the group that benefits the most from screening. Three cancer screening methods lower mortality: Pap, mammography, and colonoscopy. Mammography is simply the best of these. This is an example of a question that sidesteps controversy, since breast cancer kills more people than both cervical and colon cancer. Annual screening chest x-rays have never been found to be beneficial in any group, including smokers.

Cancer Tests that Are Never the Right Answer

- No blood test has ever been found to lower cancer mortality. This includes carcinoembryonic antigen (CEA), alpha-fetoprotein (AFP), CA-125, and PSA.
- Screening chest x-rays or high-resolution CT scans
- Pelvic examination
- Breast self-exam
- Testicular examination
- Anal Pap smear
- Skin examination for melanoma
- Any blood or radiologic test for pancreatic, ovarian, or bladder cancer

Annual screening chest x-ray is not recommended for any group.

DIABETES, HYPERTENSION, HYPERLIPIDEMIA, ABDOMINAL AORTIC ANEURYSM, AND OSTEOPOROSIS

Diabetes

Screen for Type 2 diabetes in those with blood pressure **above 135/80 mg/dL**. Diabetes is diagnosed with 2 fasting blood glucoses above 125 mg/dL or a hemoglobin A_{1c} above 6.5%. The goal of LDL cholesterol levels is <100 mg/dL in diabetics.

The BP cutoff for diabetes screening is a unique number for this circumstance, at only 135/80 mg/dL.

Hypertension

Screen for hypertension at every office visit in those over the age of 18.

Hyperlipidemia

- Screen men above age 35 every 5 years.
- Screen women above age 45 every 5 years.
- Screen persons above 20 years of age who have additional cardiovascular risk factors (HTN, DM).

Abdominal Aortic Aneurysm

- Screen all men aged 65 to 75 who have ever smoked.
- Use ultrasound above age 65.

Osteoporosis

Screening

- Screen women above age 65 (or above 60 with risk factors such as chronic steroid use or weight less than 70 kg) with bone densitometry (DEXA scanning).
- A T-score **1 to 2.5 standard deviations** below normal is **osteopenia**.
- A T-score **more than 2.5 standard deviations** below normal is **osteoporosis**.
- Screen every 2 years.

The **T-score** is a measure of a woman's bone density as **compared to that of a healthy young woman**.

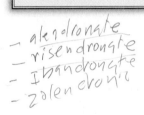

Hip fracture in an elderly woman is fatal far more often than a myocardial infarction.

TREATMENT

1. **Vitamin D** and **calcium** supplementation are routinely indicated in all patients with either osteopenia or osteoporosis.
2. **Bisphosphonates** (alendronate, risendronate, ibandronate, zolendronic acid): These medications will reduce the likelihood of hip and vertebral fracture by 50% in those with decreased bone density. Adverse effects are:
   - Osteonecrosis of the jaw
   - Esophagitis if not taken with adequate fluid intake
3. **Exercise with high-impact physical activity.** Running, stair-climbing, and weight training all increase bone density.

Alternate Therapy (Less Evidence than Bisphosphonates)

Several other therapies exist that would be the correct answer only if bisphosphonates were not in the choices or there was a contraindication or complication of bisphosphonate use.

- **Teriparatide:** an analogue of PTH that increases new collagenous bone matrix formation
- **Calcitonin:** decreases vertebral fractures, but does not clearly reduce hip fractures
- **Raloxifene:** a selective estrogen receptor modifier that also decreases the risk of breast cancer
- **Estrogen replacement:** limited benefit with severe osteoporosis
- **Denosumab:** a RANKL inhibitor that stops osteoclasts

Diseases Not to Be Routinely Screened (The Wrong Answers)

- Thyroid disease
- Hemochromatosis
- Carotid artery stenosis
- Glaucoma

IMMUNIZATIONS

Hepatitis A and B Vaccines

Although hepatitis A and B vaccinations have both been added to the routine vaccinations in childhood, adults should be vaccinated in the following circumstances:

- Chronic liver disease
- Men who have sex with men
- Injection drug users
- Household contacts of those with the active disease

Hepatitis A vaccine is recommended for those traveling to countries with an unsafe food and water supply. Routine hepatitis B vaccine is recommended in healthcare workers.

> Hepatitis vaccine is of greatest benefit to patients with chronic liver disease.

Influenza Vaccine   *(inactivate form)*

Influenza vaccine is recommended annually for **all** adults. The question, however, may account for possible reversal in this recommendation back to high-risk groups by asking: "Which of the following groups is **most likely to benefit** from influenza vaccine?" The answer to this is:

- Patients with chronic disease of the heart (CHF), lung (COPD and asthma), or kidney
- Diabetic patients
- Patients with HIV/AIDS
- Pregnant women
- Immunosuppressed patients such as those with hematologic malignancy or users of glucocorticoids
- Healthcare workers
- Obese patients

- Children age 6-23 months
- Adults age 50 years and older
- Women who are pregnant during influenza season
- Persons age 2 to 50 years who have underlying chronic medical problems
- Nursing Homes and other care facility president

Pneumococcal Vaccine

This vaccine is indicated in those above age 65. Generally healthy individuals require only a single vaccination at age 65. A second vaccine is given to those whose first injection was before age 65 and in those with underlying illness such as:

- Patients with chronic disease of the heart (CHF), lung (COPD and asthma), or kidney *} Chronic Cardiovascular Disease*
- Diabetic patients *, Chronic liver disease, Alcoholism*
- Immunosuppressed patients such as those with hematologic malignancy, *cirrhosis* users of glucocorticoids, or patients with HIV/AIDS

- asplenia patient, cochlear implant, Immunocompromised Patient

Meningococcal Vaccine

Although this vaccine has now been added to the routine age 11 visit, adults should be vaccinated if they are:

- Functionally (sickle cell) or anatomically asplenic
- Living in dormitories or military barracks
- Deficient in terminal complement

Papilloma Virus Vaccine

- Routine for all women between ages 9 and 26
- Acceptable to give in men as well

Varicella Vaccine

Shingles or the reactivation of varicella, also called herpes zoster, is extremely common in elderly patients, affecting as many as 5% of patients above age 60. Varicella vaccine is a version of the vaccine given in children, but at higher dose. This is indicated in **all individuals at the age of 60.** Contraindications are the use of steroids and AIDS with less than 200 CD4 cells/µL, pregnancy, or any immunosuppression (AIDS, malignancy, immunosuppressant medications).

LOW BACK PAIN

Low back pain is so common as to be considered an expected finding in the general population. The most frequently tested point is about in which patients x-rays are useful. The vast majority of individuals are not suffering from cord compression or spinal stenosis. Hence, unless there are additional severe findings described in the case, the most likely answer is:

- No x-rays
- No bed rest
- Yes to moderate exercise and stretching such as yoga

> **A positive straight leg raise does not count as a "focal neurological deficit."**

If there is evidence of cord compression such as focal neurological findings, vertebral tenderness, or a sensory level deficit, the "most appropriate next step in the management of the patient" is to give steroids and obtain an MRI or CT.

If there is fever in addition to focal neurological findings, vertebral tenderness, or a sensory level deficit, then you should add antibiotics that are active against staphylococcus, such as vancomycin, to the steroids. **Fever** with signs of cord compression **suggests a spinal epidural abscess**.

▶ **TIP**

Unless there are focal neurological findings, vertebral tenderness, incontinence, or a sensory level deficit, do not perform imaging studies of the spine.

Fever + cord compression = epidural abscess

Tetanus/Acellular Pertussis

> **Expect Tdap questions!**

A booster of tetanus toxoid is given every ten years. Tetanus toxoid acellular pertussus (Tdap) is the preferred form. If the wound is soiled or "dirty," the interval is 5 years. Give a booster in the form of Tdap.

The goal is to increase vaccination rates for pertussis by giving it every time a tetanus booster is needed.

ALLERGY AND IMMUNOLOGY

ANAPHYLAXIS

In anaphylaxis, the causative agent is not as important as the response of the host. Anaphylaxis is defined as:

- Hypotension
- Tachycardia
- Respiratory distress

This occurs in response to medication, chemical agents, insect venoms, or the ingestion of a food. In addition, the patient may have:

1. Rash, urticaria, itching, flushing
2. Bronchospasm
3. Swelling of the lips, tongue, or throat
4. Stridor
5. GI symptoms (diarrhea, nausea/vomiting)

The best initial steps in management are:

- **Epinephrine** intramuscularly (1:1,000 solution)
- Antihistamines (**diphenhydramine**)
- Intravenous fluids (normal saline)
- Oxygen
- **Corticosteroids**
- Inhaled bronchodilators such as albuterol
- H2 blockers

Epinephrine

Epinephrine will work the **most rapidly** and will restore central perfusion pressure. In addition, epinephrine will reverse bronchospasm and laryngospasm. When anaphylaxis occurs, especially with hypotension and any form

> Epinephrine self-injection (epi-pen) is given when repeat anaphylaxis may occur.

of respiratory distress, there are no contraindications to the use of epinephrine. Steroids will take 4 to 6 hours to work, whereas epinephrine will work instantly. Antihistamines do not have the same decrease of efficacy as steroids or epinephrine. When an insect sting may recur after anaphylaxis, the best initial management is desensitization and epi-pen.

▶ TIP

Epinephrine is used as a 1:1,000 solution intramuscularly in anaphylaxis. It is used as a 1:10,000 solution intravenously for cardiac resuscitation.

Epinephrine Use in Asthma

In an acute exacerbation of asthma, there are contraindications to the use of epinephrine. This is because in asthma there is:

> There are no contraindications to epinephrine when there is **any** concern that anaphylaxis may be life-threatening.

- Effective alternative therapy such as albuterol
- Potential harm in those with a history of coronary artery disease

URTICARIA AND ANGIOEDEMA

DEFINITION/PRESENTATION/ETIOLOGY

Urticaria is defined as eruptions of itchy, red wheals or hives with sharp borders, commonly affecting the trunk and extremities but sparing palms and soles.

> Urticaria can be caused by infection.

Acute urticaria may be caused by **bugs** (insect bites), **drugs** (e.g., penicillin), or **foods, but frequently there is no known cause.** Chronic urticaria is caused by **pressure, cold, and vibration.** Chronic urticaria is defined as lasting longer than 6 weeks. Nearly half of those with chronic urticaria never have a specific etiology identified.

> Itching is not always present with urticaria and angioedema.

Angioedema is a severe, life-threatening form of urticaria. Angioedema implies swelling of **deeper** subcutaneous tissues such as the lips, face, and eyelids. Both urticaria and angioedema can be associated with laryngeal edema and hypotension.

> Aspirin and other NSAIDs can worsen urticaria due to mast cell degranulation.

Common Causes of Acute Urticaria				
Bugs	**Drugs**	**Foods**	**Other**	**Contact**
• Bee stings	• Penicillin	• Shellfish	• Hereditary	• Latex
• Feathers	• Aspirin	• Tomatoes		
• Animal dander	• NSAIDs	• Strawberries		
	• Morphine and codeine	• Nuts, especially peanuts		
	• ACE inhibitors (presents without hives)	• Eggs		
	• Sulfa drugs	• Chocolate		
	• Contrast agents			

No response to glucocorti cord [handwritten]

DIAGNOSTIC TESTS

Acute urticaria is a clinical diagnosis and needs no diagnostic testing, and there should be no delay in administering treatment. Chronic urticaria is best managed by trying to identify and eliminate the trigger. A CBC is done to look for eosinophilia. Food, pollen, and latex allergies can be identified with radio-allergosorbent (RAST) testing. Skin testing confirms the presence of allergen-specific IgE. RAST is done when skin testing is not possible.

> Icatibant is a bradykinin antagonist used for hereditary angioedema.

TREATMENT

Severe urticaria is treated with antihistamines such as hydroxyzine or cyproheptadine, although these are sedating; occasionally a few weeks of steroids are required. Milder urticaria can be controlled with newer, nonsedating antihistamines such as:

Handwritten margin note:
Vistaryl
Hydroxyzine
Atara *
↓
Antihistamine
Anticholinergic (dry)
Sedative

- Fexofenadine
- Loratadine
- Cetirizine

Chronic Urticaria

- **Eliminate the trigger** if one is identified.
- **Doxepin** is a nonspecific histamine and serotonin blocker that is used for chronic urticaria.
- Avoid systemic steroids for chronic urticaria.
- Use venom immune therapy (desensitization)

> Venom immune therapy desensitizes patients when the insect sting cannot be avoided.

Prevention of Contrast Allergy

Radiologic procedures requiring iodinated contrast material are often unavoidable even in those with an allergy to this material. These patients should receive **corticosteroids and antihistamines** prior to receiving the contrast.

A 43-year-old man comes to the emergency department with severe swelling of his face, lips, and scrotum. No hives are found. He has recently been started on lisinopril for hypertension not responsive to hydrochlorothiazide. His complement levels, specifically C2 and C4, are decreased.

What is the best initial therapy for this patient?

a. Fresh frozen plasma
b. Loratadine
c. Diphenhydramine
d. Furosemide
e. Prednisone
f. Epinephrine

> C2: decreased in SLE
> C3: decreased in pyogenic bacterial infection
> C5–C9: Neisseria infection

CH$_{50}$ is the initial test for the complement pathway.

Answer: The correct answer is (a). Fresh frozen plasma (FFP) will replace C1 esterase inhibitor. Epinephrine will not be effective in those with C1 esterase inhibitor deficiency. This case has given clear evidence of C1 esterase inhibitor deficiency. In this condition, C2 levels are decreased during acute attacks. C4 is decreased both during acute attacks and between attacks.

C1 esterase inhibitor deficiency can also be treated with replacement with C1 esterase inhibitor concentrate and by giving anabolic steroids. Ecallantide is an inhibitor of kallikrein used for hereditary angioedema.

ALLERGIC RHINITIS

DEFINITION/ETIOLOGY

Allergic rhinitis is an extremely common hypersensitivity reaction to inhaled allergens. Inhaled allergens include pollens, grasses, ragweed, molds, household mites, or pets. Symptoms can be provoked by cold air, odors, or dust. It is associated with a history of atopic disorders such as eczema, asthma, and food allergy.

PRESENTATION

Allergic rhinitis presents with:

- Rhinorrhea
- Sneezing
- Eye irritation with redness, itching, and tearing
- Occasional cough and bronchospasm

Nasal polyps are associated with chronic rhinitis.

DIAGNOSTIC TESTS

With severe symptoms, an investigation should be made to identify specific environmental allergens in order to avoid them. The most sensitive test is allergen-specific IgE levels. RAST testing and skin testing are also useful.

TREATMENT

The best initial therapy is intranasal corticosteroids.

Intranasal steroids such as beclomethasone, flunisolide, budesonide, or fluticasone are all superior to oral antihistamines such as fexofenadine, desloratadine, or cetirizine. Steroids are also less expensive than antihistamines. There are also antihistamine eye drops for treatment of local ocular symptoms.

Recurrence of allergic rhinitis is more likely with oral antihistamines than with intranasal steroids.

A 34-year-old woman is seen in the office for a chronic runny nose, cough, and itchy eyes. She has these symptoms for several weeks every spring. On physical examination, her nasal mucosa is hypertrophic, edematous, and pale. A polyp is detected. You prescribe intranasal fluticasone. She returns 3 days later because her symptoms have not resolved. She insists she is fully adherent to the fluticasone.

What is the most appropriate management?

Rhinorrhea

a. Stop intranasal steroids and switch to oral desloratadine
b. Prescribe a short course of oral prednisone
c. Tell her to temporarily leave her home
d. Tell her to continue the fluticasone
e. Switch to oral montelukast
f. Switch to inhaled cromolyn

Answer: The correct answer is (d). Intranasal steroids will take 2 weeks to reach a full effect and she has only been using it for 3 days. Antihistamines may work acutely, but you should not stop the steroids, which are ultimately associated with fewer recurrences as well as the chance to shrink her polyp. Cromolyn and montelukast are not as effective as steroids.

Patients Not Controlled with Intranasal Corticosteroids and Oral Antihistamines

For a patient with persistent symptoms after weeks of steroids and antihistamines, the answer to the question "What is the most appropriate next step in the management of this patient?" is:

- Leukotriene inhibitors (e.g., montelukast)

or

- Intranasal anticholinergic medications (ipratropium)

or

- Intranasal mast cell stabilizers (cromolyn or nedocromil)

> Intranasal steroids need 2 weeks to work.

A patient comes to the emergency department with persistent rhinorrhea, sneezing, and ocular itching despite weeks of treatment with intranasal budesonide, ipratropium, nedocromil, oral fexofenadine, and oral montelukast. Her symptoms are worse at night and on weekends. IgE testing is specific for environmental allergens.

What is the most effective management?

a. Change jobs
b. Use dustproof covers on pillows and mattress
c. Vacuum the rugs
d. Hire a professional cleaning service
e. Begin oral steroids

Answer: The correct answer is (b). Dustproof covers on pillows and mattresses decrease exposure to environmental allergens. This is more effective than just washing these items. Vacuuming is not strong enough to remove mites from the environment. Oral steroids are never the right answer for allergic rhinitis. There is no point in changing jobs for an allergen that happens at night and weekends at home.

Management of Environmental Allergens

- Remove household items containing dust (rugs, drapes, bedspreads).
- Use air purifiers and dust filters.
- Flush out allergens using nasal irrigation with saline.
- Keep household items, such as pillows, in dustproof covers.

PRIMARY IMMUNODEFICIENCY DISEASES

Common Variable Immunodeficiency

ETIOLOGY

Common variable immunodeficiency (**CVID**) is a defect in the productive capacity of B cells. **B cells** are present in **normal numbers**, but they do **not produce effective immunoglobulins**. This leads to a panhypogammaglobulinemia, although you will find a normal number of cells on CBC. Lymph **nodes** and **adenoids are present** in either normal or enlarged size. IgG, IgM, and IgA all become decreased over time. The onset may occur at any time in adulthood, hence the word "variable" in the name.

PRESENTATION

Look for an adult of either gender with frequent episodes of sinopulmonary infections such as:

- Sinusitis, otitis media, and pharyngitis
- Bronchitis and bronchiectasis
- Pneumonia (bacterial or nonbacterial; a few develop *Pneumocystis* species or other fungal pneumonia without HIV)

Gastrointestinal disorders such as celiac disease occur, as does chronic infection with *Giardia*. *Giardia* is the classic enteric pathogen. Look for malabsorption with steatorrhea.

> CVID is associated with autoimmune diseases.

DIAGNOSTIC TESTS

The B cell count is normal, but serum protein electrophoresis SPEP shows a marked **decrease in antibody production** of all types. IgG is depressed more than IgA or IgM.

> Beware of lymphoma in CVID.

TREATMENT

Besides using antibiotics as infections arise, patients should get monthly intravenous immunoglobulin injections (IVIG). With IVIG, the patient's immune function is relatively normal.

X-Linked (Bruton) Agammaglobulinemia

Because this disorder is X-linked, it presents **exclusively in male children**. The clinical manifestations of increased sinopulmonary infection are the same as for CVID. The main difference, besides the age of onset, is that this is a **deficiency in B cells**, rather than a B cell defect in production of immunoglobulins. The CBC will show a low WBC count because of **low lymphocyte count**.

Physical Examination

Lymph nodes, spleen, tonsils, adenoids, and all other machinery for the production of B cells will be markedly **diminished**.

TREATMENT

Treatment includes antibiotics for infections and monthly intravenous immunoglobulin.

DiGeorge Syndrome

This is an isolated T cell deficiency, occurring as a result of a deletion in chromosome 22. The **thymus is hypoplastic**. There are also:

- **Cardiac** defects (classically tetralogy of Fallot)
- **Hypocalcemia** from failure of parathyroid development
- **Facial** abnormalities (including cleft palate)

Treat infections as they arise. PCP prophylaxis with trimethoprim/sulfamethoxazole is given. IVIG infusion helps.

> B cells and immunoglobulins are normal in DiGeorge syndrome.

Severe Combined Immunodeficiency

In severe combined immunodeficiency (SCID), **both B cell and T cell immunity are deficient**. Patients are profoundly immunosuppressed, leading to bacterial, fungal, and viral infections. Treat with bone marrow transplantation.

IgA Deficiency

IgA deficiency is the most common primary immunodeficiency. Patients frequently survive into adulthood and may not exhibit any symptoms. Some have frequent respiratory infections and some progress to bronchiectasis.

With IgA deficiency, look for:

- Asthma
- Atopic disease
- Autoimmune disorders
- Anaphylaxis with blood transfusion

> Blood donations to IgA-deficient patients must be from IgA-deficient donors.

Treatment is symptomatic since we do not have the ability to replace IgA.

Hyper IgE Syndrome

Look for increased number of **skin and lung infections** with *Staphylococcus*. Folliculitis and boils, or carbuncles, occur frequently. Treat the infections as they arise.

Chronic Granulomatous Disease

Chronic granulomatous disease (CGD) is a defect in the granules of neutrophils. There is a defect in the oxidative burst that allows neutrophils to destroy bacteria. It is like having a match that won't light: There is a defect in the production of hydrogen peroxidase. Patients present with infections with catalase-positive organisms such as:

- *Staphylococcus aureus*
- *Burkholderia cepacia*
- *Aspergillus*

This gives recurrent, severe infections of the skin, ears, lungs, liver, and bone.

Look for "suppurating lymph nodes" with CGD.

DIAGNOSTIC TESTS

Nitroblue tetrazolium is the test that shows decreased superoxide or hydrogen peroxide production by neutrophils.

TREATMENT

Treat infections as they arise. Use **trimethoprim/sulfamethoxazole for PCP prophylaxis** as you would in AIDS. Gamma interferon is used to prevent infection.

CARDIOLOGY

3

CORONARY ARTERY DISEASE

Risk Factors

The major, and clearest, risk factors for the development of coronary artery disease (CAD) are:

- Diabetes mellitus
- Hypertension
- Tobacco smoking
- Hyperlipidemia
- Age of the patient
- Family history

Risk factors for coronary artery disease are important because:

1. They answer the "What is the most likely diagnosis?" question when the history and physical examination are equivocal.
2. They are used to lower mortality, especially in those with established coronary artery disease.

If the question describes an older male patient with chest pain, risk factors have less importance; coronary artery disease or a myocardial infarction can be present without major risk factors. Risk factors are critical for the "what is the most likely diagnosis?" question when a patient is younger than 55 or is a premenopausal woman.

Defining the Risk Factors

Diabetes Mellitus
- Two fasting blood glucose levels above 125 mg/dL
- One fasting blood glucose above 200 mg/dL with symptoms
- Two hemoglobin A1$_c$ levels above 6.5%
- Abnormal glucose tolerance test

▶**TIP**

The question will most often simply state that the patient has a history of diabetes.

Hypertension

- Blood pressure above 140/90 mm Hg
- Blood pressure **above 130/80 in diabetic patients** or those with end organ damage such as renal insufficiency

Hyperlipidemia

Hyperlipidemia is generally defined according to the level of LDL. Although an increased triglyceride level confers some increased risk of CAD and vascular disease in general, this is not as clear as the risk associated with an increased LDL level. Questions involving high levels of LDL can be challenging because the level that is dangerous or needs to be modified varies based on the number of other risk factors present and the presence of coronary disease itself.

For example:

> A 51-year-old woman comes to the office to see her primary care provider for a routine visit. Her only past medical history is hypertension that is well controlled on hydrochlorothiazide. Her LDL level is 145 mg/dL.
>
> What is the best management of her lipid level?
>
> a. No management needed
> b. Fat-restricted diet
> c. Cholestyramine
> d. Niacin
> e. Atorvastatin
>
> Answer: The correct answer is (a). This is a difficult question for many test takers. The goal of therapy for this patient is an LDL below 160 mg/dL. The patient has only a single risk factor and no coronary artery disease equivalents such as diabetes. The risk factors that are used in terms of hyperlipidemia are hypertension, tobacco smoking, family history, and older age, defined as above age 45 for a man and above age 55 for a woman. This woman has only a single risk, hypertension, and therefore does **not** need to be maintained at an LDL below 100 mm/dL as you would with CAD or one of its equivalents.

Age of the Patient

Patients are at increased risk of CAD with increasing age. This is defined as:

- Above age 45 for a man
- Above age 55 for a woman

Family History

In order for a family history to be considered significant for a patient, it has to be a history of **premature coronary disease**. If all of the patient's relatives developed CAD at the age of 80, it is not considered significant for the patient. The age cutoff for premature disease is specifically defined as:

- Under age 55 for a male relative
- Under age 65 for a female relative

The question of age in terms of family history is one of the most frequently misunderstood issues in terms of CAD. Test takers frequently take family history into account when they should not because the question describes older family members with CAD.

> Only a family history of **premature** coronary disease is considered significant for a patient.

Minor Risk Factors

There are several risk factors that have less clear pathological significance or are hard to define.

Obesity

Obesity is a risk for increased mortality in general, but it is not universally accepted as a risk for CAD. Obesity exerts its risk for CAD primarily through increasing the prevalence of diabetes, hypertension, and hyperlipidemia. Obesity separate from these diseases exerts only a small increase in the risk of CAD. This increased risk can also be neutralized by increased physical activity and exercise.

Physical Inactivity

Just as physical activity is protective against all-cause mortality, physical inactivity increases the risk of CAD. This is predominantly through the effect that physical inactivity has in increasing obesity and its subsequent increase in hypertension, hyperlipidemia, and diabetes.

Increasing Age and Male Gender

The effect of male gender on the risk of CAD is generally helpful only in those of middle age (45 to 55). By the time a woman is 5 to 10 years postmenopausal, most of the protective effects of menstruation have worn off.

▶ **TIP**

Age is not very useful in helping to answer questions about CAD, since it is unlikely you will be presented with a 20-year-old and asked to identify CAD in that age group.

Emotional Stress

This risk is nearly impossible to measure and define.

Takotsubo Cardiomyopathy

This is a sudden ballooning of the left ventricle of the heart from severe emotional or physical stress and is sometimes called transient apical ballooning syndrome. Takotsubo cardiomyopathy is not ischemic in nature, and there is no way to predict who is at risk for the disorder. The patient develops severe chest pain or symptoms of acute congestive heart failure. The EKG shows changes consistent with anterior wall myocardial infarction. There is no clearly effective therapy, and most patients have a complete recovery over time. It is thought to occur from an unpredictable massive catecholamine release.

> Severe emotions + sudden ventricular ballooning = Takotsubo cardiomyopathy

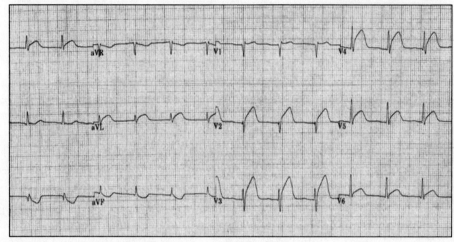

Figure 3.1: Anterior wall myocardial infarction. ST segment elevation in V2–V5.

Source: Philip Veith

PRESENTATION

CAD leading to ischemia presents with chest pain that is described as:

- Dull
- Squeezing
- Pressure-like
- Tightness or heaviness
- "Sore like being punched"

The pain of ischemia is exacerbated by physical exertion and relieved by rest. However, pain that occurs at rest can imply extremely severe ischemia.

Duration

The duration of pain that is worrisome for CAD lasts for more than a few seconds or minutes, but less than several hours. Ischemic pain can radiate to the neck, arm, or shoulder, but non-radiating pain does not exclude anything. The pain of typical ischemic episodes lasts 20 to 30 minutes.

> Pain that lasts only for seconds or persists unchanged for hours is not as ischemic in nature.

Location

The pain of ischemia from CAD localizes to being "substernal" or "retrosternal." Pain that is described as right-sided is rarely from ischemia. Even though the heart is directed anatomically more toward the left than the right, pain that is described as being on the left side of the chest is not ischemic in nature 90% of the time.

> The more lateral the pain is, the less likely it is to be ischemic in nature.

Overall, the quality and location of the pain is the most important feature that allows us to answer the "what is the most likely diagnosis?" or "what is the most appropriate next step in management?" question.

Nonspecific Features of Chest Pain

A number of associated symptoms occur with many different causes of chest pain but do not help establish a diagnosis. Many different causes of chest pain are associated with dyspnea, pallor, anxiety, diaphoresis, nausea, and fever. The presence or absence of these features will neither exclude nor prove the presence of CAD/ischemia as the cause of the patient's chest pain.

Features that Help Exclude Ischemia as the Diagnosis

Over 90% of patients coming to the emergency department with chest pain ultimately do not have a myocardial infarction. Without an EKG and cardiac enzymes, it is often impossible to know the diagnosis, either in real life or on the boards. The following features will allow you to know that the answer on the test, at least, is not ischemia. We know that the answer is **not ischemia** if the question describes pain that:

- Changes with **respiration**
- Changes with bodily **position**
- Is associated with chest wall **tenderness**

It is not necessary to have all 3 of these features present to exclude CAD. Each of them alone has a very high negative predictive value for CAD. On the boards, a 95% negative predictive value is acceptable. In clinical practice, a 5% false negative rate is not acceptable.

> Pain that changes with position, respiration, or palpation is non-ischemic 95% of the time.

Other key descriptors that help **exclude ischemia** as the cause of the chest pain:

- Knifelike or sharp
- Point-like
- Lasting for a few seconds

▶ **TIP**

The entirety of initial management is based on history + EKG in most cases.

Physical Examination

The vast majority of patients with CAD have a normal physical examination. This includes those with stable angina, unstable angina, acute coronary syndrome, and even ST segment elevation myocardial infarction.

There is a huge potential difference between "physical findings **most likely** to occur" and "complications that **may** occur."

The physical findings most likely to occur are basically **none**.

Potential complications are:

- **S4 gallop:** This is from an ischemic left ventricle that becomes stiff and non-compliant. An S4 gallop by itself is not an indication for additional therapy.
- **Murmurs of mitral or aortic regurgitation:** Myocardial infarction (MI) is associated with death of papillary muscles, which can rupture and cause acute mitral or aortic regurgitation. Patients will present with tachycardia and rales and possibly hypotension. This may need an intraaortic balloon pump and surgical repair.
- **S3 gallop:** Extension of an infarction can cause acute ventricular failure and volume overload. An S3 gallop needs afterload reduction with an ACE inhibitor or angiotensin receptor blocker (ARB).
- **Hypotension**
- **Bradycardia**
- **Rales/crepitations:** An ischemic myocardium does not pump efficiently and rales can develop due to pulmonary congestion.

Differential Diagnosis/"What Is the Most Likely Diagnosis?"

Since the majority of causes of chest pain that bring a patient to the hospital are not myocardial infarctions or even ischemic in nature, recognizing the features of the other causes of chest pain is essential. Many causes of chest pain can present with dyspnea, nausea, diaphoresis, or fever, so the best way to divide them up is by whether the pain changes with respiration or bodily position, or there is chest wall tenderness.

Pleuritic Pain (Changes with Respiration)	
Etiology	**Distinctive feature**
Pneumonia	Cough, sputum
Pneumothorax	Dyspnea, sharp pain, tracheal deviation if tension pneumothorax
Pleuritis	Friction rub
Pulmonary embolus	Sudden in onset, clear lungs
Pericarditis	Changes with bodily position: improves with sitting forward, worse when lying flat

Other Causes of Chest Pain

When a patient has chest pain and it is not from the heart, the most common etiology is in the gastrointestinal system.

Gastrointestinal Disorders

The most common gastrointestinal disorders with chest pain are reflux disease, ulcers, hiatal hernia, and gallbladder disease.

Mitral Valve Prolapse

The pain of mitral valve prolapse is atypical in nature in that:

- It is not related to exertion.
- Palpitations are common.
- It is frequently present in young women who are menstruating.
- Auscultation reveals a midsystolic click.

Aortic Aneurysm

- Pain radiates to the back in between the shoulder blades
- Difference in blood pressure between arms
- Wide mediastinum on chest x-ray

Costochondritis

Musculoskeletal pain originating from the ribs and the costochondral junctions is an extremely common cause of chest pain. Chest wall tenderness is present, and the patient is best treated with NSAIDs and other anti-inflammatory medications.

DIAGNOSTIC TESTS

EKG

The "best initial diagnostic test" for all forms of chest pain is an EKG. ST segment elevation is indicative of an infarction 75% of the time; ST segment depression is indicative of an infarction only 25% of the time. For acute coronary syndrome in the emergency department, the presence of ST segment elevation is the main feature driving the use of thrombolytics and angioplasty. If the story is typical for ischemic disease, the only truly important finding is whether there is ST elevation or not. If the EKG is abnormal and shows ST depression or T wave inversion, or is normal, it has limited importance in driving immediate therapy.

> The main drive in initial therapy is based mostly on the presence or absence of ST elevation.

Cardiac Enzymes

Cardiac enzymes such as CK-MB, troponin, or myoglobin are used in evaluating acute coronary syndromes in the emergency department. Cardiac enzymes are not useful in the stable patient in the office.

> CK-MB is the best method of confirming a reinfarction within several days.

Time Course of Cardiac Enzymes		
Name of enzyme	**First becomes abnormal**	**Duration**
Myoglobin	1–4 hours	12 hours
CK-MB	4–6 hours	1–2 days
Troponin	4–6 hours	1–2 weeks

▶ **TIP**

LDH is never the correct answer for diagnosing an acute coronary syndrome; it takes too long to become positive.

TREATMENT

Each specific coronary syndrome will be addressed separately because there is considerable variation in therapy. In the absence of contraindications, there are several medications that are used in all the syndromes. All forms of CAD are treated with:

- Aspirin
- Beta blockers (metoprolol)
- Nitrates
- Statins

Prasugrel has greater efficacy than clopidogrel in MI.

Specific Medications	
Name of medication	**Circumstances for use**
Clopidogrel, prasugrel, or ticagrelor	Acute myocardial infarction, angioplasty with stenting, intolerant of aspirin
Statins	All acute coronary syndromes, CAD to an LDL goal < 100 mg/dL
ACE inhibitors	Ejection fraction < 40%, acute ST elevation MI
ARBs	Same as for ACE inhibitors if intolerant of ACE inhibitors
Heparin, low molecular weight (LMW)	Acute coronary syndromes, especially with ST segment depression
Fondaparinux or bivalirudin	Alternative to LMW heparin
GP IIb/IIIa inhibitors	Acute coronary syndromes, especially those undergoing angioplasty
Eplerenone or spironolactone	ST elevation MI with ejection fraction < 40% and heart failure symptoms

Stable Angina

Stable angina is usually evaluated in the office or ambulatory setting. Physical examination is generally not helpful in guiding the "most likely diagnosis" or "best initial therapy" questions. Although an EKG is always performed as the best initial test, the EKG lacks sensitivity between episodes of acute ischemia.

▶ **TIP**

Do not answer CK-MB or troponin in the stable patient in an office or clinic setting.

DIAGNOSTIC TESTS

After the EKG is done, the most likely answer to the "best initial test" question is the exercise tolerance (stress) test. Imaging can be added to the EKG interpretation of a stress test either with echocardiography or by nuclear imaging (typically single photon emission computed tomography or SPECT). A standard exercise tolerance test is based on 2 features:

- The patient can exercise to a target heart rate.
- The EKG will be able to detect ischemia.

"Maximum" stress test means the patient exercises until he or she achieves a target heart rate above 80% of his or her predicted maximum level. A person's maximum heart rate is calculated by subtracting his or her age from 220. The detection of ischemia on standard exercise tolerance testing is based on being able to see ST segment depression. If the patient cannot exercise, a pharmacologic alternative to exercise is used, such as dobutamine with echocardiography, or dipyridamole or adenosine with a nuclear isotope such as thallium.

> Exercise by exertion is preferred to pharmacologic simulation of exercise.

Types of Stress Tests	
Test	**Method of detecting ischemia**
Exercise tolerance test	ST segment depression
Exercise or dobutamine echocardiography	Wall motion abnormalities
Exercise or dipyridamole thallium	Decreased uptake of the nuclear isotope during exercise

Cardiac Enzymes, Echocardiography, and Angiography

Cardiac enzymes such as troponin, CK-MB, and myoglobin are always a wrong answer for diagnosing stable angina with the case described as being in the office or clinic. Echocardiography is useful in patients with stable chest pain syndromes. It is used to determine the presence of several anatomic abnormalities that can result in pain, such as:

- Aortic stenosis
- Hypertrophic cardiomyopathy
- Mitral valve prolapse

Angiography is used to determine the need for bypass surgery.

TREATMENT

The standard of care for angina is:

- **Aspirin**
- **Beta blockers** such as metoprolol
- **Nitrates** for ongoing chest pain

> Angiography is the only way to determine if the patient has Prinzmetal (variant) angina.

> In stable angina, clopidogrel, prasugrel, and ticagrelor are used as alternatives in those intolerant of aspirin.

Additional Medical Therapy for Stable Angina	
Medication	**Indication**
ACE inhibitors	Low ejection fraction (< 35%) on echocardiography
Angiotensin receptor blockers	Low ejection fraction, intolerant of ACE inhibitors
Ranolazine	Persistent pain despite maximum medical therapy
Statin	LDL above 100 (optional with LDL above 70 with **both** DM and CAD)

▶ TIP

Anticoagulants (such as LMW heparin) other than antiplatelet medications are always wrong treatments in stable angina.

Angioplasty and Bypass Surgery

Angioplasty does not offer a mortality benefit in those with stable angina. Angioplasty does, however, help control angina in those who have persistent symptoms despite maximal medical therapy. The use of angioplasty automatically implies that a diagnostic angiography has been done, although this can certainly be done at the same time as the percutaneous coronary intervention (PCI).

The strongest indications for bypass surgery, or a coronary artery bypass graft (CABG), are:

- Three-vessel coronary disease with > 70% stenosis in each vessel.
- Left main coronary disease with > 50% stenosis
- Left ventricular dysfunction

Other potential indications are 2-vessel disease in a diabetic patient or severe left anterior descending disease.

> **Which of the following is the strongest indication for angioplasty (PCI)?**
>
> a. 80% right coronary stenosis
> b. 90% circumflex and 70% right coronary stenosis
> c. Three-vessel disease with greater than 70% stenosis
> d. Left anterior descending stenosis greater than 75%
> e. Acute ST segment elevation MI
>
> **Answer:** The correct answer is (e). The greatest mortality benefit of PCI is not based on a particular anatomy of stenosis. The greatest benefit of PCI is obtained in the particular acute presentation of an acute ST segment elevation infarction. Although PCI is frequently done in those with 1- and 2-vessel coronary disease, the main benefit of percutaneous revascularization in chronic stable angina is for more rapid relief of symptoms and not for a mortality benefit. Maximal medical therapy as the initial treatment option in chronic stable angina offers the same symptomatic and mortality benefit as percutaneous coronary intervention as an initial revascularization strategy.

> In stable angina, PCI is not better than medical therapy, which includes aspirin, beta blockers, nitrates, weight loss, smoking cessation, and statins.

Acute Coronary Syndrome

The acute coronary syndromes (ACS) are:

- Unstable angina
- Non-ST segment elevation myocardial infarction (NSTEMI)
- ST segment elevation myocardial infarction (STEMI)

The major difference in the management of ACS compared with stable angina is the use of morphine, additional antiplatelet therapy, thrombolytics, anticoagulant therapy, and revascularization. When the patient presents to the emergency department, initial treatment decisions are based primarily on the history and the EKG. Enzyme levels are not available at the time that the initial treatment decisions are made. There is nothing in the physical examination that can establish the presence of ST elevation or depression, or whether the enzymes will be elevated.

> Ticagrelor is used with aspirin for ACS; alternative to prasugrel and clopidogrel.

TREATMENT

All patients with angina should receive aspirin and beta blockers. The main difference in the management of ACS compared with stable angina is the addition of:

- Clopidogrel, prasugrel, or ticagrelor
- ACE inhibitors
- Statins
- Morphine and nitrates
- Anticoagulants
- Thrombolytics

Although morphine, oxygen, and nitrates are often given first in the temporal sequence of management, they are not as important as additional antiplatelet medications because of mortality benefit.

▶ **TIP**

Answer "What is the most appropriate next step in management?" questions based on mortality benefit. Let the mortality benefit drive you.

Unstable Angina and Non-ST Segment Elevation MI

You cannot tell the difference between unstable angina and NSTEMI from the history, physical, or EKG. The distinction is based entirely on whether the patient develops an elevated level of troponin or CK-MB. Enzymes do not begin to elevate for 4 to 6 hours after the start of chest pain and may still be normal as long as 12 to 18 hours after the onset of pain. Enzyme testing reaches greater than 95% sensitivity at 12 hours, with a handful of patients developing an elevation after that.

The main difference in treatment between unstable angina and myocardial infarction (NSTEMI or STEMI) is the use of:

- Heparin (yes in unstable angina)
- Glycoprotein IIb/IIIa inhibitors (eptifibitide, tirofiban, abciximab)

Both of these agents work rapidly to prevent the progression or development of a clot in the coronary artery. They are used routinely prior to or simultaneously with the use of PCI. Neither of them will dissolve a clot that has already formed, so neither of them is indicated in the initial management of an acute STEMI.

> Thrombolytics are not useful in NSTEMI.

> Low molecular weight heparin is superior to unfractionated heparin in acute coronary syndrome.

If the initial management of unstable angina and NSTEMI are essentially identical, what will you do differently if the development of a troponin or CK-MB elevation confirms an infarction?

a. Thrombolytics
b. Calcium channel blockers
c. Echocardiography
d. Early use of angiography/possible angioplasty (PCI)
e. Fondaparinux
f. Bivalirudin
g. Prasugrel

Answer: The correct answer is (d). The greater the severity of disease, the more likely the patient is to benefit from an early invasive strategy (ie, PCI). Calcium channel blockers don't lower mortality in anyone, although they are used in vasospastic (Prinzmetal) angina or with cocaine-induced pain. Fondaparinux is a factor Xa inhibitor that functions like heparin and is an alternative to heparin. As heparin alternatives, neither the use of fondaparinux nor that of bivalirudin is based on developing positive troponins.

Clopidogrel, Prasugrel, or Ticagrelor

These agents are used in combination with aspirin in patients with ACS. They are most beneficial for:

1. **STEMI or NSTEMI**
2. Those undergoing **angioplasty**
3. Those having **stents** placed

Prasugrel is indicated only in patients who are having ACS with either NSTEMI or STEMI. Prasugrel is contraindicated in those with an increased risk of hemorrhage. This is defined as those over the age of 75, with a low weight or a history of transient ischemic attack (TIA) or stroke.

> Prasugrel has more efficacy and more bleeding compared to clopidogrel.

ST Segment Elevation MI

The single best therapy for STEMI is primary **angioplasty** or percutaneous coronary intervention (**PCI**). Aspirin is given prior to PCI. Only 20% to 25% of hospitals in the United States have the ability to perform urgent PCI. In hospitals without PCI, thrombolytics are often the best therapy to use after aspirin. Thrombolytics should be used immediately upon presentation to the emergency department. Immediate use of thrombolytics is superior to transferring the patient for angioplasty if the transfer-related delay is greater than 60 minutes. This is because the logistics of transfer often result in a delay of PCI that pushes it beyond the expected standard of a "door-to-balloon time" of 90 minutes. Although **thrombolytics are used for up to 12 hours** after the onset of chest pain, they provide as much as a 50% decrease in mortality if they are used within the first 1 to 2 hours.

Heparin is used in STEMI after revascularization to keep the vessel from restenosing. Glycoprotein IIb/IIIa inhibitors are used in association with angioplasty and stent placement should they be performed.

Clopidogrel, prasugrel, or ticagrelor should be added to aspirin in STEMI. Prasugrel is superior to clopidogrel in STEMI provided the risk of bleeding is low (age 75 or younger; no history of TIA or stroke).

Statins, beta blockers, and ACE inhibitors should be used in STEMI. ACE inhibitors have their greatest benefit in those with a low ejection fraction and in those with large anterior wall MIs. This is because those with large infarctions are the most likely to develop systolic dysfunction (low ejection fraction).

All those with acute MI need two antiplatelet medications. Ticagrelor is an alternative to clopidogrel or prasugrel in combination with aspirin.

> Thrombolytics are indicated with:
>
> - Less than 12 hours since the onset of chest pain and either
> - ST segment elevation (1 mm) in 2 or more contiguous leads
> or
> - New left bundle branch block

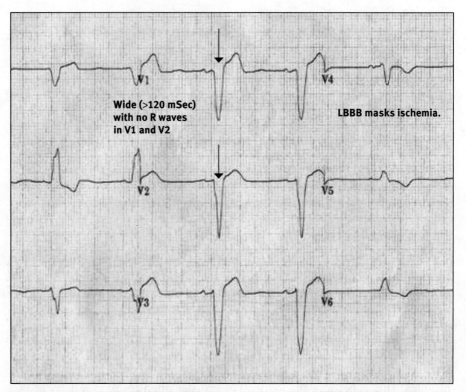

Wide (>120 mSec) with no R waves in V1 and V2

LBBB masks ischemia.

Figure 3.2: Left bundle branch block. LBBB makes it very hard to detect ischemia on an EKG. It looks like ST segment elevation.

Source: Philip Veith

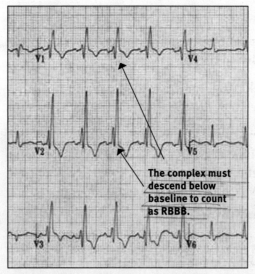

The complex must descend below baseline to count as RBBB.

Figure 3.3: Right bundle branch block. RBBB is much more benign than LBBB.
Look for two R waves in V1 and V2.

Source: Philip Veith

Contraindications to Thrombolytics

Thrombolytics cannot be used in those with major bleeding or in those with a risk of severe bleeding. Risk factors include:

- Head **trauma** within 3 to 6 months
- Intracranial **hemorrhage** *at any time* in the past
- Aortic **dissection**
- Nonhemorrhagic **stroke** within previous 3 to 6 months
- Signs of active major bleeding such as melena
- Severe **hypertension** (above 180/110)

Relative contraindications are peptic ulcer disease, recent surgery, or diabetic retinopathy.

> Heme (guaiac) positive brown stool is **not** a contraindication to thrombolytics.

Summary of Therapeutic Differences in Acute Coronary Syndromes	
Non-ST elevation MI	**ST elevation MI**
Low molecular weight heparin	Angioplasty (PCI)
GP IIb/IIIa inhibitors	Thrombolytics

All patients with ACS are best treated initially with aspirin. In addition to the treatments above, ACS patients can also be treated with:

- ACE inhibitors or ARBs (greatest benefit with anterior wall infarctions)
- Clopidogrel, prasugrel, or ticagrelor
- Statins
- Beta blockers
- Morphine, oxygen, and nitrates (no proven mortality benefit)
- Fondaparinux or bivalirudin as alternatives to heparin

> The mortality benefit of beta blockers is not dependent on time. There is no proof that it makes a difference whether they are used immediately or simply some time before hospital discharge.

▶ TIP

In an urgent case, anticoagulant and antiplatelet therapy is always the answer to "what is the most important therapy" or "what therapy is most likely to benefit this patient?"

Complications of Myocardial Infarction

All complications of MI can result in hypotension. This will not help you answer the "What is the most likely diagnosis?" question. Although some complications occur earlier (heart block, right ventricular infarction) and some later (papillary muscle rupture, ventricular septal defect, left ventricular free wall rupture), the time course is not as important as the individual presentation.

A 54-year-old woman with a recent anterior wall myocardial infarction is transferred to the intensive care unit after a sudden drop in her blood pressure from 120/76 to 86/40. Her pulse is 125 per minute. She has a 3/6 systolic murmur at the lower left sternal border. A sample of blood from the right atrium shows a pO_2 of 42 mm Hg and a sample from the pulmonary artery shows a pO_2 of 62 mm Hg.

What is the most likely diagnosis?

a. Papillary muscle rupture
b. Atrial septal rupture
c. Ventricular septal rupture
d. Third-degree AV block
e. Left ventricular free wall rupture
f. Right ventricular rupture

> All complications of myocardial infarctions give hypotension.

Answer: The correct answer is (c). The increase in oxygen saturation between the right atrium (RA) and the pulmonary artery (PA) implies the presence of a shunt of blood from the left ventricle to the right ventricle. A normal pO_2 of venous blood is about 40 mm Hg with a saturation of 75%. The murmur of a ventricular septal defect (VSD) is best heard at the lower left sternal border. Papillary muscle rupture leads to acute mitral regurgitation (MR). These murmurs will be heard at the base radiating to the axilla. This would not lead to a "step-up" in saturation from the RA to the PA. Atrial septal rupture is highly unlikely as a complication of infarction. Were it present, an atrial septal defect (ASD) would be associated with shunting into the RA, and the RA oxygen content would be higher than the usual venous pO_2 of 40 mm Hg. Even though this is much sooner than you would expect to find a VSD occurring after an MI, that is the presentation.

▶ **TIP**

Individual presentation is more important than history (e.g., time course) in answering a "most likely diagnosis" question.

Third-Degree AV Block

- Bradycardia
- Cannon "a" waves in the neck
- Recent inferior wall myocardial infarction (both the inferior wall and AV node are fed by the right coronary artery)
- Treat with atropine and pacemaker.

Free Wall Rupture/Tamponade

- Few days to a week after large anterior wall infarction
- Sudden hypotension to pulselessness
- Pulseless electrical activity
- Jugular venous distension (JVD)
- Clear lungs (no congestion)

Valve Rupture

- Severe murmur of MR (base to axilla)
- Rales and pulmonary congestion
- Intraaortic balloon pump as a bridge to surgery

Dysrhythmia

- Ectopy (premature atrial and ventricular contractions) gives an irregularly irregular rhythm with normal blood pressure.
- Ventricular fibrillation
- Ventricular tachycardia presents with everything from sudden loss of pulse to hypotension to an asymptomatic, stable patient.

Right Ventricular Infarction

- Associated with 40% of inferior wall MIs (same arterial supply: right coronary artery)
- Clear lungs
- Often with AV block
- Diagnose with right ventricular leads (flip leads to other side of chest).
- Best initial therapy is IV fluids.

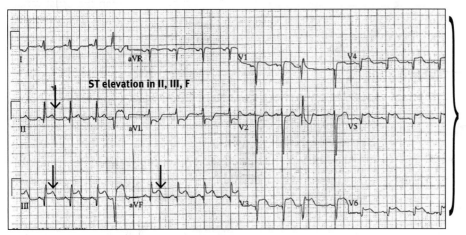

Figure 3.4: Right ventricular infarction. Right-sided leads show RV infarction in association with IWMI.

Source: Kunal Patel, MD

Reperfusion Arrhythmia

- Irritable myocardium with reestablishment of flow after thrombolytics
- Most common is accelerated idioventricular arrhythmia (wide complex with rate between 40 and 100).
- Do not treat reperfusion arrhythmias with antiarrhythmic therapy.

Pericarditis (Dressler Syndrome)

- Rare secondary to routine use of aspirin in all post-MI patients
- Occurs late after MI
- Test and treat as with any other form of pericarditis

Postinfarction Management

"The patient is going home; which of the following is most likely to benefit this patient?"

- **Stress (exercise tolerance) testing:** This test is performed in all those who did not undergo PCI in order to determine the need for revascularization. For example, if a patient has an inferior wall MI, stress testing is performed to see if there is ischemia of the anterior wall. If there is residual or persistent ischemia, the patient needs angiography to determine the need for PCI or CABG. If there is no persistent ischemia, there is no need for angiography.

> ▶ **TIP**
>
> "Reversible" ischemia is the most important thing we can find on a stress test. Those are the people we can help the most.

- **Medications:** What are the medications that should be used in patients on a long-term basis after an infarction? These medications are used in both STEMI and NSTEMI.
  - Aspirin
  - Beta blockers (e.g., metoprolol)
  - Statins
  - Clopidogrel, prasugrel, or ticagrelor
  - ACE inhibitors: The patient should leave the hospital on ACE inhibitors. They can be stopped at 6 weeks after an infarction if echocardiography shows no evidence of the development of systolic dysfunction.

> There is no point in revascularizing normal tissue or dead tissue.

> Clopidogrel, prasugrel, or ticagrelor is stopped at one year if stenting has not been done.

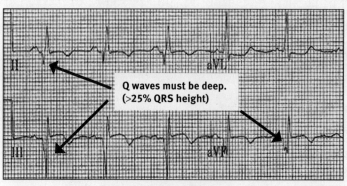

Figure 3.5: Inferior wall myocardial infarction. Q waves in II, III, aVF must be at least 25% of the total height of the QRS complex.

Source: Mahendra C. Patel, MD

CONGESTIVE HEART FAILURE

Congestive heart failure (CHF) can be from either systolic dysfunction (low ejection fraction) or diastolic dysfunction (currently called "CHF with preserved ejection fraction"). The initial management of pulmonary edema is identical for all forms of CHF. In other words, if the person comes to the emergency department with acute pulmonary edema, an echocardiogram is not needed to guide initial therapy.

Acute Pulmonary Edema

The initial management of acute pulmonary edema is to remove volume from the vascular space with diuretics and to adjust the hemodynamics by dilating the venous circulation. The veins, because they are more distensible, contain 70% of the volume of the vascular system. This is why so much of acute pulmonary edema management is based on venodilation.

> Intraaortic balloon pumps are occasionally used in severe pulmonary edema from cardiogenic shock not corrected by medical therapy.

DIAGNOSTIC TESTS

Few tests make a difference in acute pulmonary edema caused by CHF. This is because the diagnosis is essentially based on clinical findings of:

- Acute dyspnea
- Rales/congestion
- S3 gallop
- Jugular venous distension
- Orthopnea
- Paroxysmal nocturnal dyspnea

TREATMENT

The best initial therapy of acute pulmonary edema is with diuretics and preload reduction. This should lead to resolution of 90% of cases. Other initial therapies include:

- Oxygen
- Loop **diuretics** (furosemide, bumetanide, ethacrynic acid)
- Morphine and **nitroglycerin** to dilate venous circulation
- **Sitting the patient upright**

If preload reduction is not fully effective in relieving dyspnea, the "most appropriate next step in management" is CPAP or noninvasive positive pressure ventilation (NPPV) first, combined with:

- Dobutamine
- Inamrinone or milrinone
- Placing the patient in the intensive care unit

These pharmaceutical agents are identical in their effects. They are positive inotropes that are used to rapidly increase contractility and have some effect in decreasing afterload. **None of them have a proven mortality benefit**. None of them are used chronically.

Using CPAP or NPPV:

- Is definitely beneficial in cardiogenic pulmonary edema
- Decreases the need for intubation in severe illness

> CPAP or NPPV is a great way to keep severely ill people off a ventilator. Your mom would rather have a face mask (NPPV) than a tube.

Which of the following is most likely to alter initial management in a person with acute pulmonary edema?

a. Chest x-ray
b. EKG
c. Arterial blood gas
d. Echocardiography
e. Nuclear ventriculogram (MUGA scan)

Answer: The correct answer is (b). The EKG can show two of the most common causes of an acute exacerbation of CHF: ischemia and arrhythmia. Although infection and nonadherence to medication are two of the most common causes of an acute decompensation in cardiac function, ischemia and arrhythmia are more potentially dangerous and, more importantly, can alter acute management. Ischemia alters pump function and can often present with dyspnea as an "equivalent" of angina. Atrial arrhythmias can cause acute pulmonary edema by the loss of atrial contribution to cardiac output. Normally, only 10% of cardiac output is based on the contribution of atrial systole. Most ventricular filling is passive. However, in a person with left ventricular dysfunction, cardiomyopathy, or valvular heart disease, atrial systole is indispensible in "shoving" blood forward into the left ventricle to overcome the high pressure there. Hence, in an abnormal heart, atrial systole may provide as much as 20% to 30% of cardiac output. If an arrhythmia caused the pulmonary edema, the best initial therapy may be synchronized cardioversion.

Diagnostic Tests in Acute Pulmonary Edema	
Test	**What it shows**
Chest x-ray	Pulmonary vascular congestion or redistribution, cardiomegaly, effusion
Arterial blood gas	Hypoxia, most often low pCO_2 from hyperventilation
Swan-Ganz catheter	Decreased cardiac output and index; increased systemic vascular resistance and wedge pressure
B-type natriuretic peptide (BNP)	Normal levels indicate the absence of CHF; elevated levels are nonspecific

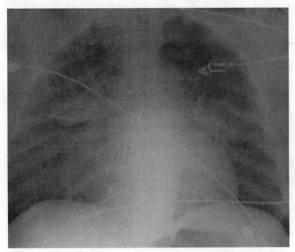

Figure 3.6: Pulmonary edema. Veins are engorged and appear white with more prominence towards the apices.

Source: Moe Sann, MD

B-type Natriuretic Peptide

When the diagnosis of CHF or pulmonary edema is obvious and treatment is clear, the BNP level adds little to the management. BNP levels are correlated with outcome; a person whose BNP remains elevated after treatment is more likely to have a worse outcome. As a diagnostic test, an elevated BNP level is highly sensitive but somewhat nonspecific in that many causes of cardiac disease can lead to dilation of the atrium and an elevation in BNP level. **A normal BNP level excludes CHF** as a cause of the person's shortness of breath.

> An elevated BNP is nonspecific. A normal BNP = no CHF.

▶ **TIP**

The Swan-Ganz catheter is not routinely indicated in anyone.

Nesiritide

Nesiritide is an analogue of atrial natriuretic peptide. There is some evidence that nesiritide will decrease symptoms in acute pulmonary edema. **Nesiritide has not been shown to decrease mortality**. The precise role of nesiritide in acute pulmonary edema is not known. It would be used in those patients not responsive to acute preload reduction, such as those who receive dobutamine. Because the benefit is not clear, if dobutamine is a choice for treatment of acute pulmonary edema, then choose dobutamine, not nesiritide.

> Nesiritide is never clearly correct.

Chronic CHF Management

The treatment of CHF is based on whether the patient has systolic dysfunction with a low ejection fraction (EF) or diastolic dysfunction with a preserved or normal EF. This is why the discussion of cardiomyopathy adds little to our ability to answer CHF questions. The etiology of the cardiomyopathy changes almost nothing in terms of short-term management. Whether the EF is low or normal changes a lot. The most common cause of dilated cardiomyopathy is from ischemia and/or infarction in the past. All forms of CHF present with dyspnea, rales, and edema. All of them can elevate the BNP. The most common way to distinguish systolic from diastolic dysfunction is by echocardiography. This is why **all patients admitted with CHF routinely have an echocardiogram** to assess left ventricular function if no recent echocardiogram is available.

Which of the following is the most accurate method of assessing ejection fraction?

a. Transthoracic echocardiogram
b. Transesophageal echocardiogram
c. Swan-Ganz catheter
d. MUGA or nuclear ventriculogram
e. Left heart catheterization

Answer: The correct answer is (d). There is an enormous difference between the questions "What would you use (or do first) to assess ejection fraction?" and "What is the most accurate?" Echocardiography is certainly what you would do "first" or "routinely," but the "most accurate" is the nuclear ventriculogram. Nuclear ventriculography is more accurate than left heart catheterization. The Swan-Ganz catheter does not assess ejection fraction.

Systolic Dysfunction

The term systolic dysfunction can be used interchangeably with the terms left ventricular dysmotility or low EF. Treatment for systolic dysfunction is:

- **ACE inhibitors** or **angiotensin receptor blockers** (ARBs)
- **Beta blockers** (metoprolol, bisoprolol, or carvedilol)
- **Spironolactone** or eplerenone
- Hydralazine with nitrates

All of these agents will lower mortality in CHF.

> Eplerenone is an aldosterone antagonist that has all the same benefit as aldosterone without the antiandrogenic effects that cause gynecomastia.

> Digoxin decreases symptoms and frequency of hospitalization but will not lower mortality.

Diuretics are used to control fluid overload. Digoxin is used if the patient is persistently symptomatic despite the use of all these other therapies. Virtually all patients a resident will see in training are in class III or IV CHF. Class III means there are symptoms with minimal exertion. Class IV means there are symptoms at rest. It is almost certain that any patient who is admitted to hospital is in class III or IV CHF.

▶ **TIP**

The single most important CHF question is "Which treatment will lower mortality?"

Beta Blockers in CHF

Not all beta blockers have been shown to have mortality benefit in CHF. Only metoprolol, bisoprolol, and carvedilol are your answers. This differs from ACE inhibitors and ARBs, in which all drugs in the class are effective. Starting beta blockers is relatively contraindicated with acute pulmonary edema. If the patient is already on them, they should be continued.

> Low ejection fraction is not a contraindication for beta blockers.

Which of the following is the most common cause of death in a person with CHF?

a. Arrhythmia/sudden death
b. Myocardial infarction
c. Fluid overload/pulmonary edema
d. Valve dysfunction
e. Embolic phenomena

Answer: The correct answer is (a). Only a very small percentage of patients with CHF are ever admitted to the hospital with pulmonary edema. Most are at home with slowly progressive disease. Even when admitted with pulmonary edema, only small percentages die. Most are relieved with diuretics, nitrates, and morphine, and ultimately discharged. CHF and low EF is a cause of arrhythmia. The lower the EF, the more likely the person is to develop an arrhythmia. Hence, most patients who die of CHF do not make it to the hospital; they die suddenly at home of an arrhythmia, which can be brought on by ischemia. Beta blockers are antiarrhythmic and antiischemic, which is why they decrease mortality in CHF.

> The lower the ejection fraction, the greater the mortality benefit from beta blockers.

Devices Used for Systolic Dysfunction

The 2 devices most useful in dilated cardiomyopathy (CHF with systolic dysfunction) are:

- Implantable cardioverter defibrillator (ICD)
- Biventricular pacemaker

The ICD is used in ischemic and nonischemic cardiomyopathy in those with an EF of less than 35% that has not improved with several months of medical therapy. The biventricular pacemaker is used in those with ischemic and nonischemic cardiomyopathy, persistent symptoms, and a QRS that is wider than 120 milliseconds. An ICD does not decrease symptoms; it simply restores normal sinus rhythm to the heart in the event of sudden death from ventricular arrhythmia, such as ventricular tachycardia or ventricular fibrillation. The biventricular pacemaker can markedly improve symptoms by resynchronizing the heart and allowing both ventricles to contract more efficiently. All biventricular pacemakers have ICD function as well.

> Biventricular pacemakers can improve severe symptoms that persist despite maximal medical therapy and delay the need for transplantation.

Test-taking Strategy for CHF Questions

The most important principle to answer the questions correctly is: "Which of the following is most likely to decrease mortality in this patient?"

The wrong answers for CHF questions will always be the same:

- Calcium channel blockers
- Warfarin
- Cardiac size reduction surgery
- Alpha blockers
- Nesiritide

The correct answer will add in ACE inhibitors, ARBs, hydralazine, beta blockers, spironolactone, a biventricular pacemaker, or ICD. You cannot be asked to choose between these therapies, so they are unlikely to appear together in the same question as answer choices. If two of these mortality-benefiting therapies do appear in the same question, it means there is a contraindication to one of them. For instance, if ACE inhibitors and hydralazine are both in the choices, you should look for the presence of hyperkalemia. If spironolactone and beta blockers are in the same question, look for severe asthma in the medical history.

▶ **TIP**

If two correct answers seem to be in the choices, you are missing a contraindication to one of them.

Diastolic Dysfunction

Diastolic dysfunction is also called "CHF with preserved EF," which may be from hypertrophic cardiomyopathy. It is impossible to distinguish this from systolic dysfunction by symptoms only. An echocardiogram is indispensible in establishing the diagnosis. The main difference between patients with systolic and diastolic dysfunction is in terms of a proven mortality benefit. None of the medications previously listed has any proven mortality benefit in heart failure with normal ejection fraction. The main goal of therapy is to:

1. Control blood pressure
2. Control fluid overload.

The medications that are *used* in diastolic dysfunction are:

- Beta blockers
- Diuretics
- Spironolactone or eplerenone
- ACE inhibitor and ARBs

None of these, however, has been proven to lower mortality.

> No drug clearly lowers mortality in diastolic heart failure.

▶ **TIP**

There is a difference between "What is the best therapy?" and "Which of the following is most likely to lower mortality?"

The treatments that do **not** have any benefit are:

- Digoxin
- ICD
- Biventricular pacemaker

> Exercise training programs really do work in CHF.

CARDIOMYOPATHY

Only a few small points about cardiomyopathy differ from the points in the previous systolic and diastolic dysfunction sections. All of them present with dyspnea, rales, and edema. All of them can cause atrial fibrillation. All of them are diagnosed with echocardiography. All of them are treated with beta blockers. Almost all of them are treated with diuretics.

Dilated Cardiomyopathy

Besides the ischemia that causes most systolic dysfunction, other causes of dilated cardiomyopathy are:

- Alcohol
- Radiation
- Chemotherapeutic agents such as daunorubicin and doxorubicin
- Thiamine and selenium deficiency
- Chagas disease

> Many "idiopathic" dilated cardiomyopathy patients have had viral myocarditis in the past.

Which of the following represents the greatest difference in the management of dilated cardiomyopathy from toxins (e.g., alcohol) as opposed to that caused by ischemia?

a. Metoprolol
b. Aspirin
c. ACE inhibitors
d. Eplerenone
e. Use of echocardiography

Answer: The correct answer is (b). Aspirin is beneficial for those with coronary artery disease. Aspirin does not directly benefit a dilated cardiomyopathy caused by toxins. The other medications decrease afterload (ACE, ARBs) or inhibit the aldosterone system (spironolactone, eplerenone), and beta blockers are used in dilated cardiomyopathy of any cause. Likewise, echocardiography is used to diagnose all cases of dilated cardiomyopathy. Another correct answer choice would have been revascularization instead of aspirin.

> Cardiomyopathy from toxins is managed in exactly the same way as that from ischemia, with the exception of direct CAD management in the latter case.

Hypertrophic Cardiomyopathy

Most hypertrophic cardiomyopathy is from hypertension or aortic stenosis. The only significant new point with regard to answering questions is in terms of hypertrophic obstructive cardiomyopathy (HOCM), a genetic disorder that presents with significant dynamic outflow tract narrowing or "obstruction."

Which of the following represents the greatest point of difference between HOCM and simple hypertrophic cardiomyopathy with a preserved ejection fraction?

a. Presence of dyspnea
b. Use of echocardiography
c. Beta blockers
d. ACE inhibitors
e. Atrial fibrillation

Answer: The correct answer is (d). ACE inhibitors and other vasodilators such as hydralazine should be avoided in those with HOCM. All forms of cardiomyopathy benefit from treatment with beta blockers and are diagnosed with echocardiography. Any cause of cardiomyopathy or valve disease increases the risk of atrial fibrillation. Digoxin would also have been incorrect as a choice; it has no place in the management of any form of hypertrophic cardiomyopathy, including HOCM.

PRESENTATION

The most common presentation of HOCM is dyspnea on exertion, not sudden death. HOCM presents with dyspnea like any other form of CHF, valvular heart disease, or cardiomyopathy.

Unique features of HOCM compared with other types of cardiomyopathy are:

- Syncope
- S4 gallop
- Sudden death (rare)

> Although rare, HOCM is still the most common cause of sudden death in healthy young athletes.

A 19-year-old college basketball player experiences his second episode of syncope while playing ball over the last several months. He reports several episodes of dyspnea. He had been found to have a 3/6 murmur at the lower left sternal border that improved with squatting and became louder with valsalva. EKG shows an S-wave in V1 and an R wave in V5 with 45 mm combined. He was placed on metoprolol after his last episode of syncope.

Which of the following is most likely to lower mortality for this patient?

a. Verapamil
b. Implantable cardioverter/defibrillator
c. Surgery
d. Diuretics
e. Biventricular pacemaker

Answer: The correct answer is (b). This patient with HOCM will benefit from the ICD because of his multiple episodes of syncope. The next episode of loss of consciousness may be sudden death. His presentation is too severe and potentially dangerous to be treated just by adding verapamil. Surgical myomectomy is performed only as the last step if maximal medical therapy (beta blocker, verapamil, ICD) does not control symptoms. In addition, surgical myomectomy would be done only if the catheter procedure to decompress the septum with the instillation of absolute alcohol was not effective. Diuretics might make it worse by diminishing the size of the left ventricular outflow tract.

TREATMENT

The best initial therapy for HOCM is with beta blockers. Alternatives as second-line agents are verapamil or disopyramide. Diuretics are generally to be avoided as they may decrease the size of the left ventricle and increase the outflow tract obstruction.

Restrictive Cardiomyopathy

Restrictive cardiomyopathy is a rare cause of dyspnea on exertion in patients with a history of:

- Sarcoidosis
- Amyloidosis
- Hemochromatosis
- Endomyocardial fibrosis
- Scleroderma
- Eosinophilic cardiomyopathy
- Radiation

Physical Findings

There is **no unique physical finding** in a person with restrictive cardiomyopathy. Many types of cardiomyopathy can present with an S3 or S4 gallop. The **Kussmaul sign** may be present and you may not be able to distinguish restrictive cardiomyopathy from constrictive pericarditis until an echocardiogram is obtained. This is also the same with **signs of right heart failure** such as edema, ascites, and hepatosplenomegaly.

> The Kussmaul sign is an increase in jugular venous distension with inspiration.

DIAGNOSTIC TESTS/TREATMENT

The diagnosis is based on the presence of restriction on echocardiography in association with one of the systemic diseases previously listed.

> Cardiac MRI is the most useful test in diagnosing restrictive cardiomyopathy.

Restrictive cardiomyopathy is the form of heart disease that is most likely to benefit from a **myocardial biopsy**. Biopsy is rarely necessary because the diagnosis is clear from a previously established diagnosis of systemic disease.

Treatment is:

1. Correcting the underlying cause, if possible
2. Diuretics and beta blockers
3. Diltiazem or verapamil

> Amyloidosis gives a "speckled pattern" on echocardiography in the septum.

Atrial Myxoma

Atrial myxoma presents in a similar fashion to endocarditis and cardiomyopathy. The patient has dyspnea, fatigue, and sometimes chest pain. Because there is a murmur and **sometimes a fever**, atrial myxoma can be confused with endocarditis. The major distinguishing point on physical examination is a murmur that **changes markedly with the position of the body**. This is sometimes called a "**tumor plop**." This is different from a simple, mild change in intensity with leaning forward. Myxoma can send emboli to the brain.

> Myxoma mimics mitral stenosis because it obstructs left atrial filling.

DIAGNOSTIC TESTS/TREATMENT

Myxoma is detected by echocardiography. The only treatment is surgical resection. The sedimentation rate can be elevated.

Peripartum Cardiomyopathy

For unclear reasons, a small number of women (fewer than 1 in 10,000) develop a dilated cardiomyopathy in the last month of pregnancy or within 6 months of delivering. Symptoms, testing, and treatment of peripartum cardiomyopathy are the same as they would be for any other form of dilated cardiomyopathy. ACE inhibitors, beta blockers, and diuretics are used as they are in general for systolic dysfunction. The patient can simply avoid breast-feeding in order to use ACE inhibitors postpartum. When the life of the mother is dependent on a medication, you must give it. Transplantation is often the only option.

> **Which of the following is the most dangerous to a woman during a second pregnancy?**
>
> a. Mitral stenosis
> b. Ventricular septal defect
> c. Peripartum cardiomyopathy with persistent left ventricular dysfunction
> d. Atrial septal defect
> e. Patent foramen ovale
>
> **Answer:** The correct answer is (c). If a woman develops peripartum cardiomyopathy and becomes pregnant again, her mortality can be as high as 50% to 70%.

VALVULAR HEART DISEASE

All valvular heart disease can present with **shortness of breath, rales, jugular venous distention**, and **edema**. In short, valve disease of any kind causes CHF. The best initial diagnostic test for all forms is an **echocardiogram**. Endocarditis prophylaxis has changed markedly. With the exception of a prosthetic valve or surgically corrected cyanotic congenital heart disease with prosthetic material, prophylaxis for endocarditis is no longer indicated for valvular heart disease.

This section emphasizes:

1. What is different in the history or the symptoms to allow you to answer "What is the most likely diagnosis?"
2. What is different in therapy?
3. Auscultation and the effects of cardiac maneuvers

Mitral Stenosis

PRESENTATION/"WHAT IS THE MOST LIKELY DIAGNOSIS?"

Mitral stenosis (MS) presents with **dyspnea in a young person** with a history of **dysphagia, hoarseness, stroke**, and atrial fibrillation. All the symptoms of MS are from dilation of the left atrium. Because MS is most often from **rheumatic fever**, you should expect to see a history that includes immigration from a country with less access to healthcare for children.

> Hemoptysis is common in MS from pulmonary hypertension.

▶ **TIP**

Worsening of symptoms during pregnancy is the big clue to mitral stenosis.

Etiology of Symptoms in Mitral Stenosis	
Symptom	**Etiology**
Dysphagia	Dilated left atrium presses against the esophagus
Hoarseness	Pressure of the atrium against the recurrent laryngeal nerve
Atrial fibrillation	From marked dilation of the left atrium
Exacerbation during pregnancy	From a 50% increase in plasma volume with no change in the size of the stenotic mitral orifice

Auscultation

MS gives an opening snap just after S2 followed by a diastolic rumbling murmur. The murmur of MS is **decreased in intensity by Valsalva and standing,** and increased by squatting and leg raise.

> As mitral stenosis worsens, the opening snap happens earlier: It moves closer to S2.

DIAGNOSTIC TESTS

The best initial test is an echo and the most accurate test is left heart catheterization. Catheterization is performed only if the echocardiogram is inconclusive. Transesophageal echocardiography is much more accurate than transthoracic echo because the left atrium is the most posterior structure in the heart and is right next to the esophagus. Severe mitral stenosis on echocardiography is defined by a valve area of less than 1.0 cm^2.

EKG: Left atrial hypertrophy (biphasic P wave in V_1 and V_2)

Chest x-ray: Straightening of the left heart border and elevation of the left mainstem bronchus

Catheterization: Although this is the answer to the "most accurate diagnostic test" question, routine catheterization should not be performed for most valvular disease. Echocardiography is usually sufficient and catheterization is only needed if the echo is not sufficiently diagnostic.

TREATMENT

> You can't "balloon" when a mitral valve is heavily calcified or when thrombus is present.

The best initial therapy is **sodium restriction** and a **diuretic** to decrease pulmonary congestion and the sensation of breathlessness. The question should describe a patient, often pregnant, with worsening symptoms despite this preload reduction. The "most appropriate next step in management" is **balloon valvuloplasty** (or **valvotomy**). Surgical repair or replacement of the valve is done if valve morphology is not amenable to balloon valvuloplasty.

Digoxin is best to control heart rate in atrial fibrillation. Rate control is extremely important in controlling symptoms.

Which of the following is the strongest indication for mitral valve balloon valvuloplasty in MS despite medical therapy?

a. Presence of atrial fibrillation
b. Emboli
c. Single episode of pulmonary edema
d. Murmur of mitral regurgitation
e. Asymptomatic woman planning a pregnancy

Answer: The correct answer is (c). The strongest indication for a balloon intervention is the development of symptoms directly related to pressure/volume overload. Emboli can occur from dilation of the atrium, and balloon valvuloplasty will not, unfortunately, directly reverse left atrial (LA) dilation. A murmur is not as important as being unable to breathe. Although atrial fibrillation may suggest a need for an intervention, it is not as severe as fluid accumulating in the lungs.

► **TIP**

Questions for which MS is the answer:

- Which is most likely to be associated with stroke (or atrial fibrillation)?
- Which of the following is the worst in a pregnant woman?
- Which of the following is most likely to be associated with hemoptysis?

Mitral Regurgitation (MR)

PRESENTATION/"WHAT IS THE MOST LIKELY DIAGNOSIS?"

MR presents with all the signs and symptoms of CHF. There is nothing in the history or physical to allow you to answer the "most likely diagnosis" question without either the description of the murmur or the echocardiogram.

MR is caused by:

1. Ischemic heart disease leading to cardiac dilation
2. Endocarditis
3. Mitral valve prolapse

> Neither MS, MR, AS, nor AR needs endocarditis prophylaxis with antibiotics.

Auscultation

MR:

- Presents with pansystolic or holosystolic murmur that obscures both S1 and S2
- Radiates to the axilla
- Increases with squatting, leg raise, and handgrip
- Decreases with standing, Valsalva, and amyl nitrate

[handwritten: → ↑ after load; ↓ after load; don't matte]

[handwritten right margin: Hand grip, squatting, legraise) ↑ after loud; ↑ regurgitation Mitral Aortic]

DIAGNOSTIC TESTS/TREATMENT

Echo is the best initial test. Catheterization is the most accurate test. The best initial therapy is based on the acuity of symptoms.

► **TIP**

There is a difference between the "most accurate test" and "what test should be routinely done." Catheterization is the most accurate, but is not to be routinely done.

1. **Acute valve rupture with pulmonary edema:** The answer is diuretics, after-load reduction, and urgent valve repair or replacement.
2. **Chronic disease:** The best initial therapy is a vasodilator such as an ACE inhibitor, ARB, hydralazine, or nifedipine.

When is surgery the answer?

- Ejection fraction dropping below 60%

and/or

- Left ventricular end systolic diameter greater than 40 mm

When valve repair and replacement are both in the choices, the answer is repair. Valve repair means placing clips or sutures at the ends of the overly loose mitral valve leaflets in order to tighten up the valve.

Valve Replacement: Bioprosthetic versus Metal Valves		
Valve type	**Advantages**	**Disadvantages**
Bioprosthetic	No need for anticoagulation, fewer thrombotic/embolic complications	Needs replacement in 10 years
Metal valves	Longer-term durability	Lifelong anticoagulation, very high INR needed (2.5 to 3.5), extremely thrombogenic

In general, bioprosthetic valves are the answer in an older person (age 70 or above) who is not likely to live long enough to need a second valve.

Aortic Stenosis

PRESENTATION/"WHAT IS THE MOST LIKELY DIAGNOSIS?"

Although aortic stenosis (AS) is extremely common in the elderly secondary to sclerosis or calcium accumulating in the aortic valve with age, an enormous percentage of cases are caused by a congenital bicuspid aortic valve. AS presents with:

- Angina
- Syncope
- Signs and symptoms of CHF

Angina is common secondary to hypertrophy of the left ventricle (increased demand) and the concomitant presence of CAD. Since the ostia that feed the coronary arteries are obstructed by the stenotic valve, this will decrease supply into them.

Auscultation

AS:

- Presents with a "diamond-shaped" (crescendo/decrescendo) systolic murmur that radiates to the carotids.
- Standing/Valsalva: Decreased intensity

Handgrip increases afterload by compressing the arteries of the arm. This makes it harder for blood to exit the ventricle in systole and will therefore decrease the intensity of the AS murmur.

- Squatting/leg raise: Increased intensity
- Handgrip: Decreased intensity

DIAGNOSTIC TESTS/TREATMENT

The diagnosis is confirmed with echocardiography as with all forms of valvular disease.

The "best initial therapy" for severe AS is **surgical replacement** of the valve. It is very unusual for a surgical procedure, rather than medications or catheter procedures, to be the first step. Although diuretics are useful in any patient with fluid overload or congestion, they are of very limited benefit in AS. Neither balloon valvuloplasty nor catheter replacement is effective for AS. This is because the calcification that leads to worsening disease is not well treated with a balloon or catheter replacement procedure. Anyone with **severe AS** and symptoms should **have the valve replaced**.

> There is no effective medical therapy for AS.

> A 72-year-old man presents with chest pain and shortness of breath. He has a 3/6 systolic murmur radiating to his carotid arteries. An echocardiogram shows an aortic valve diameter of 0.6 cm^2 and a transvalvular gradient of 70 mm Hg.
>
> Which of the following is most important to perform prior to valve replacement surgery?
>
> a. Nuclear stress test
> b. Dobutamine echocardiography
> c. Coronary angiography
> d. Electrocardiogram
> e. Troponin level
> f. Holter monitor
>
> **Answer:** The correct answer is (c). CAD is so frequently associated with AS that stress testing has little value. In addition, stress testing in symptomatic patients with AS can cause complications such as syncope or hypotension. It is essential to perform coronary angiography in anticipation of bypassing the coronary arteries at the same time as the valve replacement.

Aortic Regurgitation

ETIOLOGY

Aortic regurgitation (AR) has the greatest variety of causes of any of the valvular diseases. AR can be caused by:

- Hypertension and ischemia
- Rheumatic heart disease
- Connective tissue diseases such as Marfan syndrome, cystic medial necrosis, and Ehlers-Danlos syndrome
- Ankylosing spondylitis and Reiter syndrome (HLA B27)
- Syphilis

PRESENTATION/"WHAT IS THE MOST LIKELY DIAGNOSIS?"

As with all valve diseases, AR presents with the signs and symptoms of CHF. There are several unique physical findings in addition to the murmur. These help you find the answers to both the "most likely diagnosis" and the "which physical finding is most likely to be associated with this patient?" questions.

- **Quincke pulse:** nailbed capillary pulsations
- **Musset sign:** head bobbing in time with systole
- **Hill sign:** leg BP 40 mm Hg greater than arm BP
- **Duroziez sign:** pulses auscultated in the femoral area
- **Corrigan or water-hammer pulse:** a high-amplitude carotid pulse

Auscultation

AR gives a diastolic decrescendo murmur heard best at the lower left sternal border. It worsens (gets louder) with maneuvers that increase venous return, such as squatting or leg raise, and improves with standing or Valsalva. **Handgrip makes it markedly worse**, since handgrip increases afterload.

DIAGNOSTIC TESTS/TREATMENT

Echocardiography is the best initial test as with all other valvular disease.

The best initial treatment is with vasodilators such as **ACE inhibitors**, **ARBs**, hydralazine, and nifedipine. They do not reverse the valve damage. They serve only to decrease the rate of progression or deterioration of the cardiomyopathy.

The most effective therapy is valve replacement; however, repair is often done first.

> There is nothing specific enough on EKG or chest x-ray in AR to make them useful tests.

A 64-year-old woman comes to the office for routine follow-up. She has a history of hypertension and a 3/6 diastolic decrescendo murmur that radiates down her lower left sternal border. Her last echocardiogram a year ago showed an ejection fraction of 52% and a left ventricular end systolic diameter (LVESD) of 60 mm. She has remained asymptomatic since that time.

Which of the following is most likely to benefit this patient?

a. Transthoracic echocardiogram
b. Transesophageal echocardiogram
c. Surgical repair
d. Warfarin to an INR of 2–3
e. Digoxin

> Surgical repair is always preferable to replacement of regurgitant lesions. Repair needs no warfarin.

Answer: The correct answer is (c). The operative criteria for AR are EF below 55% **or** LVESD greater than 55 mm. Operative replacement of the aortic valve is done based on echocardiographic criteria in an asymptomatic patient. If the left ventricle starts to dilate, nothing can be done to reverse the dilation, so operative repair must be done prior to the dilation. Since the EF was below 55% and the LVESD was greater than 55 mm last year, there is no point in repeating one now since she has already met the criteria for operative repair. Warfarin is not indicated for only a dilated cardiomyopathy or regurgitant valve disease. Digoxin has no benefit in aortic regurgitation.

Mitral Valve Prolapse

Mitral valve prolapse (MVP) is perhaps the most common valvular condition, existing in as many as 10% of healthy young women. As such, MVP is not considered a disease unless symptoms are present.

PRESENTATION/"WHAT IS THE MOST LIKELY DIAGNOSIS?"

MVP, when symptomatic, presents with:

- Atypical chest pain (ie, not related to exertion)
- Palpitations
- Fatigue

▶ **TIP**

The auscultatory findings of MVP are markedly different from the other valvular disorders.

Auscultation

MVP gives a midsystolic **"click" followed by a murmur** of mitral regurgitation. The major issue for MVP, however, is that the effects of the maneuvers are the opposite of what occurs with the other forms of valve disease.

Squatting and leg raise decrease MVP.

Standing and Valsalva increase MVP.

Handgrip may decrease MVP. Handgrip increases afterload and decreases emptying.

In general, left-sided murmurs will **increase** in intensity with increased blood return, but in **MVP murmurs will decrease**.

DIAGNOSTIC TESTS/TREATMENT

After echocardiography, no further testing is generally required. When the patient is asymptomatic, no therapy is required. Patients, however, come to the doctor because they have symptoms. For a patient who is symptomatic with chest pain and palpitations, the best initial therapy for MVP is with beta blockers. It is rare for patients to develop symptoms of mitral regurgitation with MVP. If this does occur, the "best therapy" for either MVP or MR is with valve repair, such as tightening up the leaflets with sutures or shortening the chordae tendineae. **Endocarditis prophylaxis is not used with MVP.**

> Endocarditis prophylaxis is indicated for dental procedures only with: Prosthetic valves
>
> - Unrepaired cyanotic heart disease
> - Previous endocarditis
> - Cardiac transplant recipients with valvopathy

PERICARDIAL DISEASE

Pericarditis

ETIOLOGY

Pericarditis is caused by events that inflame the pericardium.

- **Infection:** Any infection can cause pericarditis, although viral infection is the most common.
- **Connective/tissue disease:** Any inflammatory disease can cause pericarditis, although SLE is the most common. Rheumatoid arthritis, Wegener granulomatosis, polyarteritis nodosa, Goodpasture syndrome, uremia, and scleroderma are examples of connective tissue or collagen vascular disorders that cause pericarditis.
- **Chest wall trauma** of any kind can lead to pericarditis.
- **Cancer** that is anatomically near the heart, such as lung, breast, or esophageal cancer, or a thoracic lymphoma, can result in pericarditis.

> Anything that causes pericarditis can also cause pericardial tamponade if enough fluid accumulates.

PRESENTATION/"WHAT IS THE MOST LIKELY DIAGNOSIS?"

Pericarditis presents with fever, and with chest pain that is:

- Pleuritic (changes with respiration)
- Positional (improves with sitting forward, worsens with lying back)

> A friction rub is a triphasic abnormal sound found in one-third of patients.

DIAGNOSTIC TESTS

The best initial test is an EKG. The EKG shows ST segment elevation in virtually every lead except aVR.

The most specific finding of pericarditis is PR segment depression.

> Echocardiogram does not show anything in pericarditis.

TREATMENT

The best initial therapy is NSAIDs.

▶ **TIP**

Recurrent pericarditis is treated with aspirin and colchicine.

Pericardial Tamponade

Tamponade means that fluid has accumulated to the point where the heart is compressed. The right side of the heart will compress first because the walls of the right side are thinner and will compress more easily. The right chambers are also at a lower pressure compared to the left chambers.

> Pericardial effusion does not automatically mean tamponade.

PRESENTATION/"WHAT IS THE MOST LIKELY DIAGNOSIS?"

Hypotension + tachycardia + distended neck veins = tamponade

Tamponade presents with clear lungs because fluid cannot get into the lungs if it cannot get into the right side of the heart. The most specific physical finding in tamponade is a pulsus paradoxus, a **decrease in blood pressure of more than 10 mm on inhalation**. Everyone's blood pressure decreases when they inhale because there is a decrease in intrathoracic pressure, leading to greater venous blood return to the right side of the heart, but it does not normally decrease more than 10 mm.

Pulsus Paradoxus

During normal inhalation, venous return increases to the right side of the heart, and the heart expands in external diameter. In tamponade, fluid surrounds the heart, compressing it. When the patient inhales and blood enters the right side of the heart, it cannot increase in external diameter. However, the right ventricle (RV) is still increasing in size. The only way this can happen is for the interventricular septum to shift to the left and compress the left ventricle (LV). This is why blood pressure decreases more than usual in pulsus paradoxus. Inhalation increases RV size. Increased RV size compresses the LV.

> Pulsus paradoxus is found most often in **tamponade**. Kussmaul sign is found most often in **constrictive pericarditis**.

DIAGNOSTIC TESTS

The most accurate test is echocardiography. The earliest finding is RA and then RV diastolic collapse.

EKG: Electrical alternans is an **alteration between big complexes and small complexes**. This is from a movement of the heart backward and forward in the pericardium. The closer the heart is to the anterior chest wall, the larger the complexes. "Low voltage," which is a generalized decrease in the height of the QRS complexes, occurs, but this is nonspecific. Other causes of **low voltage** are obesity, the barrel chest of COPD, and large breasts.

Cardiac catheterization: Equalization of pressures during diastole in all 4 chambers from the abnormally expanded level of pericardial fluid compressing the heart.

▶ **TIP**

Although catheterization is not needed if the echo shows RA/RV diastolic collapse, the "equalization of diastolic pressures" is a highly tested point.

TREATMENT

The best initial therapy is needle **pericardiocentesis**. The most effective therapy is a surgically placed **pericardial window**.

The removal of as little as 50 to 100 mL of fluid from the pericardial space can be life-saving if the patient is hemodynamically unstable. In a number of circumstances, such as in chronic conditions like hypothyroidism, large pericardial effusions may ensue, and the fluid will reaccumulate after removal of the needle. In this case, a hole must be placed in the pericardium so that the fluid will drain into the pleural space and be absorbed through the normal lymphatic drainage of the pleural space. This is called a pericardial window.

Constrictive Pericarditis

Any of the causes of pericarditis can potentially cause constrictive pericarditis if the condition lasts long enough for fibrosis and calcification of the pericardium to occur. Because chronic illness of that type is unusual, the most likely cause of constrictive pericarditis is tuberculosis.

PRESENTATION/"WHAT IS THE MOST LIKELY DIAGNOSIS?"

Constrictive pericarditis makes the normally compliant pericardium into a thickened, hard, immobile "box." It presents with signs of the chronic inability of the right side of the heart to fill, such as:

- Edema
- Ascites
- Hepatosplenomegaly
- JVD

These findings are not unique to constrictive pericarditis and would be identical in cor pulmonale and restrictive cardiomyopathy. Physical findings more specific to constrictive pericarditis are:

- **Kussmaul** sign (increase in JVD on inhalation)
- Pericardial "**knock**" (third heart sound from sudden impact of the filling heart with a noncompliant pericardium)

DIAGNOSTIC TESTS

The best initial test is a chest x-ray, which will show calcifications over the heart. A chest CT scan is more sensitive, and an MRI is more accurate. The echocardiogram will show a thickened pericardium. Mitral inflow will **decrease** on inspiration, and tricuspid inflow will **increase**.

> Constrictive pericarditis is diagnosed with imaging tests showing a thickened, calcified pericardium.

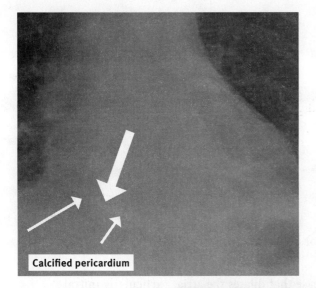
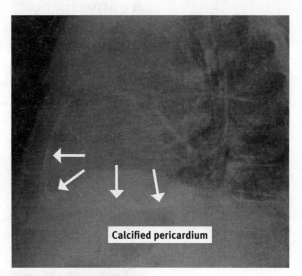

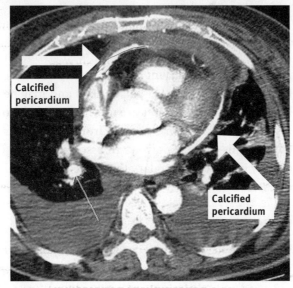

Figures 3.7–3.9: Constrictive pericarditis. Note the white calcification surrounding the heart.

Source: Mohammad Babury, MD and Mahendra C. Patel, MD

TREATMENT

The best initial therapy is a **diuretic**. The most effective therapy is **surgical removal** of the pericardium.

ARRHYTHMIA

Atrial Fibrillation

ETIOLOGY

Atrial fibrillation (A-fib) is most commonly associated with advanced age. Causes are:

- Hypertension
- Hyperthyroidism
- Caffeine
- Alcohol
- Drugs such as cocaine or amphetamines
- Pulmonary emboli
- Any valvular heart disease that dilates the atria, particularly mitral stenosis

PRESENTATION

> A-fib most often gives an irregularly irregular heart rate.

A-fib can often be asymptomatic. It is unusual for the blood pressure to be low. Patients complain of palpitations and may be short of breath. When the heart rate is rapid, patients are much more likely to be symptomatic. A-fib can result in acute pulmonary edema from the loss of atrial contribution to cardiac output. This is almost always in association with CHF, in which the heart is already inefficient secondary to ventricular dysfunction or from valvular heart disease.

DIAGNOSTIC TESTS

The EKG is the best initial test and will show an **irregularly irregular rhythm** without P waves. When A-fib is paroxysmal, the initial EKG may be normal. The most accurate tests are either an ambulatory continuous EKG monitor (the Holter monitor) or, **for inpatients, telemetry monitoring**.

Echocardiography is performed to evaluate the etiology of the arrhythmia and to see if a clot is present in the atrium. TTE is first but TEE is needed to truly exclude a clot.

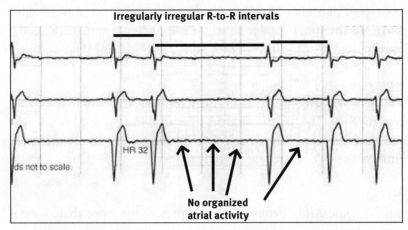

Figure 3.10: Atrial fibrillation. There is no organized atrial activity. Atrial fibrillation does not have to be rapid.

Source: Harman Chawla, MD

TREATMENT

The best initial therapy is to control the heart rate with:

- Beta blockers
- Calcium channel blockers (only diltiazem or verapamil)
- Digoxin

Once the **heart rate is controlled**, anticoagulation with **warfarin** is started to keep the INR between 2 and 3. Unless a clot is present, **heparin is not needed prior to starting warfarin**. Anticoagulation is continued as long as the A-fib persists. Dabigatran and rivaroxaban are alternatives to warfarin with equal or greater benefit in preventing stroke.

Cardioversion of Atrial Fibrillation

About 50% of patients with atrial fibrillation will spontaneously convert in the first few days. This is why anticoagulation should not be initiated until you are sure the patient is not going to convert on his or her own, eliminating the need for the risk of anticoagulation. Wait at least 48 hours.

In general, **routine conversion of A-fib should not be performed**. This is because patients will not stay in sinus rhythm. The mechanism that drives the development of chronic A-fib is largely based on an anatomic abnormality in the left atrium (dilatation and fibrosis). This is from dilated cardiomyopathy, ischemic heart disease, or valvular heart disease. Despite the use of electrical cardioversion or medications to convert the patient into sinus rhythm, patients will often not stay in sinus rhythm because you cannot eliminate the anatomic defect that caused the A-fib in the first place. After a year, only about 7% of patients who undergo vigorous attempts at chemical and electrical cardioversion will remain in sinus. This number is about equal to the amount that would convert spontaneously.

There is no overall mortality benefit to the routine attempt to convert stable patients into sinus rhythm. Unstable patients must undergo immediate electrical cardioversion.

Anticoagulation in Atrial Fibrillation

The risk of stroke per year with atrial fibrillation ranges from 1% to 18%, with an average risk of 6%. The use of warfarin with an INR of 2 to 3 reduces the risk by 65%, taking it from 6% to 2%. Warfarin, dabigatran, and rivaroxaban do not eliminate the risk of stroke; they only reduce it.

CHADS$_2$ Score

Patients with chronic A-fib, defined as being present for more than 2 days, should be anticoagulated if 2 or more points of the following scale are present:

- **Congestive failure** (defined as an EF below 35%)
- **Hypertension**
- **Age 75 or older**
- **Diabetes mellitus**
- **Stroke/TIA = 2 points**

This risk assessment is called a CHADS$_2$ score because each of these factors is given a value of 1, except for stroke or TIA, which is given 2 points for either. Low-risk persons with a CHADS score of 0 or 1 are at such a small risk of stroke that warfarin is not mandatory; they can be managed with aspirin alone.

Risk of Warfarin

The risk of major bleeding with warfarin is about 1% a year. "Major" bleeding means:

- Intracranial
- Requiring a transfusion

That means even if warfarin causes a gastrointestinal hemorrhage resulting in melena and a 10-point drop in hematocrit from 45 to 35, but no transfusion is necessary, it does not constitute a "major" bleeding episode by this definition.

The risk of stroke with A-fib is about 6% a year. The "cost" of using warfarin is about 1% a year in terms of the danger to the patient. If the CHADS$_2$ score is very low (0 or 1), the risk of stroke is less than 6% a year. It may be only 2%. The reduction in risk of stroke with warfarin from 2% to 1% a year would not then be worth the cost of anticoagulation with warfarin.

Unnecessary Risk of Heparin While Waiting for a Therapeutic INR

If a patient is being anticoagulated only for stroke prevention from atrial fibrillation, there is more harm in treating the patient with heparin than in waiting for the INR to be therapeutic. The risk of stroke per year is only about 6%. This is about 0.1% risk per week, which is the amount of time it takes to become therapeutic on warfarin. This is such a small risk of stroke that the risk of acute anticoagulation with heparin is greater than the risk of a stroke.

This is very different from using heparin with a DVT or pulmonary embolism. Those patients have a clot that is dangerous to them now. Mechanical heart valves have a much higher risk of emboli/clotting than A-fib does. Use heparin with an existing clot or a mechanical heart valve while waiting for a therapeutic INR. Do not use heparin while waiting for a therapeutic INR just for atrial fibrillation.

> Dabigatran and rivaroxaban produce full anticoagulation in hours.
> Their efficacy is equal to or greater than warfarin, with no INR monitoring.

▶ TIP

Do not use heparin while waiting for an INR of 2 to 3 for A-fib. Heparin use is the most common wrong answer when the only reason for anticoagulation is A-fib.

There are several advantages to the use of dabigatran and rivaroxaban:

- Oral anticoagulants
- Prevent stroke in A-fib or A-flutter
- Efficacy equal to or greater than warfarin
- Efficacious on first day of treatment
- No heparin is needed

Atrial Flutter

Atrial flutter is managed in the same way as atrial fibrillation, including rate control and anticoagulation with warfarin, dabigatran, or rivaroxaban. Anticoagulation is not necessary unless the arrhythmia is chronic, meaning it has been present for more than 2 days. Transient atrial arrhythmias, such as those that occur with alcohol, cocaine, or other transient cardiac insults, do not need chronic anticoagulation with warfarin.

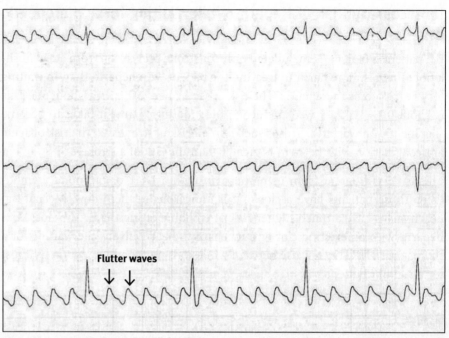

Figure 3.11: <u>Atrial flutter.</u> Atrial flutter is extremely regular in both the R-R intervals and the appearance of the flutter waves. Management is nearly identical to atrial fibrillation.

Source: Mahendra C. Patel, MD

Multifocal Atrial Tachycardia

Multifocal atrial tachycardia (MAT) is an atrial arrhythmia often occurring in association with COPD. MAT is usually associated with a normal width of QRS complex and has at least three distinct P wave morphologies. Treatment for MAT is the same as that for A-fib except that **beta blockers are often avoided**, since their use is associated with COPD. Some patients may tolerate beta blockers, but since calcium channel blockers are just as effective, there is no particular reason to use beta blockers. If your test question shows you two answers with equal efficacy, there is probably a contraindication to one of them, such as beta blockers in MAT from COPD.

Supraventricular Tachycardia

ETIOLOGY/PRESENTATION

Supraventricular tachycardia (SVT), unlike A-fib or atrial flutter, is not associated with hypertension or disorders that dilate the atria. SVT is associated with an abnormal conduction tract around the AV node. Patients present with palpitations and are rarely hemodynamically unstable. The **heart rate in SVT is always rapid**, usually around 160 beats per minute. This is very different from A-fib or flutter, in which the heart rate can be fast or slow.

SVT is not a common finding of myocardial ischemia. It is often a result of abnormalities in cardiac conduction pathways.

DIAGNOSTIC TESTS

SVT is found on EKG with a QRS complex that is usually normal in the absence of fibrillatory waves or flutter waves. The most accurate test is an **electrophysiology (EP) study**. The EP study is used to determine the etiology of the SVT and to map out the location of the aberrant conduction pathway that is resulting in the reentry around the AV node.

> SVT can sometimes have a wide complex, but is usually narrow.

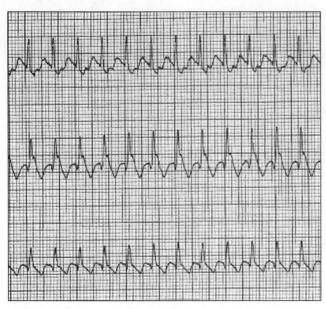

Figure 3.12: Supraventricular tachycardia. SVT has a QRS <120 mSec with no flutter waves, or fibrillatory waves at 160–180/minute.

Source: Harman Chawla, MD

TREATMENT

The best initial treatment for SVT is with:

1. **Vagal maneuvers:** Carotid sinus massage, Valsalva, ice water immersion, and cough can increase vagal tone and convert the SVT into normal sinus rhythm.
2. **Adenosine:** Adenosine can be both diagnostic and therapeutic. This is because adenosine has no meaningful effect on any arrhythmia except for SVT. In the event of an unclear presentation, if the arrhythmia converts to sinus with adenosine, it is essentially diagnostic of SVT.
3. **Beta blockers, calcium channel blockers, or digoxin:** If adenosine is unsuccessful, these agents can be used to slow down and convert the rhythm. They are equal in efficacy.
4. **Radiofrequency catheter ablation:** This is the answer to the question "What is the best long-term management of this patient?" Ablation is curative.

Ventricular Tachycardia

Ventricular tachycardia (V-tach) is a **wide complex** arrhythmia that is caused by ischemia, drug toxicity, hypokalemia, hypocalcemia, tricyclic antidepressant overdose, and dilation of the myocardium. As the ejection fraction lowers, and the ventricle becomes more dilated, the frequency of V-tach increases. This is why an ICD is used in those with persistent dilated cardiomyopathy. V-tach and ventricular fibrillation are the ultimate cause of death in myocardial infarction and CHF.

Patients present with a wide complex tachycardia on EKG. The presentation can vary from asymptomatic nonsustained runs of V-tach to palpitations, hypotension, and sometimes sudden death and pulselessness.

> The presence of V-tach does not imply a single presentation or clinical picture.

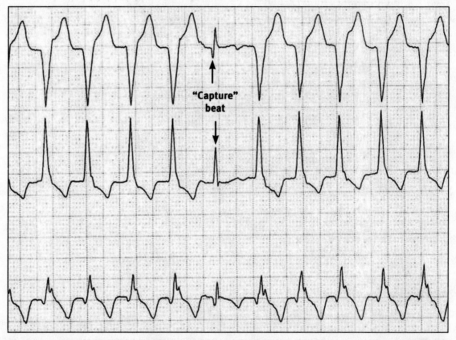

Figure 3.13: Ventricular tachycardia. Ventricular tachycardia is characterized by "fusion" beats or "capture" beats, which are occasional normal-appearing beats.

Source: Mahendra C. Patel, MD

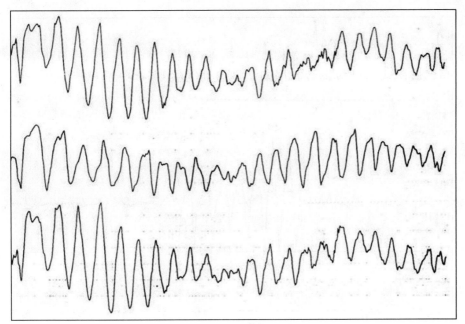

Figure 3.14: Torsade. Torsade has a characteristic undulating amplitude.

Source: Eduardo Andre, MD and Giselle Debs, MD

TREATMENT

Treatment of V-tach is based on the hemodynamic status of the patient. Those with minimal symptoms, such as palpitations, can be managed with medical therapy such as:

- Amiodarone
- Sotalol
- Procainamide
- Lidocaine

After resolution, long-term management with a beta blocker may be all that is required.

Hemodynamically **unstable V-tach is managed with synchronized cardioversion**. Hemodynamic instability is defined as:

- **Hypotension** with systolic blood pressure below 90 mm Hg
- **Chest pain** from insufficient coronary artery perfusion
- **Dyspnea** from CHF
- **Confusion** from insufficient cerebral perfusion

Any one of these is all that is necessary to define a patient as being unstable; you don't need to have all of them.

V-tach without a pulse is managed in the same way as ventricular fibrillation: Immediate unsynchronized shock is given.

> Asystole is no longer treated with atropine.

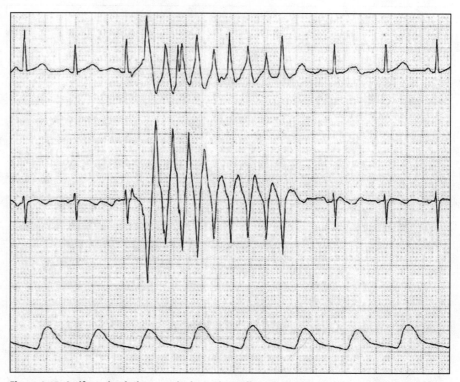

Figure 3.15: Artifact-simulating ventricular tachycardia. V-tach is present in all leads; an artifact is often limited to the leads being moved.

Source: Mahendra C. Patel, MD

Ventricular Fibrillation

V-fib is caused by the same things that cause V-tach. The management of V-fib is much simpler because there is only one presentation: The patient is pulseless.

The best initial therapy of V-fib is with unsynchronized cardioversion. Cardiopulmonary resuscitation (CPR) of chest compressions and ventilation are continued the entire time, except for the actual moment of delivering the shock.

The patient is shocked twice, followed by several cycles of CPR. Epinephrine or vasopressin is then given in an attempt to constrict the peripheral blood vessels and shunt blood into the central circulation. This is followed by another attempt at cardioversion and more CPR. If this is unsuccessful at restoring a normal rhythm, another shock is given followed by CPR and amiodarone or lidocaine.

Route of Medication Administration

Acceptable routes of medication administration are:

- Intravenous
- Through the endotracheal tube
- Intraosseous

> Amiodarone is superior to lidocaine for V-fib.

> ▶ **TIP**

Intracardiac administration of medications is always incorrect.

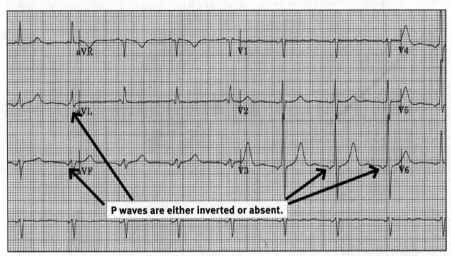

Figure 3.16: Junctional rhythm. Junctional rhythm originates at the AV node or bundle of HIS, which is the "junction" between the atrium and ventricle. P waves are absent or inverted.

Source: Danny Guillen, MD

Wolff-Parkinson-White Syndrome

Wolff-Parkinson-White (WPW) is an abnormal conduction tract between the atrium and ventricle. This can result in a sudden derangement of conduction.

PRESENTATION/"WHAT IS THE MOST LIKELY DIAGNOSIS?"

WPW presents with:

- SVT alternating with V-tach
- SVT that suddenly decompensates with the use of calcium channel blockers, beta blockers, or digoxin

Which of the following is the most distinctive physical finding of WPW?

a. Wide S2

b. Parodoxically split S2

c. Loud S1

d. Fixed splitting of S2

e. Palpable thrill

f. Displaced point of maximal impulse

Answer: The correct answer is (c). A loud S1 is heard when the left ventricle contracts while the mitral valve is still partially open. It is like slamming a door shut. Fixed splitting of S2 is heard with atrial septal defect (ASD). A palpable thrill is felt with very severe, high-volume murmurs. A thrill is the definition of a murmur being graded as 4/6. A displaced point of maximal impulse (PMI) is felt with CHF. A paradoxically split S2 is heard when the closure of the aortic valve is delayed. A widely split S2 is heard when closure of the pulmonic valve is delayed.

Causes of Abnormal Splitting of the Second Heart Sound (S2)	
Wide split S2	**Paradoxically split S2**
Pulmonic stenosis	Aortic stenosis
Pulmonary hypertension	Hypertension
Right bundle branch block	Left bundle branch block

DIAGNOSTIC TESTS

The best initial test of WPW is an EKG, which will show:

- **Delta wave**
- **Short PR** interval less than 120 milliseconds

The most accurate test is **electrophysiology studies,** which are done to pinpoint the precise location of the bypass tract. EP studies are very useful in the management of symptomatic WPW.

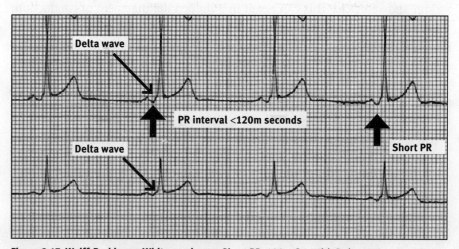

Figure 3.17: Wolff-Parkinson-White syndrome. Short PR<120 mSec with Delta wave.
Source: Eduardo Andre, MD and Giselle Debs, MD

TREATMENT

The most effective therapy for WPW is with **radiofrequency catheter ablation**. This is a catheter with the tip placed directly against the abnormal conduction pathway. The tip is heated by radiofrequency waves until the abnormal conduction pathway has been destroyed.

If WPW is presenting with an arrhythmia such as SVT and/or V-tach, the best initial therapy is with procainamide or amiodarone.

> Catheter ablation is curative for WPW.

Bradycardia

Most cases of sinus bradycardia are managed by treating the underlying cause if the patient is asymptomatic. **Symptomatic bradycardia** is treated initially with **atropine**. If the patient remains symptomatic after atropine, a transcutaneous pacemaker is used while awaiting a permanent pacemaker.

First-degree AV block and Mobitz I (Wenckebach) are managed in the same way. A patient who has a Mobitz II second-degree AV block or a third-degree (complete) heart block will always need a pacemaker, even if he or she is asymptomatic.

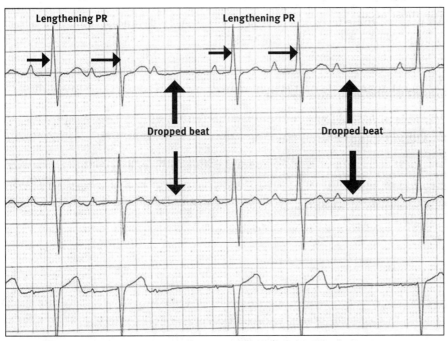

Figure 3.18: Mobitz I second-degree AV block (Wenckebach). Notice the progressively lengthening PR interval followed by a dropped beat.

Source: Mahendra C. Patel, MD

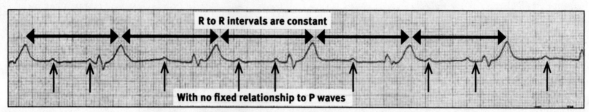

R to R intervals are constant

With no fixed relationship to P waves

Figure 3.19: Third-degree AV block. No fixed relationship of R to P waves.
Source: Philip Veith

AORTIC DISEASE

Aortic dissection presents with chest pain that can radiate to the back in between the shoulder blades. EKG excludes myocardial infarction. The best initial test to diagnose a dissection of the thoracic aorta is a chest x-ray, which will show a widened mediastinum.

The next best step in management is to confirm the diagnosis with either:

- Transesophageal echocardiography (TEE)
- Magnetic resonance angiography (MRA)
- CT angiogram (CTA)

All three of these tests have a 90% to 95% sensitivity and specificity. None of them is clearly superior to the others.

If TEE, MRA, or CTA confirms the presence of a dissecting aortic aneurysm, the "most appropriate next step in management" is to start therapy with:

1. Beta blockers (first)
2. Nitroprusside

The most accurate test is an angiogram with a catheter and contrast. However, an angiogram with contrasted aortography would only be done if the other noninvasive studies were not diagnostic. Definitive therapy is surgical resection.

> After x-ray, CT angiogram is often first simply because of availability.

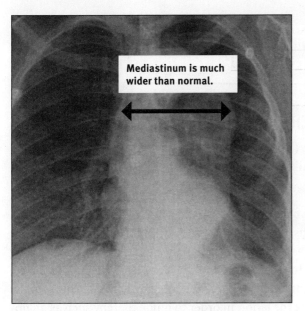

Figure 3.20: Aortic dissection. Look for a widened mediastinum on the chest x-ray as the first clue.

Source: Mahendra C. Patel, MD and Mohammad Babury, MD

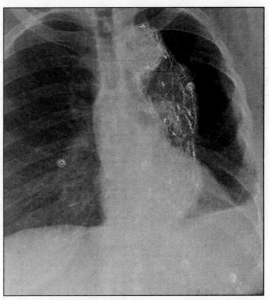

Figure 3.21: Repaired aortic dissection. Repair of the aneurysm does not mean compressing it to normal size. The multiple white markings are sutures and clips.

Source: Kunal Patel, MD

Abdominal Aortic Aneurysm

Abdominal aortic aneurysm (AAA) is diagnosed with ultrasound. Although CT angiogram and MR angiogram can assess an AAA, if ultrasound, CT, and MR are all in the answer, the correct answer is ultrasound. **Aneurysms greater than 5.5 centimeters in diameter should be repaired either surgically** or with a catheter-placed stent. Endovascular procedures should be tried first.

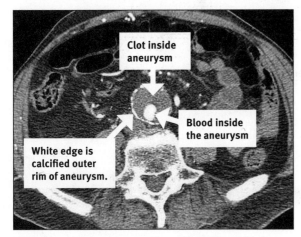

Figure 3.22: Aortic aneurysm. The outer wall is calcified. The patent lumen is white from contrast surrounded by a dark gray–appearing clot inside the aneurysm.

Source: Kunal Patel, MD

Screening for AAA

A single screen for AAA with an ultrasound is recommended in men between age 65 and 75 if they have ever smoked.

PERIPHERAL ARTERIAL DISEASE

Peripheral arterial disease (PAD) is diagnosed in older patients who develop pain in their legs while walking that is relieved by rest, which is the definition of claudication.

The **best initial test is an ankle/brachial index** (ABI). A normal value for ABI is 0.9 or above. This means that the blood pressure in the lower extremities should be within 10% of the pressure in the upper extremities. A value below 0.9 implies an obstruction to the flow of blood into the legs. The most accurate test is an angiogram. Angiography is not done to diagnose PAD. Angiography is done to identify the site of the lesion in order to guide therapy such as angioplasty, stenting, or bypass.

The best initial therapy for PAD is:

- **Aspirin**
- **Statins** to keep the LDL below 100 mg/dL
- **Stopping smoking**

The single most effective therapy is **cilostazol**, which is both antiplatelet and antispasmodic.

▶**TIP**

The most common wrong answers in PAD are:

- Pentoxifylline
- Calcium channel blocker

These agents do not help PAD.

DERMATOLOGY

4

BLISTERING DISEASES

The blistering diseases are all, in a sense, **idiopathic** or **autoimmune** disorders. Some represent a hypersensitivity reaction to medications such as ACE inhibitors or NSAIDs. Why some people react to these medications with a simple maculopapular (morbilliform) rash and some get erythema multiforme, Stevens-Johnson, or pemphigoid is not known. The minor, non-life-threatening versions of drug hypersensitivities do not need a biopsy, and there is no specific therapy. When bullae, or blisters, occur, it is important to biopsy because these disorders are potentially life-threatening. When blisters occur and a large surface area of the body is involved, the patient will follow the clinical course of a patient who has a burn. This specifically means:

- Fluid loss
- Infection

Serious blistering diseases are treated with glucocorticoids such as prednisone. Serious forms of **Stevens-Johnson** or **toxic epidermal necrolysis** are treated with **intravenous immunoglobulin (IVIG)** in addition to rehydration and local wound care. As with treatment of all serious autoimmune disorders, when long-term steroids are used, alternative treatment (steroid-sparing) regimens are used to avoid the adverse effects of steroids.

Pemphigus Vulgaris

ETIOLOGY

Pemphigus vulgaris is most often autoimmune. It can sometimes occur secondary to predictable allergenic substances (e.g., penicillin) or ACE inhibitors. Autoantibodies attack the epidermis and split the already thin epidermal layer in half. This is why the lesions of pemphigus vulgaris do not stay intact as bullae. They are too thin. If the skin split at a deeper layer, as **in bullous pemphigoid, the lesions would be able to stay intact**.

> Oral lesions are the most specific finding for pemphigus vulgaris.

PRESENTATION/"WHAT IS THE MOST LIKELY DIAGNOSIS?"

Presentation characteristics include:

- Diffuse, desquamating lesions over most of the body
- Broken bullae; they do not stay intact
- Oral involvement
- Extremely ill person
- Possibly infection and severe fluid/volume loss

DIAGNOSTIC TESTS

> The Nikolsky sign (skin removed in sheets with slight pressure) is present in pemphigus.

Biopsy, both routine and with direct immunofluorescence, is both the "best initial test" and the "most accurate test." There really is no other way to confirm the diagnosis. Antibodies will be seen splitting the epidermal junction.

TREATMENT

Steroids (glucocorticoids) such as prednisone are the best initial therapy. Steroid-sparing treatments to try to wean a patient off of steroids are:

> Untreated pemphigus vulgaris has a mortality rate exceeding 50%.

- Cyclosporine
- Azathioprine
- Tacrolimus
- Pimecrolimus

Bullous Pemphigoid

As with pemphigus vulgaris, bullous pemphigoid is usually an **autoimmune** blistering skin lesion that can sometimes arise **secondary to medications** and often with no identified reason. Because the antibodies attack the skin at a layer deeper than pemphigus, a lesion of bullous pemphigoid is able to stay intact as a bulla. This is because the skin is split at the dermal/epidermal junction, which is deeper than the extremely superficial split in pemphigus vulgaris. Bullous pemphigoid differs from pemphigus in that:

> Lesions in bullous disease are **painful**, but **not** pruritic.

- Bullae remain intact.
- There is no oral involvement.
- Fluid loss is much less common.
- Infection is much less common.

DIAGNOSTIC TESTS/TREATMENT

The skin biopsy is essentially the only test. Steroids are the best initial therapy.

Porphyria Cutanea Tarda

Porphyria cutanea tarda (PCT) is a hypersensitivity reaction of the skin to light, reacting with abnormal porphyrins seen in:

- Chronic liver disease (hepatitis C)
- Iron overload
- Estrogen use
- Alcoholism

PRESENTATION

Bullous skin lesions occur almost exclusively on **sun-exposed areas**. The question will describe involvement of the face and the backs of the hands, which are the two most reliably sun-exposed areas. These lesions are fragile and are associated with hypertrichosis.

DIAGNOSTIC TESTS

The most accurate test is an abnormally elevated level of **uroporphyrins** found in a 24-hour urine collection. Abnormal uroporphyrins are not reliably detected by blood tests.

TREATMENT

Besides **eliminating alcohol and estrogen use**, the most effective therapy is phlebotomy. Antimalarials are effective. When you remove the abnormal blood along with the abnormal porphyrins, the disorder resolves. If the porphyrins are not present in the bloodstream, there is nothing to react with sunlight.

> Severe infection and volume depletion are much less common with pemphigoid.

> Hydroxychloroquine is an option when phlebotomy cannot be done.

HYPERSENSITIVITY REACTIONS

Morbilliform Rash

A morbilliform rash means one that looks like measles. When sulfa drugs were introduced in the 1930s, physicians had never seen a sulfa drug reaction before. When it occurred, it suggested to them the reddish, maculopapular eruption characteristic of measles. The rash is diffuse and will resolve on its own when the medication is stopped.

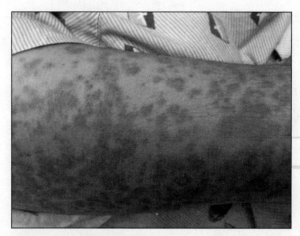

Figure 4.1: Morbilliform rash. This patient reacted to sulfa drugs.
Source: Mayurkumar Gohel, MD

ETIOLOGY

Drug hypersensitivity reactions are characteristic of certain medications such as:

- Penicillin, cephalosporins, and rifampin
- Sulfa drugs: antibiotics, hydrochlorothiazide, NSAIDs
- Phenytoin, carbamazapine, and lamotrigine
- Allopurinol
- Quinidine

These same medications are also the medications associated with the development of drug-induced allergic interstitial nephritis and hemolysis. Some drugs cause allergies and some medications, like calcium channel blockers, beta blockers, or SSRIs, do not cause rash, hemolysis, or interstitial nephritis.

Erythema Multiforme

Erythema multiforme (EM) is a more severe form of hypersensitivity reaction that can occur from the same **medications** previously described, as well as infections with **herpes simplex** and *Mycoplasma*. Small, circular, target-shaped lesions occur. There may be some very minor involvement of mucous membranes. EM is managed by stopping the offending agent and potentially treating the infection that caused it. **Prednisone is of unclear benefit.**

Stevens-Johnson Syndrome

Stevens-Johnson means a drug reaction so severe that there is damage to mucous membranes.

Stevens-Johnson syndrome (SJS) is a more severe form of drug hypersensitivity reaction. The etiology does not differ from the medications previously described, but the lesions are more severe in the sense that there is mucous membrane involvement. Less than 10% of the total body surface area is involved as a matter of definition. The **conjunctiva of the eyes** is involved as well as the **oral mucosa** and the **respiratory tract**. SJS may be so severe as to cause sloughing of the respiratory tract and result in marked hypoxia and respiratory failure. The most severe cases require mechanical ventilation. Steroids have no clear benefit. **Intravenous immunoglobulins** may be useful.

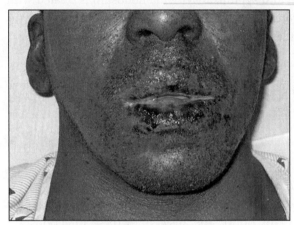

Figure 4.2: Stevens-Johnson syndrome. Steroids are not reliably helpful in Stevens-Johnson.

Source: Moe Sann, MD

Toxic Epidermal Necrolysis

Toxic epidermal necrolysis (TEN) is the most severe form of drug hypersensitivity reaction. There is:

- **Greater than 30% body surface area involved**
- Mucous membrane involvement (conjunctiva, oral, respiratory)
- Sloughing of the skin that comes off in sheets (Nikolsky sign)

TEN is generally a clinical diagnosis based on a history of the ingestion of a characteristic toxin and the pattern of cutaneous involvement just described. The most accurate diagnostic test is a skin biopsy. **Steroids are not clearly beneficial**. Use **intravenous immunoglobulins**. These patients are best managed in the intensive care unit or a burn unit.

▶**TIP**

The boards will avoid controversial issues such as the use of steroids in drug hypersensitivity reactions like SJS and TEN.

Fixed Drug Reaction

This is a limited form of drug hypersensitivity reaction. When it occurs, it is limited to a single area of the skin. It is treated with local, topical steroids.

Erythema Nodosum

These are tender, reddish-brown, slightly raised skin lesions that represent an inflammatory reaction of local subcutaneous tissues. They usually appear on the legs. The cause is not known. We know that it is associated with **streptococcal infection**, **coccidioidomycoses**, **histoplasmosis**, sarcoidosis, pregnancy, inflammatory bowel disease, and syphilis. Erythema nodosum is treated with aspirin, NSAIDs, and in severe cases, corticosteroids. The most essential management is to control the underlying cause.

CUTANEOUS INFECTIONS

Fungal Infections

DEFINITION

Fungal infections of the skin are also referred to as dermatophytes, or "tinea" followed by the name of the body part in Latin: e.g., corporis (body), capitis (head), manum (hand), or pedis (foot). The answers to these infections are generally the same no matter what body part is involved: The best initial test for all of them is a scraping of the skin for a **potassium hydroxide (KOH) preparation**. KOH, when added to a scraping of the skin and heated slightly, will melt away epithelial cells while leaving the fungal hyphae behind to be easily visualized. The most accurate test is a **fungal culture**. If the scraping shows hyphae, it is never a correct answer to wait for the results of the fungal culture in order to initiate therapy.

TREATMENT

Cutaneous fungal infections are treated with topical antifungal medications as long as there is no involvement of hair (tinea capitis) or nail (onychomycosis). Topical antifungal medications are:

- Clotrimazole
- Ketoconazole
- Miconazole
- Terbinafine
- Ciclopirox
- Naftifine
- Butenafine

Systemic antifungals for onychomycosis and tinea capitis are:

- Terbinafine
- Itraconazole
- Fluconazole weekly for 3 to 6 months

▶ **TIP**

Griseofulvin is rarely the right answer to anything in adult medicine because of the need to use it for a prolonged period of time.

Tinea Versicolor

Tinea versicolor is caused by the organism *Malassezia furfur*. The only difference between tinea versicolor and the other superficial fungal infections is:

- It is **diffuse**, covering large areas of the body.
- KOH shows a unique "**spaghetti and meatball**" pattern.
- **Selenium sulfide** is used as a topical lotion in order to cover large surface areas.
- Occasional very widespread or recurrent cases are treated with a single dose of oral ketaconazole.

Oral and Vaginal Candidiasis

Both oral and vaginal candidiasis present with large white plaques that easily scrape away. Both readily reveal fungal hyphae on KOH prep. Neither requires a fungal culture result in order to initiate therapy. Both can be treated with topical clotrimazole. Both readily respond to short courses of oral fluconazole.

> Fluconazole is an excellent drug for yeasts such as *Candida*, but is weak for molds on the skin and nails.

Bacterial Skin Infections

Impetigo

Impetigo is the most **superficial** of the **bacterial** skin infections. Impetigo means that the infection is largely limited to the epidermis. The most common organisms are *Staphylococcus aureus* and *Streptococcus pyogenes*. Because it is so superficial, it is characterized by weeping, crusting, oozing, and draining of purulent material from the skin.

> Bacterial skin infections are rarely confirmed by a specific diagnostic test.

TREATMENT

Impetigo can be treated with topical antibiotics such as:

- Mupirocin
- Retapamulin
- Neomycin
- Bacitracin

> Streptococcal skin infections can lead to glomerulonephritis, but not rheumatic fever.

Erysipelas

Caused by *Streptococcus pyogenes*, erysipelas is a deeper infection than impetigo and can involve the lymphatic channels in the dermis. This can lead to systemic spread of the infection, and 5% of patients with erysipelas develop bacteremia. As with most skin infections, the diagnosis is made on visual appearance and a specific bacterial organism is rarely identified. Erysipelas is particularly bright red and hot to the touch.

> Topical therapy will not work for erysipelas.

Cellulitis

This infection is deeper than erysipelas and involves the subcutaneous tissues as well as the dermis. Because cellulitis is an infection well underneath the dermal/epidermal junction, purulent material rarely rises to the top and there is usually no weeping, crusting, oozing, or draining. As with all infections, the area is red, warm, swollen, and tender (rubor, calor, tumor, and dolor).

▶ **TIP**

Exclude deep venous thrombosis with most cases of cellulitis.

Folliculitis, Furuncles, Carbuncles

When *Staphylococcus* begins as an infection of the skin starting from around a hair follicle, the infection is known as folliculitis. The terms furuncle and carbuncle imply a larger, deeper infection. There is no precise demarcation in size between a furuncle and a carbuncle. They are essentially small skin abscesses; because they are too small to be drained, however, the term "abscess" is not used. They are staphylococcal skin infections that are centered around a hair follicle and may be small (folliculitis), medium (furuncle), or large (carbuncle). They are staphylococcal skin infections with multiple ineffective drainage points around a hair follicle, usually in areas of thick skin (e.g., back of neck). They may be small.

Treatment of Bacterial Skin Infections

Because of the rapid spread of methicillin (or oxacillin)-resistant *Staphylococcus aureus* (MRSA), it is difficult to give a precise single therapy for skin and soft tissue infections (SSTIs) with bacteria. Treatment precision is further complicated by the usual custom of empiric treatment. Only rarely is a specific organism obtained from the skin to guide therapy.

> Ceftaroline is the only cephalosporin covering MRSA.

▶ **TIP**

Swab of superficial lesions for culture is never a correct answer. You cannot distinguish colonization from the true causative organism by this method.

Sensitive Organisms

Treatment is divided according to the severity of the infection. Minor infection is treated with oral therapy. Severe infection is treated with intravenous therapy. "Severe" is defined as:

- Fever and severe pain
- Hypotension
- Rapidly spreading and bullae
- Lymphangitic streaking

- Large area of involvement
- Associated with lymphadenitis

Treatment of Bacterial Skin Infections	
Minor infection (oral)	**Severe infection (intravenous)**
Dicloxacillin, cloxacillin	Oxacillin, naficillin
Cephalexin	Cefazolin
Clindamycin	Clindamycin
Trimethoprim/sulfamethoxazole (TMP-SMZ)	Vancomycin
Doxycycline	Linezolid
Azithromycin, clarithromycin	Daptomycin, ceftaroline

> Beta-lactam antibiotics (penicillins and cephalosporins) have the best efficacy. Empiric treatment with trimethoprim/ sulfamethoxazole or doxycycline for minor skin and soft tissue infections will adequately cover MRSA.

Penicillin Allergy

Rash: Cephalosporin antibiotics are safe to use if the allergic reaction to penicillin was only a rash (i.e., no angioedema, anaphylaxis, or hypotension as in a type 1 reaction). The amount of cross-reaction between penicillins and cephalosporins is considerably under 5%.

> Gas formation and high CPK is a sign of very severe disease.

Anaphylaxis: Doxycycline, TMP-SMZ, or clindamycin should be used for minor SSTIs if the reaction to penicillin was life-threatening such as anaphylaxis. For severe infections requiring hospitalization, use vancomycin, daptomycin, or linezolid. There is no cross-reaction at all between penicillin and these classes of antibiotics.

Resistant Organisms (MRSA)

Minor SSTIs can be treated with:

- Doxycycline
- TMP-SMZ
- Clindamycin (add for necrotizing fasciitis)

> Treatment of minor SSTIs with resistant organisms is a rapidly changing area of medicine.

Severe SSTIs with Resistant Organisms

This is a clearer area in which to answer questions because vancomycin, linezolid, and daptomycin are all reliable intravenous therapies for resistant organisms.

Necrotizing Fasciitis

Because necrotizing fasciitis is associated with **anaerobic infection** or **streptococci** that produce toxin that dissects through tissue layers, clindamycin should be added to the usual therapy for cellulitis with either a penicillin (nafcillin or oxacillin) or a cephalosporin (cefazolin). Debridement should also be performed to surgically remove necrotic tissue.

> Surgical debridement can be life-saving in necrotizing fasciitis.

For this indication give clindamycin for 3–4 days. Linezolid, with its protein synthesis inhibition (preventing further toxin production), has similar function and can be used instead of clindamycin.

Viral Skin Infections
Herpes Simplex

Oral and genital infection with herpes simplex presents with multiple painful vesicular lesions. When the vesicles are clearly identifiable, no testing is needed and the answer to the question "What is the most appropriate next step in management?" is to start antiviral therapy with **acyclovir**, **famciclovir**, **or valacyclovir**. The efficacy of all three of these agents is equal.

> Topical therapy is useless for herpes infections; use oral therapy.

DIAGNOSTIC TESTS

If the roof comes off of the vesicles, as often happens with genital lesions, then a diagnostic test may be necessary to distinguish herpes from other forms of ulcerative genital lesions. The best initial test is a Tzanck prep. A Tzanck prep is very similar to a Pap smear. Freshly swabbed tissue is obtained, placed on a slide, and fixed in order to identify multinucleated giant cells. These cells cannot distinguish the specific type of herpesvirus. The "most accurate test," and the only way to tell the specific organism, is with a viral culture. Herpes virus is fast growing and the viral culture can give a definite answer in as little as two days.

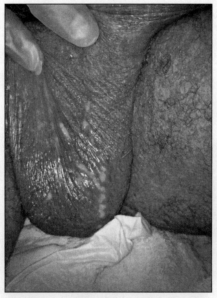

Figure 4.3: Herpes simplex. When the roofs come off of vesicles they can be hard to distinguish from other STDs. Herpes is smaller and multiple lesions are present.

Source: Farshad Bagheri, MD

▶ **TIP**

Boards do not test dosing, but they do test route of administration.

Varicella Zoster Virus (Shingles)

Varicella zoster virus (VZV) infections reactivate along a dermatomal distribution. They present as multiple vesicular lesions and can be associated with extremely severe pain. Immunocompromise and increasing age predispose to reactivation of VZV infections. If the vesicles are clear, no further testing is needed. As with herpes simplex infections, the "most appropriate next step in management" is to start antiviral therapy; acyclovir, famciclovir, and valacyclovir are equal in efficacy and topical therapy is useless.

When the diagnosis is not clear, **Tzanck prep** and **viral culture** are the most accurate tests to perform.

The differences between VZV and herpes simplex are:

- Dosing of medications is higher with VZV
- Culture takes longer to grow
- **Vaccination** should be given to all those **above age 60** to prevent VZV reactivation

Steroids do not clearly decrease the risk of postherpetic neuralgia.

TREATMENT

The best initial therapy for reactivation of varicella or shingles is acyclovir, valacyclovir, or famciclovir. All three are essentially equal except in terms of dosing. There is no fundamental difference in efficacy. They can decrease the risk of herpes zoster–related pain.

Intravenous therapy is used for:

- Disseminated disease (lung, liver)
- Ocular disease
- Central nervous system involvement
- Immunocompromised patients with greater than one dermatome involved

Prevention

Varicella vaccine should be given routinely to all adults over the age of 60. The varicella vaccine to prevent shingles is essentially the same vaccine as that used in children to prevent the primary infection, except that it is at higher dose. Vaccination reduces the risk of shingles by two-thirds.

> Herpes zoster is synonymous with the term "shingles."

> There is no clear role for steroids in shingles.
>
> Foscarnet is the drug of choice for acyclovir-resistant herpes.

A pregnant nursing student comes to you after she discovers that a patient developed chicken pox the day after she was in his room. The skin lesions were not present on the day she was in the room. She is very clear that she did not touch the patient, but she was in the room for nearly an hour. She never had chicken pox as a child and her varicella antibody is undetectable.

What is the most appropriate action in this case?

a. No action required
b. Varicella vaccine
c. Varicella immune globulin (VZIG) now with varicella vaccination after delivery
d. VZIG only
e. VZIG and varicella vaccination now

Answer: The correct answer is (c). VZIG is indicated in the prophylaxis of exposures to chicken pox or shingles within 96 hours (four days) of exposure. VZIG will do nothing to treat an established infection. The source patient is considered capable of transmitting the infection from 1 to 2 days before the development of a rash through the first week of rash, which is when the lesions begin to dry and crust over.

Physical contact with the source patient is not necessary to develop the infection. Varicella is transmitted by the airborne route. Varicella vaccine is an attenuated live vaccine and is contraindicated in pregnant women, users of glucocorticoids, severely immunocompromised patients, and those with AIDS with less than 200 CD4 cells/µl.

> Healthcare workers should be screened for varicella and vaccinated if not immune.

Complications of Shingles
- Postherpetic neuralgia: occurs in 60% to 70% of those above age 60
- Bacterial superinfection
- Seventh cranial nerve (Bell) palsy

Postherpetic Neuralgia
This can be extremely painful and difficult to treat. The best therapy is with **pregabalin**, **gabapentin**, or lidocaine patch. Alternate treatment is with tricyclic antidepressants, opiates, or capsaicin cream.

Sexually Transmitted Diseases

Human Papillomavirus or Condyloma Acuminatum
Human papillomavirus (HPV)-associated **genital warts** can occur at any time in a person's lifetime as a complication of the sexual transmission of HPV. The lesions are flesh colored and are often asymptomatic. They can become enormous and cauliflowerlike in appearance.

There is **no routine test** to diagnose genital warts. They are diagnosed by their appearance. Wrong answers are: stain, smear, serology, and biopsy.

Sometimes lesions are difficult to identify, and biopsy is indicated. It is also possible to type human papillomavirus to assess the risk of cervical cancer.

Treatment of HPV-associated genital warts is with **mechanical removal** by almost any method such as:

- Cryotherapy with liquid nitrogen
- Podophyin (podophyllotoxin) or trichloroacetic acid to dissolve or "melt" the lesion
- Curettage
- Electosurgery or laser oblation
- Imiquimod, a self-administered immunomodulator

Syphilis

Primary syphilis presents as a painless, firm (indurated) genital lesion with surrounding lymphadenopathy. The most accurate test of primary syphilis is a dark-field examination. The most common wrong answer for diagnosis of primary syphilis is a VDRL or RPR test of the blood. These serologic tests are 75% to 80% sensitive and will therefore miss 20% to 25% of patients.

Secondary syphilis almost always presents with a skin lesion such as:

- Maculopapular rash
- Mucous patches
- Alopecia areata
- Condylomata lata

The most accurate test for secondary syphilis is with a VDRL or RPR confirmed with an FTA-ABS or MHA-TP. The sensitivity of these tests in secondary syphilis is nearly 100%.

Both primary and secondary syphilis are treated with a single intramuscular dose of penicillin. Those with a penicillin allergy are treated with doxycycline.

> **▶ TIP**
>
> The most common wrong answer for treating a penicillin-allergic patient with syphilis is to desensitize the patient. Desensitization is used for pregnant patients or those with neurosyphilis.

Scabies and Pediculosis

Scabies presents with pruritic lesions described as occurring in the **web-spaces** of the hands, feet, and joints. They also occur around the nipples and in the groin. Because *Sarcoptes scabiei* is much smaller than *Pediculus humanus* (lice), the diagnosis of scabies is made by **scraping** the skin for magnification. Lice are larger, and do not burrow under the skin as do scabies. Pediculosis can be diagnosed upon visual inspection of the skin in the groin, axilla, or other hair-bearing areas.

> Imiquimod stimulates the immune system against:
>
> - warts
> - actinic keratoses
> - molluscum
> - basal cell abnormalities

> Pediculosis is synonymous with "lice" or "crabs."

TREATMENT

Both scabies and pediculosis are treated effectively with topical **permethrin**.

Alternate therapy is with:

- **Ivermectin** orally
- Benzyl benzoate
- Lindane

Norwegian Scabies

The term "Norwegian" refers to scabies that is:

- Severe and widespread
- Associated with severe crusting
- Associated with immunocompromised patients

Norwegian scabies is diagnosed with scraping for microscopic identification in the same way as routine scabies in web spaces. Because it is widespread, it should be treated with oral ivermectin.

▶ **TIP**

The clue to the diagnosis of Norwegian scabies is a question describing an "institutionalized" patient or a debilitated patient in a nursing home.

LYME

Lyme presents as a circular, target-shaped lesion with a pale center. This is sometimes called erythema migrans. Patients may have a history of fever, arthralgia, myalgia, and fatigue. When a characteristic lesion of Lyme is described or shown, the answer is to give doxycycline, amoxicillin, or cefuroxime. The wrong answer is to do serology. An obvious Lyme rash is more specific than serologic testing.

Only 20% of patients with Lyme remember a tick bite.

▶ **TIP**

Camping or hiking in the history is the clue to Lyme and tick bites.

TOXIC SHOCK SYNDROME AND STAPHYLOCOCCAL SCALDED SKIN SYNDROME

Staphylococcus aureus produces a toxin that can lead to a severe, life-threatening desquamative disorder that leads to the skin coming off in sheets. When the disorder is limited to the skin alone, it is known as staphylococcal scalded skin syndrome (SSSS). When it involves multiple internal organs and drastically decreases the blood pressure, it is toxic shock syndrome (TSS). SSSS presents in a manner similar to TEN: Greater than 30% of the body surface area is involved and the skin will come off in a sheet with gentle pressure (Nikolsky sign).

TSS leads to:

- Hypotension and high fever
- Elevation of **liver function tests**
- Elevation of **BUN** and **creatinine**
- Confusion and **CNS** abnormalities
- Diarrhea

TSS develops when *Staphylococcus* grows in an abnormal focus such as:

- Nasal packing
- Wounds around sutures
- Abscesses
- Vaginal canal around high-absorbency tampons, particularly those left in place for prolonged periods of time

In addition to the skin manifestations, *Staphylococcus* is grown from the blood or at the site of accumulation. Treatment is with antistaphylococcal medications such as:

- Oxacillin or nafcillin
- Cefazolin
- Vancomycin (particularly when the sensitivity of the organism is not known)
- Linezolid, daptomycin, ceftaroline

TSS is also managed with dopamine, levarterenol, (norepinephrine) and other pressors used to maintain blood pressure. A burn unit is used for those with large surface area involvement.

> Add clindamycin as a second drug for toxic shock treatment.

> Don't forget to remove the site of the growth of *Staphylococcus*.

SEBORRHEIC KERATOSIS

This is a hyperpigmented skin lesion that has a characteristic "stuck on" appearance. Early mild lesions are referred to commonly as "liver spots." When they become large and elevated above the skin, they are seborrheic keratosis. They have **no premalignant potential**. They are treated with various forms of **mechanical removal** such as cryotherapy or curettage. Since they are never premalignant, the major driver of the need for removal is cosmetic.

MALIGNANT SKIN DISEASES

Actinic Keratosis

Actinic keratosis is a premalignant lesion that has the potential to develop into squamous cell cancer. The word "actinic" specifically means "related to the sun." The case will describe extensive sun exposure in a light-skinned person. Look for a person who works outdoors, such as on the roofs of houses. **Biopsy** is the most accurate test, although many cases can be diagnosed simply from their appearance.

Treatment of actinic keratosis is to **remove them** before they have time to transform into squamous cell cancer. Any mechanical method of removal such as previously described for HPV-associated warts is useful. Examples include curettage, liquid nitrogen, topical 5-fluorouracil, and imiquimod.

Melanoma

Malignant melanoma presents with a hyperpigmented lesion in virtually any area of the body. The lesions also have a predilection for:

- Eyes
- Nails
- CNS metastases

This feature is part of what distinguishes melanoma from the other cutaneous malignancies.

▶ **TIP**

The most important points for the internist in terms of skin cancer are:
1. When do I refer?
2. What differentiates a malignant/aggressive malignancy from benign disease?

Presentation of Malignant Disease

Skin lesions that need biopsy are:

ABCDE

Asymmetric, Borders are uneven, Color changes, Diameter changes, Evolution

DIAGNOSTIC TESTS

Excisional biopsy is the one and nearly only test for all skin cancers. The most important prognostic factor for melanoma is the **thickness** of the lesion. This is why shave biopsy is inappropriate to determine the extent of disease. Lesions less than 0.5 mm in thickness are generally cured by resection, need little additional therapy, and do not metastasize. Lesions more than 4 mm in thickness will almost always go into the regional lymph nodes.

Sentinel Lymph Node Biopsy

Similar to breast cancer, the sentinel node is the first node "downstream" from the lesion. If the sentinel node is free of cancer, an extensive regional lymph node dissection is not necessary.

▶ **TIP**

The most important question is: What type of biopsy is indicated for melanoma? The answer is full thickness excisional biopsy.

> Thickness determines the likelihood of metastases to regional lymph nodes.

TREATMENT

Excision is the best initial therapy. Metastatic disease is treated with:

1. • Impilimumab, IL2, vemurafenib
2. • **Interferon**
3. • **Radiation** to regional lymph nodes
4. • Brain metastases should be resected or radiated

> Chemotherapy is not useful for melanoma.

Squamous Cell Carcinoma

Squamous cell carcinoma (SCC) is related to sun exposure and pale skin, which will most likely be in the case.

▶ **TIP**

Look for the word "ulcerated" to suggest SCC as the diagnosis.

DIAGNOSTIC TESTS/TREATMENT

Biopsy is the "best initial test" and the "most accurate test." Physical removal of the lesion is the "best initial therapy" and the "most effective therapy." The questions will center more on the method of removal.

Smaller lesions, especially on areas not exposed to sunlight, are treated with:

- Topical 5-fluorouracil
- Topical imiquimod
- Cryotherapy
- Electrosurgery
- Radiation

Large lesions on sun-exposed areas such as the neck, face, or hands are treated with surgical resection.

Mohs Microsurgery

This is a method of removing skin cancer such as SCC or basal cell. **Very thin slices are removed** around the lesion. The thin slices are examined under a microscope as they are removed. This allows the dermatologist/surgeon to stop resecting normal tissue as soon as they know the surrounding area is clear of even microscopic metastases. This is more accurate than, and certainly **cosmetically superior** to, simply removing a wide margin irrespective of the presence of disease in the local tissue.

Basal Cell Carcinoma

As with all skin cancers, basal cell carcinoma (BCC) occurs on sun-exposed areas. **Biopsy** is the most accurate test, and **removal** is the most effective therapy. Low-risk lesions can be treated with 5-FU or imiquimod.

Kaposi Sarcoma

Kaposi sarcoma (KS) is a purplish-colored skin cancer that is associated with human herpesvirus 8. There is a "classic KS," found as a very slowly progressive skin lesion in older men of Mediterranean origin, and there is the form found in association with AIDS and less than 100 CD4 cells/µl. Classic KS in HIV-negative persons generally does not require specific therapy. In KS associated with AIDS, the most important management is to treat the HIV. **If the CD4 count increases, the KS will go away.**

Although KS can be treated with doxorubicin or vinblastine, this often proves unnecessary if the HIV is adequately treated.

Psoriasis

Psoriasis is extremely common. The questions will almost always be about treatment.

Local Disease/Limited Surface Area

The best initial therapy for psoriasis involving small amounts (less than 10%) of body surface area is:

- **Salicylic acid topically** to remove scaling and loose skin
- **Topical corticosteroids**

The salicylic acid allows the topical steroids to come in contact with the skin. The problem with the chronic use of glucocorticoids is that they will lead to skin atrophy.

If the questions describes a patient whose disease recurs every time steroids are discontinued, the answer is:

- **Vitamin D topically** (calcipotriene)
- **Vitamin A topically** (tazarotene, adapalene)
- And, as second-line agents, **calcineurin inhibitors** (tacrolimus, pimecrolimus)

These agents can be effective in allowing the patient to discontinue the use of topical steroids. There are few adverse effects when used topically. If they are not effective, topical coal tar (anthralin, dithranol) can be used. Coal tar is a local therapy and is very difficult cosmetically because it stains skin, bedding, and clothing.

Extensive Disease/Extensive Surface Area

Extensive psoriasis that covers large amounts of surface area is difficult to cover with topical steroids, calcipotriene, or tazarotene. Therapy is with:

- **Ultraviolet light**
- Biological agents such as **anti-TNF agents** (etanercept, adalimumab, infliximab)

Ultimately, for extensive disease not responsive to any other therapy, the treatment is methotrexate. Methotrexate is also used for psoriatic arthritis.

> Methotrexate causes lung and liver fibrosis.

ATOPIC DERMATITIS (ECZEMA)

Atopic dermatitis is characterized by:

- Severe **pruritus**
- Red plaques, especially on flexor surfaces
- Complications of scratching such as **infection** (impetigo)

TREATMENT

- **Topical steroids:** used for local disease and typically the "best initial therapy" for acute flares of disease

- Control of itching with:

  - **Antihistamines** such as fexofenadine, cetirizine, or loratadine
  - Avoiding harsh soaps
  - Avoiding skin trauma during washing
  - Avoiding hot water or skin dryness
  - Use of skin moisturizers

- **Phototherapy** for extensive disease

- **Immune modulators** such as tacrolimus or pimecrolimus for those with extensive disease and those not responding to phototherapy. These agents inhibit T cells and modify the immune system without the adverse effects of steroids or the cosmetic staining of coal tars.
- Treating impetigo with antistaphylococcal medications as it arises. This is critically important since the more a patient's skin itches, the more the patient scratches. Impetigo leads to more itching and scratching.

PAPULOSQUAMOUS DISORDERS

Asteatotic Dermatitis

Asteatotic dermatitis is the loss of sebum from the skin leading to severe dryness and itching. This is managed with lubricants and moisturizers of the skin such as petroleum jelly, ammonium lactate lotion, oatmeal baths, mineral oil, or oil-based creams. The specific brand does not matter as long as the skin is kept moisturized and itching and scratching is avoided.

> The moisturizers for asteatotic dermatitis are the same as should be used in atopic dermatitis.

Seborrheic Dermatitis

> Never biopsy seborrheic dermatitis unless the disease is unresponsive to treatment.

Also called dandruff, seborrheic dermatitis is a hypersensitivity reaction of the skin to a minor cutaneous fungal infection with *Malassezia furfur* (formerly known as *Pityrosporum ovale*).

The diagnosis is based on its appearance. Scraping or biopsy is rarely done. The question will describe "flaky white (or yellow) greasy (or oily) scales."

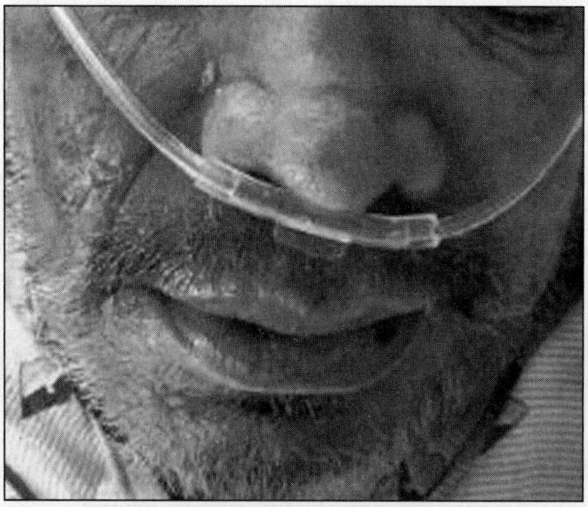

Figure 4.4: Seborrheic dermatitis. There is hypersensitivity to infection of the skin with fungus.

Source: Farshad Bagheri, MD

▶ **TIP**

Nasolabial fold involvement is a strong clue to the diagnosis.

The best initial therapy is either with:

- Topical steroids (when on a face)

or

- Topical antifungal medications such as ketoconazole, clotrimazole, or ciclopirox

> Selenium sulfide is used only because it can cover large surface areas.

Venous Stasis

This is a complication of venous insufficiency in the lower extremities. There is no specific therapy to reverse venous stasis ulcers. The management consists entirely of keeping the legs elevated and using supportive care such as elastic stockings. Hyperpigmentation is common because blood extravasates; the metabolic end product of the blood is hemosiderin, which ends up discoloring the skin.

Pityriasis Rosea

Pityriasis rosea begins with a single large lesion, or **herald patch**, on the chest, back, or abdomen. This is followed a short time later by dissemination that still predominates on the trunk. The lesions:

- Are maculopapular
- Resemble secondary syphilis
- Resolve spontaneously over a few days to weeks

There is **no specific diagnostic test** for pityriasis rosea. Use the VDRL or RPR to exclude secondary syphilis. Treat with topical steroids.

> "Christmas tree" pattern = pityriasis rosea

Pressure (Decubitus) Ulcers

This is an extremely difficult subject clinically; however, in terms of board questions, that makes it easier, since there are only a few clear points that can be tested.

- Only relief of pressure will prevent these ulcers.
- Any time "improve nutritional status" is a choice, it is the right answer. However, relief of pressure is the single most effective management.
- "Swab the ulcer" and "culture the wound" are always wrong answers.

> Foley (urinary) catheters do not prevent pressure ulcers.

▶ **TIP**

Debridement of necrotic tissue helps, but this is so obvious that it is usually in the question, not an answer choice.

> Pressure relief with frequent turning beats all other answers.

ACNE

Mild, noncystic acne with no inflammatory changes is treated with topical cleansers or antimicrobials such as benzoyl peroxide. Besides killing the bacteria that cause acne, benzoyl peroxide is also comedolytic and can have some effect in controlling the disease process.

If benzoyl peroxide is not controlling the disease or the question describes "mild inflammatory changes," the answer is:

- **Topical vitamin A** derivatives (tazarotene, adapalene, tretinoin), also known as retinoids
- **Topical antibiotics** (clindamycin, erythromycin, dapsone, azelaic acid)

> Both antibiotics and vitamin A are effective alone, but the combination is more effective.

▶ TIP

If the question asks you to choose between topical antibiotics and retinoids (vitamin A), the answer is retinoids. If the question describes "moderate inflammatory lesions not controlled with topical medications," the answer is to use oral antibiotics such as minocycline or doxycycline.

Severe cystic acne should be treated with oral vitamin A (isotretinoin). Also look for words like "scarring," "nodular," or "recalcitrant" as the clue to using oral isotretinoin.

> Beware of teratogenicity with oral vitamin A derivatives (isotretinoin).

Acne treatment is a 5-step sequence:

1. Topical benzoyl peroxide
2. Add topical antibiotics: clindamycin or erythromycin
3. Add topical vitamin A: tazarotene, tretinoin, adapalene
4. Add oral antibiotics: minocycline, doxycycline
5. Add oral vitamin A: isotretinoin

ENDOCRINOLOGY

PITUITARY DISORDERS

Hyperprolactinemia

ETIOLOGY

Prolactin originates from the anterior lobe of the pituitary. It should be inhibited at all times, except during normal pregnancy and breastfeeding. During pregnancy, rising estrogen levels drive the increase in production of prolactin by inhibiting the release of dopamine from the hypothalamus into the pituitary.

Very **high prolactin levels** (above 200 ng/mL) are essentially diagnostic of a **pituitary adenoma**. In general, it is important to exclude other causes of hyperprolactinemia prior to scanning the brain with an MRI. Pituitary lesions (incidentalomas) are so common that it is critical to prove the existence and location of an endocrinopathy prior to performing a scan.

Causes of High Prolactin Levels Other than Pituitary Adenoma

- Pregnancy
- Medications (antipsychotic medications, metoclopramide, tricyclic antidepressants, SSRIs, methyldopa)
- Illicit drugs (cocaine, opiates)
- Chest wall/nipple stimulation (nipple piercing, shingles of the chest wall)
- Brain lesions that compress the pituitary stalk (craniopharyngioma, meningioma, empty sella syndrome, metastatic tumors)
- Primary hypothyroidism (thyrotropin releasing hormone (TRH) from the hypothalamus will stimulate the release of prolactin at pathologically increased amounts)
- Renal insufficiency (decreased urinary clearance of prolactin)
- Cirrhosis

> Multiple causes of hyperprolactin outside the pituitary make this disorder complex.

> Hyperprolactinemia can be idiopathic.

PRESENTATION

Men present with **erectile dysfunction** and decreased libido. **Women present with amenorrhea and galactorrhea.** Prolactin inhibits the release of gonadotropin-releasing hormone (GnRH) from the hypothalamus. Prolactin will also inhibit follicle-stimulating hormone (FSH) and luteinizing hormone (LH). Without FSH, LH, or GnRH, the body cannot ovulate or release testosterone or estrogen. Visual field testing is mandatory.

> Hyperprolactinemia causes bone abnormalities in both genders. Sex hormones normally increase bone density.

DIAGNOSTIC TESTS

1. After an elevated prolactin level is found, the "best initial test" is a pregnancy test.
2. After you exclude pregnancy, the most appropriate next step is to exclude all the other causes of hyperprolactinemia previously described.
3. MRI of the brain is done last to confirm the presence of a pituitary lesion.

▶ **TIP**

Never start with a scan in endocrinology.

TREATMENT

1. The "best initial therapy" is a dopamine agonist such as cabergoline or bromocriptine, to which 90% will respond. Eventually, many patients can stop the dopamine agonists after the lesion has been controlled.
2. Transsphenoidal surgery is used to remove the pituitary.
3. Radiation is used in those not responsive to either dopamine agonists or surgery.

> Dopamine agonists are associated with heart valve abnormalities.

Acromegaly

DEFINITION/ETIOLOGY

Acromegaly is the oversecretion of growth hormone (GH) from a pituitary lesion. Oversecretion of GH is associated with increased mortality even if obvious abnormalities of physical features are not present.

PRESENTATION

The oversecretion of GH leads to abnormally increased amounts of insulinlike growth factor (IGF-1). Patients present with:

- Coarsening of facial features with enlarging hat, ring, and shoe size
- **Carpal tunnel** syndrome (soft tissue grows in the wrist and compresses the median nerve)
- Obstructive **sleep apnea** (soft tissue grows in the neck)
- Increased **colonic polyps**

- Bad body **odor** (hypertrophy of sweat glands) and skin tags
- Teeth grow out of alignment from jaw enlargement
- **Arthropathy** (joints grow out of alignment)
- Cardiomyopathy

> Growth hormone excess in adults does not result in an extra-large person, but it can cause giantism if the onset occurs in childhood.

DIAGNOSTIC TESTS

The best initial test is elevated **IGF-1 level**. The most accurate test is failure of GH to decrease in response to infusing glucose.

After these tests are done, an MRI of the brain is done to confirm the presence of a pituitary lesion.

Other laboratory abnormalities are:

- Elevated glucose levels
- Hyperlipidemia

What is the most common cause of death in a person with acromegaly?

a. Colon cancer
b. Congestive heart failure
c. Brain metastases
d. Respiratory failure
e. Pancreatic insufficiency

Answer: The correct answer is (b). Acromegaly leads to abnormal growth of the heart. In addition, the antiinsulin qualities of GH result in elevated glucose and lipid levels, which accelerate the development of coronary artery disease.

> Patients with giantism or acromegaly can become wheelchair-bound and immobile by the age of 50.

TREATMENT

The best initial treatment is surgery with transsphenoidal resection of the pituitary. The majority of patients will be cured.

Alternate therapies to surgery:

- Somatostatin analogues (octreotide, lanreotide)
- Pegvisomant, a GH receptor antagonist
- Dopamine agonists such as cabergoline
- Radiation if surgery and all the medical therapies fail

> Surgical cure rates:
> Microadenomas: 90%
> Macroadenomas: 50%

Panhypopituitarism

DEFINITION/ETIOLOGY

Panhypopituitarism is the deficiency of all of the hormones originating from both the anterior and posterior pituitary. Because of the proximity of the hormone-producing cells in the pituitary, it is nearly impossible to have a mass

Anosmia, Renal Agenesis 508

> Kallmann syndrome is one of the only causes of an isolated deficiency of a single pituitary hormone (FSH/LH).

> The cause of panhypopituitarism is best summarized as "any brain damage."

> Kallmann syndrome = loss of FSH/LH + anosmia

lesion or cancer-impairing production of just one of the pituitary hormones. Panhypopituitarism is caused by any disease that involves the area of the brain anatomically near the pituitary such as:

- Tumors (e.g., craniopharyngioma, meningioma, glioma, germinoma)
- Radiation of the brain
- Hemochromatosis
- Infection (e.g., encephalitis)
- Stroke
- Head trauma
- Traumatic childbirth (Sheehan syndrome)

PRESENTATION

Symptoms are related to the individual hormone deficiencies.

Anterior Pituitary

ACTH: Hypocortisolism with weakness, fatigue, fever, headache, abdominal pain, and hypoglycemia. Hyponatremia occurs from decreased free water clearance.

TSH: Symptoms of hypothyroidism (slow everything)

FSH/LH: Infertility, anovulation, and amenorrhea in women; erectile dysfunction and loss of libido in men

Growth hormone: Very limited, almost undetectable symptoms such as low energy and decreased lean muscle mass

Prolactin: Inability to lactate. No symptoms except for women wanting to breastfeed.

Posterior Pituitary

Antidiuretic hormone (ADH): Diabetes insipidus with polyuria, polydipsia, and hypernatremia.

Oxytocin: Impaired breastfeeding. Oxytocin normally helps in parturition to increase uterine contractions. Women are still able to give birth.

A patient comes to the hospital after a motor vehicle accident in which she sustains head trauma that transects the pituitary stalk.

Which of the following is most likely to occur?

a. Hypernatremia
b. Fatal hypotension
c. Loss of energy from loss of TSH, growth hormone, and ACTH
d. Galactorrhea
e. Hyperkalemia

Answer: The correct answer is (c). Thyroxine regulates the energy metabolism of virtually every organ in the body except for the brain, testes, and uterus. Growth hormone in the postpubertal adult is a stress hormone that raises the glucose and free fatty acid levels. ACTH controls cortisol levels. Cortisol has a nearly identical function to growth hormone as a "stress hormone" that increases energy levels with increased glucose and free fatty acid levels.

Presentation of Panhypopituitarism: Why Don't We Die When We Lose the Pituitary?

Hypotension and hyperkalemia do not occur because aldosterone is not under the control of the pituitary. Angiotensin II and hyperkalemia control the zona glomerulosa, which is the site of production of aldosterone. Aldosterone will maintain blood pressure. In addition, norepinephrine is produced at the synapse of neurons and this is not affected by loss of the pituitary.

> Hypothyroidism has decreased free water clearance.

Blood pressure may be low because of loss of cortisol:

1. Cortisol has some mineralocorticoid activity.
2. Cortisol has a permissive effect on the ability of catecholamines to cause vascular reactivity.

Even if epinephrine and norepinephrine levels are normal, a person who does not have cortisol has a lower blood pressure than someone who does have cortisol. A bolus of glucocorticoids can have an immediate effect in raising blood pressure. Arterioles constrict more when catecholamines are present and the cortisol level is normal. This may be why glucorticoids seem to benefit septic shock.

Hypernatremia does *not* occur for two reasons:

> The adrenal medulla is not controlled by the pituitary. Epinephrine and norepinephrine levels are intact when the pituitary is lost.

- ADH is still produced in the hypothalamus. It will simply be released directly into the bloodstream.
- **Hypothyroidism** from loss of the pituitary tends to lower sodium levels. This is from **impaired free water clearance**. Thyroxine normally helps clear or excrete free water.

▶ **TIP**

The fact that loss of the pituitary does not result in immediate cardiovascular collapse is the most reliably tested point in panhypopituitarism. Aldosterone keeps the body alive.

Diagnostic Tests

The best initial tests for panhypopituitarism are:

- TSH and free T4; ACTH and cortisol level; FSH/LH and testosterone level in men; estrogen in women; insulinlike growth factor (IGF) and growth hormone level.

> Giving insulin to induce hypoglycemia should increase both GH and cortisol in patients without panhypopituitarism.

The most accurate test for panhypopituitarism is:

- **Growth hormone:** Give insulin to provoke hypoglycemia, and observe for a rise in GH level. Give arginine and look for a rise in GH level. Because GH causes protein synthesis, giving an amino acid like arginine should lead to a rise in GH.
- **Cortisol and ACTH:** Test for adrenal gland function by measuring cortisol levels before and after injecting cosyntropin, which is artificial ACTH. The adrenal gland is normal if there is a rise in cortisol level. **Metyrapone should raise ACTH levels in a healthy patient.** Metyrapone is an inhibitor of 11-hydroxylase. If you inhibit 11-hydroxylase, cortisol should not be produced. If cortisol is not produced, feedback inhibition on the pituitary is removed; in an unaffected person, the ACTH level should rise.

▶ **TIP**

Provocative testing such as giving insulin, arginine, or metyrapone is rarely necessary. These are, however, the answers to the question, "What is the most accurate diagnostic test?"

TREATMENT

Replace deficient hormones.

Which of these is <u>least</u> important to replace?

a. Thyroxine
b. Testosterone or estrogen
c. Hydrocortisone or prednisone
d. Growth hormone
e. Desmopression (artificial ADH)

Answer: The correct answer is (d). Although growth hormone is deficient in panhypopituitarism, replacing it is not critical in an adult. Children must have GH replaced in order to ensure normal stature. In adults, GH is one of four stress hormone systems (along with glucagon, cortisol, and catecholamines). Hence, if the other hormones are replaced, there should never be episodes of hypoglycemia.

POSTERIOR PITUITARY DISORDERS

Diabetes Insipidus

DEFINITION

Diabetes insipidus (DI) is the loss of free water from the body because of a decrease in the amount of antidiuretic hormone that is produced, or a decrease in the effect of ADH at the kidney tubule. Decreased production or release is central DI (CDI) and decreased effect at the kidney is nephrogenic DI (NDI). Any form of DI presents with polyuria and polydipsia. (The word "diabetes" means "fountain.")

▶ **TIP**

You cannot distinguish between CDI and NDI clinically without specific lab testing.

ETIOLOGY

Central diabetes insipidus: Virtually **any cause of damage to the central nervous system can lead to CDI.** The most common causes are:

- Head trauma
- Hypoxia
- Stroke (destroying the hypothalamus)
- Tumors that compress the pituitary
- Infections and radiation

Nephrogenic diabetes insipidus: NDI is caused by disorders and medications that interfere with the effect of ADH on the collecting duct. The most common causes are:

- **Hypercalcemia**
- **Hypokalemia**
- Lithium, demeclocycline
- Sickle cell disease
- Amyloidosis, myeloma, chronic pyelonephritis, Sjögren syndrome

PRESENTATION

The presentation of both CDI and NDI is the same. The patient has **polyuria** and **polydipsia** (greater than 3 liters of intake and urine output). Because thirst mechanisms are intact, the patient will not have symptoms unless the ability to match urinary output with oral intake is impaired. This can be quite voluminous since maximum urine output can be as much as 20 to 24 liters per day.

If oral intake of fluid does not match urine output, the patient's serum sodium will rise. When the sodium level rises, the patient will develop symptoms related to CNS abnormalities; these can range from mild confusion to lethargy, coma, and seizures. **Hypernatremia** is a cause of delirium, not dementia.

> Water deficit causes CNS problems.

DIAGNOSTIC TESTS

The best initial test in DI is a urine sodium level. The urine will show:

- **Low urine sodium concentration** due to dilution by water due to decreased ADH effect or levels
- **Low urine osmolality**

Normal urine osmolality ranges from 50 to 1,200 mOsm/L. In DI, the urine will come out very close to 50 mOsm/L.

▶ **TIP**

Urine specific gravity approximates urine osmolality. The patient will have a very low specific gravity (below 1.005).

The most accurate test is a water deprivation test. A healthy person, when deprived of fluids, will do two things. First, the urine volume will decrease; second, the urine osmolality will increase. In DI, the urine volume will stay high and the urine osmolality will stay low despite the massive volume loss.

The most accurate method of distinguishing CDI from NDI is the response to the administration of ADH (vasopressin).

> ADH is given as desmopressin, which has the effect of vasopressin on the kidney tubules without the vasoconstrictive effects.

- **CDI:** Urine volume will decrease and osmolality will increase in response to giving ADH.
- **NDI:** There will be no change in volume or osmolality in response to giving ADH.

A man with a history of bipolar disorder comes to the emergency department during an episode of mania. He says he takes lithium. In addition to buying 10 televisions and 5 MP3 players and working 27 hours straight at his job, he is also drinking 17 liters of water per day. His urine output is 17 liters per day. His serum sodium is precisely normal at 140 mEq/L (normal 135 to 145 mEq/L).

What is the best initial way of determining the etiology of his problem?

a. Determine presence of massive nocturia
b. Urine osmolality
c. Serum osmolality
d. Urine sodium
e. Urine volume

Answer: The correct answer is (a). If the patient is having NDI from lithium, he will have massive nocturia. NDI does not stop just because he goes to sleep. If this is psychogenic polydipsia from a manic episode from bipolar disorder, urine volume will decrease at night because he will not be drinking when he goes to sleep. The serum and urine values in terms of sodium level and osmolality will be the same in both NDI and psychogenic polydipsia. Everything will be low. This patient's serum sodium is normal because his oral intake is equal to his urine output. If the serum sodium is high, then it is NDI. If the serum sodium is low, it is psychogenic polydipsia.

> Water deprivation tells if DI is present. Response to vasopressin differentiates CDI from NDI.

TREATMENT

The best initial therapy for any patient with severe hypernatremia leading to mental status changes, seizures, or coma is to **replace fluids**. Do not correct sodium levels too rapidly (more than 1 mEq/L per hour). Over-rapid lowering of hypernatremia can lead to cerebral edema. This is from a shift of fluid into brain cells if the serum suddenly becomes hypotonic compared to the brain cells. Cerebral edema can itself lead to altered mental status, seizures, and coma.

CDI: Replace ADH by giving desmopressin. Use desmopressin intravenously for acute cases. Use it orally, intranasally, or intramuscularly for chronic cases.

NDI: Correct the underlying cause such as stopping lithium or correcting hypercalcemia or hypokalemia. In those in whom there is no correctable cause, use NSAIDs or hydrochlorothiazide.

> Tested point: Amiloride is the drug of choice for lithium-induced NDI not resolving after the lithium is stopped.

▶ **TIP**

Both CDI and NDI will benefit from thiazide diuretics; they increase proximal tubule water reabsorption, which is independent of ADH.

Syndrome of Inappropriate ADH

ETIOLOGY

Syndrome of inappropriate ADH (SIADH) can arise for many unidentified reasons with disorders involving:

- Brain
- Lung
- Cancer
- Drugs (vincristine, clofibrate, carbamazepine, SSRIs, sulfonylureas)

Any abnormality of the brain such as stroke, tumor, trauma, or infection can cause SIADH. **Any abnormality of the lung** such as pneumonia, PE, tuberculosis, or atelectasis can cause SIADH.

> The mechanism of most cases of SIADH is never identified.

PRESENTATION

All disorders of serum sodium concentration present with abnormalities of the CNS. This ranges from mild confusion to seizures and coma. The speed at which the sodium level drops, not the serum sodium level itself, is the most important factor determining symptoms. A sudden drop from a normal sodium level of 140 to 120 mEq/L over a few hours can cause seizures. A slow drop over days to weeks can give a patient a sodium level of 110 mEq/L with no symptoms.

> The speed at which the sodium level drops is the most important factor in the development of symptoms of hyponatremia.

DIAGNOSTIC TESTS

A healthy person with a low serum sodium level has a low urine sodium concentration and low urine osmolality.

A person with SIADH has a high urine sodium concentration and high urine osmolality due to water reabsorption.

▶**TIP**

With hyponatremia, anything except the most maximally dilute urine (osmolality less than 100 mOsm/L) is SIADH.

TREATMENT

Mild hyponatremia is managed by simply **restricting fluid**. Since SIADH is entirely a problem of excess free water, limiting free water will raise the sodium level. "Mild" in terms of SIADH is not a specific sodium level; rather, it refers to the severity of symptoms. Mild SIADH essentially describes a person with an asymptomatic decrease in sodium level. *800mL /day.*

Moderate SIADH is managed with saline and a loop diuretic. If you give saline alone, it will worsen the sodium level. You must give a loop diuretic as well in order to remove free water from the body and impair renal concentrating ability. Moderate disease can be defined as a person who exhibits mental status changes but is not seizing or comatose.

Patients with severe SIADH, such as those with **seizures** or very profound obtundation or lethargy, are managed with **hypertonic saline**.

> ADH antagonists (conivaptan, tolvaptan) inhibit ADH effect on the kidney.

ADH Antagonists

ADH antagonists such as conivaptan and tolvaptan are used in those not responding well to the treatments previously described, or in those who have an uncorrectable cause of the SIADH in whom the symptoms will recur once treatment is stopped. An example of this would be metastatic cancer or a CNS or lung lesion that cannot be fixed.

Demeclocycline can also be used for chronic SIADH. Demeclocycline works by preventing the action of ADH at the collecting duct—ie, by causing NDI.

THYROID DISORDERS

Hypothyroidism

Most hypothyroidism is caused by Hashimoto thyroiditis that has resulted in a "burnt out" gland that no longer produces hormone. Other causes are:

> Pregnancy increases the need for iodine by 50%. Lactation increases the need for iodine by 100%.

- Lithium, amiodarone, interferon, or after radioactive iodine use
- Pituitary insufficiency (rare)
- Iodine deficiency
- Hepatitis C treatment with interferon
- Subacute thyroiditis (transient)

PRESENTATION

Hypothyroidism presents with signs of decreased metabolic activity. Hyperthyroidism presents with signs of increased activity. The exception is menstruation: Hypothyroidism presents with menorrhagia and hyperthyroidism gives amenorrhea.

Presentation of Thyroid Disorders	
Hypothyroidism	**Hyperthyroidism**
Weight gain	Weight loss
Bradycardia	Tachycardia
Constipation	Increased number of bowel movements
Depression	Anxiety
Cold intolerance	Heat intolerance
Dry skin	Sweating
Delayed, diminished reflexes	Tremor
Hypothermia	Fever
Decrease in angina with coronary disease	Increase in angina with coronary disease

Hypertension is seen in both hyperthyroidism and hypothyroidism.

Findings Specific to Hypothyroidism

- Carpal tunnel syndrome
- Galactorrhea from stimulation of prolactin by thyrotropin releasing hormone (TRH)
- Thinning of the outer half of the eyebrows
- Pericardial effusion
- Hoarseness, smell, taste, and hearing disturbance

Pathologically high TRH levels stimulate prolactin release.

▶ **TIP**

The presence of an enlarged gland or goiter does not indicate how the thyroid is functioning.

Diagnostic Tests	
Hypothyroidism	**Hyperthyroidism**
High TSH	Low TSH (most cases)
Decreased T4	Increased T4
Increased LDL	Decreased LDL

T3 is not a reliable measure of thyroid hormone activity level. T3 levels are maintained at normal even with profoundly low thyroid activity.

Lab Abnormalities Unique to Hypothyroidism
- **Hyponatremia** from decreased free water clearance at the kidney
- Anemia

Autoimmune (Hashimoto) thyroiditis may be associated with:

- Antithyroperoxidase antibodies
- Antithyroglobulin antibodies
- Positive ANA

▶ **TIP**

Imaging studies such as MRI of the head are never correct answers for diagnosing hypothyroidism.

TREATMENT

Hypothyroidism is simply treated with replacement of levothyroxine in the majority of cases to normalize TSH. Replace iodine in the occasional case secondary to nutritional deficiency.

> Beware of precipitating angina with thyroxine replacement.

Hyperthyroidism

ETIOLOGY

There are far more causes of hyperthyroidism than there are of hypothyroidism. This is a much more frequently tested topic for "What is the most likely diagnosis?" questions.

Graves disease: Only Graves disease is associated with:

- Ophthalmopathy with exophthalmos/proptosis
- Skin abnormalities such as pretibial myxedema
- Digital clubbing (acropachy)

> Only Graves has eye and skin findings.

Silent (painless) thyroiditis: An autoimmune thyroiditis with lymphocytes infiltrating the thyroid. Transient hyperthyroidism may be followed by transient hypothyroidism.

Subacute (de Quervain) thyroiditis: The thyroid is acutely inflamed resulting in a very painful, tender thyroid gland. It is thought to be viral in etiology. The ESR may be elevated. Transient hyperthyroidism may be followed by transient hypothyroidism.

> Only subacute thyroiditis is painful.

Pituitary adenoma: This is the only form of hyperthyroidism associated with an elevated TSH level.

Amiodarone: This drug can give either high or low function of the thyroid.

Lithium and interferon can alter thyroid function.

Thyrotoxicosis factitia: These are patients who are abusing levothyroxine replacement, usually in an attempt to lose weight. On physical examination the thyroid gland will have involuted and there is no palpable gland. This is from feedback inhibition on the thyroid shutting off TSH production.

Struma ovarii: A small percentage (less than 5%) of patients with ovarian dermoid tumors will secrete thyroid hormone.

Reidel thyroiditis: This is fibrosis of the thyroid from an unknown cause. Most patients have normal thyroid function, but 30% become hypothyroid and a smaller number become hyperthyroid. It can be associated with mediastinal or retroperitoneal fibrosis. **Treat with prednisone or tamoxifen.**

DIAGNOSTIC TESTS

The best initial test to detect hyperthyroidism is an **elevated free T4 level.** The best initial test to confirm the etiology of the disorder is the TSH. All of the forms of hyperthyroidism previously described will have a decreased TSH, except for a pituitary adenoma, which produces TSH. If the TSH and T4 are elevated, the most appropriate next step in management is an MRI of the pituitary looking for a pituitary lesion (very rare).

Also look for **osteoporosis** and **hypercalcemia.** This is from increased bone turnover from an elevated thyroid hormone level.

Look for cardiac dysfunction, especially in high-risk patients.

Graves Disease Diagnostic Tests

When the TSH is low, only Graves disease gives an increase in activity in the radioactive iodine uptake. This is because of the presence of thyroid-stimulating antibodies (immunoglobulin) that mimic the activity of TSH. These are also known as thyroid receptor antibodies. Graves disease is, essentially, a hyperfunctioning gland on the basis of an autoimmune condition.

Thyroid Related Antibody Testing

From a practical standpoint, antithyroperoxidase antibodies, thyroid-stimulating immunoglobulin, and serum thyroglobulin tests are occasionally used in patients in whom the diagnosis is not clear.

On the boards, they are the answer to the question: "Which of the following is most likely to be found in immune-related hyperthyroidism?"

Specific Thyroid Autoantibodies	
Antibody test	**Disease**
Thyroid-stimulating immunoglobulin	Graves disease
Serum thyroglobulin	Subacute thyroiditis
Antithyroperoxidase antibody	Hashimoto thyroiditis

TREATMENT

Hyperthyroidism is treated initially with:

- Thiourea drugs (**propylthiouracil, methimazole**): These agents inhibit the production of thyroid hormone and PTU decreases the peripheral conversion to T4 to the more active T3. Methimazole is first except in pregnancy.
- **Radioactive iodine:** This is only for a hyperfunctioning gland as occurs with Graves disease. This is a different from the radioactive iodine that is used as a diagnostic test for Graves disease.

> Methimazole acts faster than PTU.

Specific Therapy

Aspirin: Subacute thyroiditis is painful and self-limited. Aspirin and antiinflammatory medications will decrease the pain. Beta blockers can be used to treat symptoms of hyperthyroidism.

Surgical resection:

- Pituitary removal in the rare case of a TSH-producing adenoma
- Thyroidectomy in those with a large gland that is compressing the airway, or in pregnant women with Graves disease; radioactive iodine should be avoided due to concerns about the use of radioactive material in pregnant patients

Graves ophthalmopathy:

- Glucocorticoids such as prednisone
- Radiation of the orbits

Thyroid Storm or Acute Thyrotoxicosis

Treatment is aimed at every step in the production, conversion, and target organ effect.

> PTU is the best choice for pregnant patients.

- **Propranolol** (and other beta blockers): These drugs provide a symptomatic benefit most rapidly because they block tissue response to hormone that has already been produced.
- **Thiourea drugs:** Propylthiouracil (PTU) and **methimazole** block the production of the hormone. Methimazole is preferred.
- **Iodinated contrast agents** (iopanoic acid, ipodate): These agents block the uptake of iodine by the thyroid and also inhibit peripheral conversion of T4 to T3. They also block release of preformed hormone.
- Hydrocortisone: This blocks peripheral conversion.
- Radioactive iodine: This ablates the gland for a definitive treatment.

> PTU and methimazole are associated with neutropenia.

Treatment Differences Between Graves Disease, Toxic Multinodular Goiter, and Toxic Adenoma

Generally all three of these causes of hyperthyroidism are treated the same way as previously described. The only differences are:

- Graves disease will permanently resolve in 30% to 60% of cases after a year of PTU or methimazole.
- Toxic multinodular goiter (TMG) and toxic adenoma will recur after these thiourea drugs are stopped.
- TMG and adenoma require much larger doses of radioiodine than Graves disease since the uptake is low with TMG and adenoma.
- Surgery is more frequently used for toxic adenoma.

> T3 is much more active than T4, so blocking T4 to T3 conversion controls hyperthyroidism.

Thyroid Nodules

Thyroid nodules are far more common than most people think, even physicians. Nodules are palpable in as much as 5% of female patients over a lifetime. They are less common in men. You are expected to know four basic questions.

The Four Basic Questions

1. What is the best initial step in management of a thyroid nodule?

   Answer: Thyroid function tests (TSH and T4). Malignancy is rarely (<1%) found in a hyperfunctioning lesion. **Cancer is generally nonfunctional.** This means the cancer displaces normal tissue, but it does not make normal hormone and certainly not in increased amounts. A toxic adenoma is different. A toxic adenoma is, by definition, not malignant. This is why a toxic adenoma presents in an identical fashion to Graves disease in terms of having hyperthyroidism, but it is without the eye and skin findings of Graves disease.

2. When is radioactive iodine scan as a diagnostic test the answer?

   Answer: Never. Hot nodules can have cancer. Cold nodules might not have cancer.

   "Hot" = Hyperfunctioning
   "Cold" = Nonfunctioning

   A radioactive iodine scan of a nodule does not eliminate the need for a biopsy.

> "Hot" nodules *usually* are not cancerous. "Cold" nodules *usually* are cancerous. This is not precise enough to definitively exclude or prove the presence of cancer.

▶ TIP

In nodule evaluation, radioactive iodine scan is the most common wrong answer.

3. When is biopsy the answer?

   Answer: Always. This, of course, refers to a nodule that is not hyperfunctioning.

4. **When is thyroid ultrasound the answer?**

   Answer: To guide the placement of the biopsy needle. The ultrasound helps locate lesions that are small in order to make sure you do not miss the tissue for a false negative on biopsy. Lesions under a centimeter can be hard to feel with just the fingers for a precise location. The ultrasound is not a substitute for biopsy.

Bonus Question for the Test Taker Seeking the Top Decile

5. **What is the answer when the words "follicular neoplasm" are in the question?**

   Answer: Surgery for removal of the entire nodule. Follicular neoplasm is a histologic pattern that essentially means you cannot make a determination of malignancy or benign tissue from a needle biopsy alone. The question may say "suspicious for follicular neoplasm" or "cannot exclude follicular neoplasm." The phrasing does not matter: When the words "follicular neoplasm" are in the question, remove the whole lesion in order to exclude malignancy.

Thyroid Cancer

In the event that cancer is found on the fine needle aspirate/biopsy of the thyroid, the management is surgical removal. Large tumors may be radiated prior to surgery, but this will not eliminate the need for surgery.

When to Answer "Cancer" as the Most Likely Diagnosis

- Recent or rapid growth
- Neck irradiation in the past
- Lymphadenopathy
- Hoarseness
- Fixation to surrounding tissues

Tested Facts about Thyroid Cancer

- The most **common** type of thyroid cancer is **papillary carcinoma**.
- The cancer with the **worst prognosis** is **anaplastic** carcinoma.
- **Medullary** carcinoma is associated with multiple endocrine neoplasia type II (MENII).
- The type of thyroid cancer associated with **calcitonin** is **medullary**.

CALCIUM DISORDERS

Hypercalcemia

ETIOLOGY

Hyperparathyroidism and **malignancy** account for **90%** of cases of hypercalcemia. Other causes of hypercalcemia are:

- Increased vitamin D from ingestion or granulomatous disease producing vitamin D such as sarcoidosis

- **Familial hypocalciuric hypercalcemia** (genetically related undersecretion of calcium)
- Hyperfunctioning of the **parathyroid** gland, caused by lithium
- **Immobilization** leading to increased bone turnover (hyperthyroidism also dissolves bone)
- **Thiazide** diuretics preventing urinary excretion of calcium
- Milk-alkali syndrome
- Vitamin A excess
- Acidosis: hydrogen ions displace calcium from albumin leading to increased free calcium; acidosis also "leaches" calcium out of bone

> Bone biopsies are softened by soaking them in acid. The same effect happens in the blood of people with prolonged metabolic acidosis.

▶ **TIP**

When the question describes a high calcium level in an otherwise healthy person, the answer is hyperparathyroidism.

PRESENTATION

High calcium levels inhibit normal neuromuscular function. This leads to:

- Gastrointestinal: nausea, vomiting, constipation, anorexia, pancreatitis
- Neurological: lethargy, stupor, coma, and weakness
- Renal: nephrolithiasis, nephrogenic diabetes insipidus, acute tubular necrosis
- Cardiac: arrhythmia, ectopy, hypertension

> High calcium levels cause ulcers. Calcium stimulates gastrin release.

> Hypercalcemia is associated with profound volume depletion from osmotic diuresis and nephrogenic diabetes insipidus.

DIAGNOSTIC TESTS

The "best initial test" when the diagnosis is not clear from the history is always a parathyroid hormone (PTH) level.

Other lab abnormalities are:

- EKG with short QT interval
- Elevated BUN-to-creatinine ratio from volume depletion
- Increased urinary calcium
- Phosphate levels may be low (usually with high PTH levels)

> Loop diuretics are needed only if urine flow is insufficient after hydration.

TREATMENT

The best initial therapy for severe hypercalcemia is always normal saline at very high volume. This will correct the volume loss from NDI and should resolve most CNS symptoms.

After hydration, furosemide is used if urine output is not sufficient. Loop diuretics such as furosemide cause urinary calcium loss, but also lead to low potassium and magnesium levels.

> Bisphosphonates cause esophageal ulceration and osteonecrosis of the jaw (rare).

> Calcitonin rapidly lowers calcium levels while waiting for bisphosphonates to work over a few days.

Bisphosphonates (pamidronate, zolendronate): These agents are very effective in returning calcium to the storage pool in the bone. They inhibit osteoclasts and **need 2 to 4 days to work.**

Calcitonin: If the calcium level is still very high after saline infusion, the "most appropriate next step in management" is calcitonin. Calcitonin has a very rapid onset of action and also wears off rapidly. Calcitonin inhibits the action of osteoclasts on bone.

Glucocorticoids: Prednisone is effective in only a few circumstances such as:

- Cancers like myeloma, lymphoma, and breast cancer
- Sarcoidosis
- Vitamin D intoxication

Dialysis: This is the answer if the patient has renal injury and diuretics are unlikely to be effective. Bisphosphonates will still be effective; however, dialysis is useful in the short term while waiting several days for them to take effect.

▶ **TIP**

Plicamycin and gallium are always wrong answers in treating hypercalcemia.

> Tachyphylaxis means the effect of the drug wears off.

Hyperparathyroidism

ETIOLOGY

Primary hyperparathyroidism is the single most common cause of hypercalcemia. This is especially true in a person who is asymptomatic. When there are symptoms, they are of the GI, renal, CNS, and cardiac systems as previously described.

Causes of Primary Hyperparathyroidism	
Cause	**Frequency**
Single-gland adenoma	85%
Four-gland hyperplasia	14%
Parathyroid malignancy	1%

▶ **TIP**

Look for a person with hypercalcemia on "routine" testing in an asymptomatic outpatient.

DIAGNOSTIC TESTS/TREATMENT

Besides an elevated PTH level, look for a decreased phosphate level. PTH causes increased urinary excretion of phosphate. Disorders that cause hypercalcemia from increased vitamin D will also increase the phosphate level, since vitamin D drives the GI absorption of both calcium and phosphate.

Besides the measures previously described to decrease calcium levels, hyperparathyroidism is treated with surgical removal of the parathyroid glands.

Indications for Parathyroidectomy

Since so many patients with hyperparathyroidism are asymptomatic, many patients will not need surgical removal of the glands.

Parathyroidectomy is definitely indicated if there is:

- **Renal injury** from the hypercalcemia (creatinine clearance less than 60 mL/min)
- Any **symptoms** (GI, CNS, bone, nephrolithiasis, or cardiac)
- Markedly elevated calcium levels, defined as more than 1 mg/dL above normal
- Age below 50

> Cinacalcet is used to inhibit PTH release in those who are symptomatic and are not surgical candidates.

> Ultrasound or parathyroid scan is used to localize the abnormal gland to guide surgical removal.

Hypocalcemia

ETIOLOGY

Hypocalcemia is caused by:

- Vitamin D deficiency (nutritional, renal failure, malabsorption)
- Increased loss of calcium (alcoholism, loop diuretics)
- Hypoparathyroidism (from surgical removal)
- **Hypomagnesemia (prevents PTH release and effect)**
- Hyperphosphatemia (causes increased binding of calcium)
- Calcitonin release from medullary thyroid cancer (very rare)
- Pancreatitis
- Rhabdomyolysis (damaged muscle binds free calcium)

> Infiltration of the parathyroid glands is caused by:
> - Copper (Wilson disease)
> - Iron (hemochromatosis)
> - Granulomas (sarcoidosis)
> - Amyloidosis

A man is brought to the emergency department with massive hematemesis and black stool. He is an alcoholic. He has splenomegaly and spider angiomata. His prothrombin time is elevated. Upper endoscopy reveals varices, which are treated with band ligation. He also receives pantoprazole and octreotide. He receives ten units of packed red blood cells and six units of fresh frozen plasma. He develops a generalized seizure. The head CT is normal.

What is the most likely cause of his seizure?

a. Hypocalcemia from the blood transfusion
b. Hypocalcemia from fresh frozen plasma
c. Hypoxia
d. Hepatic encephalopathy
e. Octreotide decreasing free calcium
f. Pantoprazole decreasing PTH release

Answer: The correct answer is (a). Packed red blood cells are typically kept from coagulating with a citrate anticoagulant. Citrate inhibits the clotting cascade by chelating the calcium, which is necessary to start the process of clotting. Fresh frozen plasma does not use the same anticoagulant. Octreotide and proton pump inhibitors such as pantoprazole do not have any effect on calcium levels.

Medication-induced Hypocalcemia

- Citrate buffer
- Fluoride
- Foscarnet
- Calcitonin and bisphosphonates

Pseudohypocalcemia

A low albumin level decreases the total calcium level. For every point of albumin below normal levels, there is a 0.8 point decrease in the total calcium. Look for a patient with low calcium and no symptoms. The free calcium level will still be normal so there are no symptoms.

> 1 decrease in albumin = 0.8 decrease in total calcium

PRESENTATION

Low calcium levels leads to neuromuscular hyperexcitability. Hypocalcemia presents with:

- Spasm of skeletal muscle with cramps and tetany
- Laryngospasm leading to stridor
- Seizures
- Perioral numbness
- Abdominal pain
- Chvostek sign: facial spasm on tapping the facial nerve (nonspecific)
- Trousseau sign: carpal spasm with occlusion of the brachial artery with a BP cuff

Laboratory EKG Abnormalities

- Prolonged QT interval on EKG
- Evaluate magnesium, PTH, and albumin levels
- Hypoparathyroidism increases phosphate levels

TREATMENT

Replace calcium.

Use **intravenous** calcium chloride or calcium gluconate if there are:

- Seizures
- EKG abnormalities
- Acute symptoms
- GI malabsorption of oral calcium or vitamin D

Pseudohypoparathyroidism

This is from an **abnormal G-protein** attached to the PTH receptor on the target organ cell. The PTH will bind, but there will be no effect. This leads to hypocalcemia and hyperphosphatemia in association with a high PTH level. Look for:

- **Short fourth** digit
- **Round face** and obesity
- Mental **retardation**
- Short stature
- Subcutaneous calcifications

It is treated like hypoparathyroidism with calcium and vitamin D replacement.

> Autoimmune hypoparathyroidism is associated with:
> - Vitiligo
> - Addison disease
> - Hashimoto thyroiditis
> - Type 1 diabetes

A 47-year-old woman with a history of bipolar disorder comes to the emergency department extremely anxious with palpitations and chest pain. She has circumoral numbness. Her respiratory rate is 32 per minute and pulse is 115 per minute. The EKG is normal.

What is most likely to be found?

a. Normal total and free calcium
b. Normal total calcium and low free calcium
c. Increased urinary calcium
d. Decreased PTH level

Answer: The correct answer is (b). Anxiety and panic attack leads to an acute respiratory alkalosis. Alkalosis decreases free calcium. This is from increased protein binding of the free calcium. Alkalosis removes hydrogen ions from albumin. They are replaced on the albumin with calcium, which is another cation.

DIABETES MELLITUS

ETIOLOGY

Nearly 95% of diabetes mellitus (DM) is Type 2. The number of people with Type 2 is going up because of an explosive increase in obesity. The average American grows 2 to 4 ounces heavier each year. The pancreas is not able to

> Type 2 DM has a greater genetic correlation than Type 1.

> Adipose tissue and resting muscle must have insulin to allow glucose to enter.

produce enough insulin to support this much added weight. Type 2 DM was formerly called non-insulin dependent diabetes, but this is not a good term since many of these patients do start using insulin eventually. Type 1 DM (also known as juvenile diabetes) has generally remained constant in incidence.

Comparison of Type 1 and Type 2 Diabetes	
Type 1	**Type 2**
Juvenile onset usually before age 10–20	Adult onset after age 40
Thin	Obese
Immune mediated destruction of islet cells	Peripheral insulin resistance
Not related to physical activity	Strongly correlated with physical inactivity
Strong HLA association, DR3, DR4	No HLA association
Associated with Graves, Addison, Hashimoto, vitiligo, pernicious anemia	No specific disease associations
Prone to ketoacidosis	Resistant to ketoacidosis
Weight loss ineffective	Weight loss and exercise highly effective
Insulin necessary from the beginning of therapy; oral agents not effective	Oral agents first; many never need insulin

PRESENTATION

The most common presentation of diabetes is related to hyperglycemia and the effects of urinary loss of glucose. Patients present with **polyuria**, **polydipsia**, or **polyphagia**.

Type 2 diabetics are far more likely to be asymptomatic at presentation. Both types are associated with vulvovaginal candidiasis, blurry vision, peripheral neuropathy, erectile dysfunction, and generalized fatigue and weakness.

Screening for Diabetes Mellitus

Asymptomatic adults should be screened for DM if they have a BP greater than 135/80, obesity, proteinuria, or family history.

DIAGNOSTIC TESTS

The screening methods and the criteria for the diagnosis are the same:

- Two fasting blood glucose levels above 125 mg/dL
- One blood glucose above 200 mg/dL found in association with symptoms
- Elevated level of blood glucose 2 hours postprandial on an oral glucose tolerance test
- Hemoglobin A_{1c} above 6.5%

TREATMENT

Treatment of Type 1 Diabetes

The best initial therapy for Type 1 diabetes is with a combination of long-acting insulin and rapid-acting insulin.

Long-acting insulin (glargine, detemir): The most frequently used long-acting agent is insulin glargine. This is because of a unique pharmacokinetics that allows a rapid peak level followed by a steady state until the dose wears off at 24 hours.

Rapid-acting insulin (aspart, lispro, glulisine): These are given with meals. These agents reach an onset of activity within 10 minutes. They will wear off after 3 to 4 hours. Regular insulin is an alternative to this rapid-acting insulin.

> NPH insulin is intermediate in duration. NPH does not have the constant levels that glargine does and there is more fluctuation in action.

Treatment of Type 2 Diabetes

1. Diet, exercise, and weight loss: The best initial management of Type 2 diabetes is with diet, exercise, and weight loss. At least **25% of patients will never need drug therapy if lifestyle modifications are successful**. Weight loss alone can completely resolve Type 2 DM. The effects of 15 minutes of aerobic exercise on improving glycemic control can last for as long as 24 hours.

2. Metformin: The best **initial drug therapy for Type 2 DM is with metformin**. Metformin works by blocking gluconeogenesis. Metformin does not increase insulin levels; consequently, there is no hypoglycemia. Insulin drives glucose and free fatty acid into cells. Because there is no insulin release with metformin, there is no increase in weight.

3. Sulfonylureas (glyburide, glipizide, glimepiride): If the patient is not controlled with metformin or there is a contraindication to metformin, the "most appropriate next step in management" is to use a sulfonylurea, an incretin drug, or thiazolidinedione. Because sulfonylureas increase insulin release from the pancreas, they provoke further weight gain. They can also cause hypoglycemia.

> Resting muscle needs insulin. Exercising muscle does not require insulin for glucose to enter.

> Metformin should not be used with renal insufficiency. There is a risk of metabolic acidosis.

> Sulfonylureas can cause SIADH.

What Is the Treatment of Type 2 Diabetes Not Responsive to Both Metformin and Sulfonylureas?

1. If the glucose level is close to tight control (under 200 mg/dL), add a third oral agent.

The third agent can be:

- **Thiazolidinedione (rosiglitazone or pioglitazone):** These agents increase peripheral insulin sensitivity but can lead to fluid overload.

or

- Incretin modulator (exenatide or liraglutide), amylinomimetic (pramlintide), or DPP inhibitor (sitagliptan, saxagliptin, or linagliptin): These agents **decrease glucagon release**, **delay gastric emptying**, and **increase insulin release** from the pancreas.

> Insulin use = additional needle sticks for monitoring and treatment of elevated glucose levels between doses

> Beware of rosiglitazone and pioglitazone in CHF. They increase edema and risk of CHF exacerbations.

> Exenatide and pramlintide have a marked effect on increasing weight loss!

or

- **Alpha-glucosidase inhibitor (acarbose, miglitol):** These agents block the absorption of glucose in the bowel. They are rarely used because of diarrhea and GI distress.

Each oral agent lowers the average glucose level by 50 to 100 mg/dL. The alpha-glucosidase inhibitors are the least potent in lowering glucose levels. However, if two agents get you almost to the tight control you are aiming for, it is preferable in terms of comfort for the patient to try to keep them off the multiple injections and risk of hypoglycemia that comes with the use of insulin. Not only are there several injections a day for the insulin, there is also the need for additional "sticks" for blood sugar monitoring.

2. If the glucose level is still very high (above 200–250 mg/dL) despite the use of metformin, sulfonylureas, and an incretin drug such as sitagliptin, add or switch to insulin.

Use insulin as a combination of long (glargine) and short (aspart, lispro, glulisine) as previously described under "Treatment of Type 1 Diabetes."

> A patient with diabetes is about to undergo coronary angiography for an acute coronary syndrome. His BUN and creatinine are normal. He is on multiple medications for diabetes. Which of the following should be stopped prior to undergoing the angiography?
>
> a. Insulin glargine
> b. Metformin
> c. Sulfonylurea
> d. Rosiglitazone
> e. Exenatide
>
> Answer: The correct answer is (b). *Metformin* is associated with the rare complication of *metabolic acidosis*. This complication is more likely in those with *renal insufficiency*, in whom the drug will accumulate. It is standard to stop metformin prior to any procedure that requires iodinated contrast material. This is because of the concern that the contrast agent may cause renal insufficiency and the renal insufficiency precipitates metabolic acidosis because of the metformin. Rosiglitazone is a concern with congestive failure.

Adverse Effects of Diabetes Medications	
Medication	**Adverse effect**
Metformin	Lactic acidosis, contraindicated with renal insufficiency
Sulfonylureas	SIADH, weight gain
Thiazolidinediones (glitazones)	CHF exacerbation from fluid overload
Alpha-glucosidase inhibitors	Flatulence, diarrhea, and abdominal pain. They cause the same effects as lactose intolerance.

> Second and third agent for type 2 diabetes: Either sulfonylurea *or* incretin (sitagliptin, saxagliptin, linagliptin) *or* thiazolidinedione (rosiglitazone or pioglitazone).

> Nateglinide and repaglinide have the same mechanism of action as sulfonylureas and add nothing when a patient is on a sulfonylurea.

Prevention of Complications of Diabetes

The prevention of diabetic complications is similar for both Type 1 and Type 2 diabetes.

Retinopathy

An **annual screening ophthalmologic examination** should be performed to detect the presence of proliferative retinopathy. If proliferative retinopathy is detected, the patient should undergo laser photocoagulation to prevent progression.

Proliferative retinopathy is defined as:

- **Neovascularization** (new blood vessel formation)
- **Vitreal hemorrhages**

The only effective management to prevent the progression from nonproliferative (background) retinopathy to proliferative retinopathy is tighter glucose control. Although control of hypertension is important, controlling the blood pressure does not prevent neovascularization or vitreal hemorrhages. Aspirin is effective for macrovascular disease, but not on microvascular disease such as diabetic retinopathy. Macrovascular disease is coronary, carotid, cerebral, and peripheral arterial disease.

> Use at least 3 or 4 oral agents before going to insulin.

> VEGF inhibitors (ranibizumab, bevacizumab) inhibit the progression of diabetic retinopathy.

▶ **TIP**

In controlling diabetic retinopathy, wrong answers are lipid-lowering therapy and aspirin use.

A 62-year-old woman with long-standing diabetes comes for her annual comprehensive health maintenance visit. Blood pressure is 110/70 mm Hg. Dilated examination of the eye reveals some flame hemorrhages. The urine dipstick is negative for protein.

What is the most appropriate next step in the management of this patient?

a. Ramipril
b. Spironolactone
c. Urine for microalbumin
d. No further action required, return in one year
e. Losartan

> Don't do things for patients you wouldn't want for yourself.

Answer: The correct answer is (c). A routine urine *dipstick* will *detect protein* once it has reached a level of *300 mg per 24 hours*. At that level the dipstick will read positive at *"trace."* *Microalbumin is between 30 and 300 mg.* It means there is albumin, but at a level lower than could be found on a dipstick. ACE inhibitors and angiotensin receptor blockers (ARBs) are indicated in diabetes management if there is hypertension or proteinuria. Spironolactone has no benefit for diabetes. Flame hemorrhages are not proliferative retinopathy. They are background (or nonproliferative) retinopathy.

Nephropathy

Annual **urine evaluation for proteinuria** should be done in all diabetic patients. Start with a urine dipstick. If it shows proteinuria, the patient should be placed on an ACE inhibitor (ACEI) or an ARB. Both of these medications decrease intraglomerular hypertension and will delay or decrease the rate of progression of renal insufficiency.

If the dipstick does not show protein, the "most appropriate next step in management" is urine evaluation for microalbumin. If this is present, start an ACEI or ARB. If both choices are in the answer, then choose the ACEI.

▶ **TIP**

An ACEI and an ARB in combination is always a wrong answer.

> A 62-year-old woman with diabetes is found to have microalbuminuria. She is started on lisinopril. On a follow-up visit a week later her creatinine is found to have risen from 0.8 mg/dL to 1.2 mg/dL.
>
> What is the most appropriate management?
>
> a. No change in management
> b. Reduce the dose of lisinopril
> c. Hydrate the patient
> d. Switch the lisinopril to telmisartan
> e. Switch the lisinopril to hydralazine

Answer: The correct answer is (a). A small increase in creatinine is expected after the start of an ACEI or ARB. This is because dilation of the efferent arteriole will decrease GFR. You do not have to alter therapy because of this. This is the same mechanism by which these medications protect the kidney. They prevent damage to the nephrons by decreasing intraglomerular hypertension. If there were a need to switch, then hydralazine would be a better choice because the mechanism is different.

Hyperlipidemia

All diabetic patients should be screened for the presence of hyperlipidemia annually. **The goal for LDL in a diabetic patient is 100 mg/dL or lower.** All diabetic patients with an LDL above 100 mg/dL should be started on a statin.

If there is coronary artery disease **in addition** to DM, the **goal of LDL is 70 mg/dL or less.** If a statin alone does not control the LDL, a second agent should be added. Although niacin is relatively contraindicated in diabetes because it has some adverse effects on glucose control, the benefit of controlling the LDL exceeds the risk of a slight elevation in glucose.

In terms of LDL, **diabetes is considered equivalent to coronary disease** (ie, goal 100 mg/dL or less).

Ezetimibe lowers the LDL but has no mortality benefit.

Hypertension

The goal of BP in a person with diabetes is below 130/80. If the BP in a diabetic is above 130/80, treatment with an ACEI or ARB is the best initial therapy. The dose should be raised until the target is reached.

The Diabetic Foot

A specific examination of the foot by a physician **should be performed at least annually to detect neuropathy.** The proper tool is a 10-g monofilament. If neuropathy (defects in sensory input) is detected, the patient should increase his or her level of attention to inspection of the feet on a daily basis. Referral to a podiatrist is also the answer.

There is no specific treatment to reverse diabetic neuropathy of the feet. Management is based on making sure minor injury does not become a source of skin breakdown, ulceration, and amputation.

> Do not use rosiglitazone in CHF.

▶ TIP

Diabetic foot neuropathy is one of the only times, ever, that "referral" may be the correct choice on a board exam. Usually "referral" is automatically a wrong answer.

Summary of Diabetic Complications		
Potential complication	**Screening method**	**Therapeutic intervention**
Retinopathy	Annual dilated retinal examination	Laser photocoagulation for proliferative retinopathy
Nephropathy	Annual urine for albumin/microalbumin	ACEI or ARB for any degree of proteinuria
Hyperlipidemia	Annual LDL	Statin for LDL >100 mg/dL (>70 mg/dL if coronary disease is present)
Hypertension	BP check at every visit	ACEI if BP > 130/80; use an ARB if intolerant of ACEI (e.g., cough)
Foot care	Annual physician exam of feet	Meticulous foot care; refer to podiatrist.

Treatment of Complications of Diabetes

Coronary Artery Disease

The **goal of BP is below 130/80 in DM**. The goal of LDL is below 70 mg/dL when DM is present in those also with coronary artery disease (CAD). CAD is the most common cause of death in diabetic patients. There are two further issues:

- "Silent" myocardial infarction: Those with DM are more likely to have an MI without symptoms of chest pain.

- Once having occurred, the standard for coronary bypass surgery is different in a diabetic patient. Coronary bypass is usually indicated for those with greater than 70% stenosis of the left main coronary artery or in three other vessels. In those **with diabetes, bypass surgery is considered for only two or more vessels with more than 70% stenosis.**

Peripheral Neuropathy

Diabetes is damaging to the microvasculature throughout the body. This is also true for the vaso nervorum, the microvascular supply around the peripheral nerves. Manifestations are:

> Coronary bypass for only 2 vessels is limited to diabetics.

- **Diffuse, symmetrical peripheral neuropathy** in a "glove and stocking" pattern. This can be either with loss of sensation (numbness) or with pain that can be very uncomfortable.
- **Mononeuritis:** involvement of single large nerves such as the radial, ulnar, or cranial nerves. When cranial nerves are involved, the third cranial nerve is most common.
- Radiculopathy can produce the same symptoms of pain as would occur from a herniated vertebral disk.

DIAGNOSTIC TESTS/TREATMENT

The most accurate tests of peripheral neuropathy are nerve conduction studies. The best initial therapy of a painful peripheral neuropathy is with:

> Capsaicin and topical lidocaine help when others fail.

- Gabapentin or pregabalin
- Amitriptyline

Autonomic Neuropathy

Diabetes can damage the afferent sensory connections to the bowel. This results in diabetic gastroparesis. The major stimulant to gastric motility is the stretch or distention of the bowel. If this stretch is not detected, motility is inhibited. This leads to bloating, abdominal cramping, and a sense of fullness that presents with either constipation or diarrhea.

Although the most accurate test is a barium/nuclear gastric emptying study, the diagnosis is most often determined on clinical presentation.

The best initial **therapy is with metoclopramide or erythromycin**, both of which increase gastrointestinal motility.

Erectile Dysfunction

Prolonged diabetes will often lead to erectile dysfunction (ED). Patients will most often not volunteer this information, so it is important to ask. Treat ED from diabetes with sildenafil or tadalafil as you would anyone with ED. Bypass surgery of the vasculature supplying the penis may be effective if medical therapy fails.

Diabetic Ketoacidosis

ETIOLOGY

Although diabetic ketoacidosis (DKA) is more frequent in Type 1 DM, it can still occur in Type 2 DM. **DKA is precipitated by:**

- **Infection**
- **Nonadherence to medications**
- **Alcohol intoxication**

Anything that increases cortisol output as a stress hormone can lead to DKA because cortisol makes the peripheral tissues insensitive to insulin and drives up the glucose level. If the cells cannot take in glucose as a fuel, then the cells seek an alternate fuel such as ketoacids.

PRESENTATION

DKA presents with a profoundly ill person ranging from mild confusion to coma. Patients are hyperventilating because of the compensatory response to metabolic acidosis. As with all forms of uncontrolled diabetes, there is polyuria and polydipsia.

A diabetic patient comes into the emergency department with uncontrolled diabetes. He is slightly sleepy, and hyperventilating with a fruity odor on his breath. His blood pressure is normal. You are uncertain about the severity of his condition and whether he should go to the regular floor or to the intensive care unit.

Which of the following would you choose to determine where the patient should be placed?

a. Serum glucose
b. Urine ketones
c. Blood ketones
d. Serum bicarbonate
e. Urine glucose
f. BUN and creatinine

Answer: The correct answer is (d). Serum bicarbonate level is essentially equivalent to the anion gap in terms of determining the level of metabolic acidosis. Glucose level is not reliable since patients can have a very high glucose, but not have become ketotic. Glucose levels can be corrected rapidly and the patient discharged if there is no acidosis. The presence or absence of acidosis is the main way of determining the seriousness of hyperglycemia. Urine ketones can happen with very mild disease, and can occur even from skipping a few meals. Blood ketones can be negative even in severe DKA because the test does not accurately assess all forms of ketoacids. That is, the serum ketones can be falsely normal.

The correct answer could also have been:

- pH on a blood gas
- Anion gap

DIAGNOSTIC TESTS

Although the glucose level will likely be handed to you, the **most accurate way to assess DKA is with the serum bicarbonate, pH, and anion gap**. There is no need to do an arterial puncture to assess the degree of acidosis if there is no respiratory illness. The pH on the venous blood gas is essentially equal to the pH on an arterial puncture. Because of transcellular shift, the cells will take in hydrogen ions to prevent death from metabolic acidosis. In exchange, the cells release potassium.

▶ **TIP**

Beware the question "How will the patient die?" The answer to this in DKA can also be hyperkalemia.

Potassium Levels in DKA

When the acidosis is still severe, the **serum potassium level will be elevated**. This will lead to urinary loss of potassium. Hence, the blood potassium level will be elevated, **but the body will be depleted of potassium**. As the acidosis is corrected, potassium will move back into the cells and hypokalemia may develop.

▶ **TIP**

Potassium questions are one of the most frequently tested aspects of DKA.

TREATMENT

The **best initial therapy for DKA is high-volume fluids** (normal saline) and intravenous insulin.

When the potassium level comes to a normal value, it is important to add potassium to the fluids in order to correct the total body deficit of potassium.

> Add potassium to fluids when level comes to normal.

ADRENAL DISORDERS

Hypercortisolism

DEFINITION/ETIOLOGY

Hypercortisolism is defined as the presence of an increased level of serum cortisol from any cause. This can be from overproduction or exogenous administration such as the chronic use of prednisone. The clinical manifestation of hypercortisolism is the same regardless of the etiology, so we cannot use the following "Presentation" section to help answer the question "Which of the following is the most likely diagnosis?"

▶ **TIP**

Most endocrine questions, especially the ones on hypercortisolism, will be about diagnostic tests.

The term "Cushing syndrome" (or disease) is often used interchangeably with the term "hypercortisolism." This is probably because they are all clinically indistinguishable.

Which of the following is the most common cause of hypercortisolism?

a. Pituitary (Cushing disease)
b. Adrenal (Cushing syndrome)
c. Ectopic ACTH production
d. Prednisone use
e. Ectopic corticotropin releasing hormone (CRH)

Answer: The correct answer is (d). Cushing syndrome is a rare disease. There are about 10 cases per million people per year, or about 3,000 cases nationally. Now think about how many patients you have each week on prednisone, or methylpred-nisolone, or another form of therapeutic glucorticoid. So clearly, many more cases of hypercortisolism originate in the physician's prescription pad.

Let us look at the question again.

Which of the following is the most common cause of hypercortisolism?

a. Pituitary (Cushing disease)
b. Adrenal (Cushing syndrome)
c. Ectopic ACTH production
d. Ectopic corticotropin releasing hormone (CRH)

Answer: The correct answer is (a). These two questions are a good example of how the answer to a given question can change based on what the other choices are. Although Cushing disease is not *the* most common cause of hypercortisolism, it is the most common within this group.

Causes of Hypercortisolism	
Etiology	**Frequency**
Pituitary adenoma	65%–70%
Ectopic ACTH	10%–15%
Adrenal adenoma	10%
Adrenal cancer	5%–10%

ACTH Dependent vs. ACTH Independent

This is an excellent way of naming these disorders rather than being tortured by the names "disease" or "syndrome."

> Ectopic ACTH comes from the lung, pancreas, and thymus most often.

ACTH dependent Cushing syndrome:

- Pituitary adenoma
- Ectopic ACTH production (often in the lung)

ACTH independent Cushing syndrome:

- Adrenal adenoma
- Adrenal cancer
- Adrenal hyperplasia

Other **causes of hypercortisolism**:

- **Depression**
- **Alcoholism**

Presentation of Hypercortisolism

Cortisol causes lipolysis, increases gluconeogenesis, and is immunosuppressive. Why cortisol causes fat to be produced in the trunk of the body, the back of the neck ("buffalo hump"), or the face ("moon face") is unknown. Because of gluconeogenesis, hypercortisolism will be damaging to protein, like muscle, causing weakness. **Cortisol breaks down the amino acids in muscles to use them for gluconeogenesis**. The same is true of dissolving the protein matrix of skin and bones, causing striae, bruising, and osteoporosis, respectively.

Permissive Actions of Cortisol

Cortisol has a permissive action on glucagon and on catecholamines. This is why hypercortisol patients present with:

- Hypertension
- Hyperglycemia and glucose intolerance sometimes with polyuria and polydipsia
- Hyperlipidemia
- Leukocytosis

Cortisol Has Some Androgen Effects

ACTH stimulates the zona reticularis, which makes androgens like DHEA. In addition, cortisol has a small amount of androgen effects. This is why patients with hypercortisolism also present with:

- Acne
- Virilization
- Oily skin and acne (androgens increase sebum production; this is why acne is common at puberty)

> It is not clear why cortisol breaks down fat in some places and forms it on the trunk, neck, and face.

DIAGNOSTIC TESTS

The first tests of hypercortisolism establish whether hypercortisolism is present. If they are positive, only then is the answer "ACTH level" or "dexamethasone suppression testing."

▶ **TIP**

First confirm Cushing is present, then later find the source.

Is Hypercortisolism Present?

Random cortisol levels can be falsely elevated. Almost any cause of physical or emotional anxiety will stimulate the adrenals to release cortisol. This is why **depression and alcoholism can both cause high cortisol levels.** Cortisol goes up normally if the body is being attacked ("fight or flight"). The body doesn't actually have to be attacked in order for the adrenal gland to feel attacked.

▶ **TIP**

Random cortisol levels are always a wrong answer.

The **best initial test** for hypercortisolism is the **24-hour urine cortisol.** If this test is equivocal, the "most appropriate next step in management" is 1 mg overnight dexamethasone suppression test or late-night salivary cortisol level.

Late-night Salivary Cortisol Level

Cortisol levels are normally highest in the morning and lowest at 10 or 11 at night. **If the cortisol level is markedly elevated at night, hypercortisolism is present.** This normal diurnal variation is kept intact even in depressed patients or those with other physical or psychological stressors. Saliva samples are useful because:

- They can be collected by the patient.
- Cortisol level stays intact and does not degrade in saliva.

What Is the Source of the Hypercortisolism?

Only after you have confirmed the presence of hypercortisolism by:

- Elevated 24-hour urine cortisol (the "most accurate test")
- Failure of cortisol to suppress after dexamethasone
- Increased late-night salivary cortisol level

Which of the following would you do first to confirm the etiology of hypercortisolism?

a. ACTH level
b. Inferior petrosal sinus sampling
c. MRI of the pituitary
d. CT of the adrenals
e. High-dose dexamethasone suppression testing
f. Corticotropin-releasing hormone stimulation and petrosal sinus sampling

Answer: The correct answer is (a). This is a very clear question. ACTH levels are unequivocally first to determine the origin of the hypercortisolism.

Let's try the question again.

Which of the following would you do first to confirm the etiology of hypercortisolism *in a person with an elevated ACTH level?*

a. Inferior petrosal sinus sampling
b. MRI of the pituitary
c. CT of the adrenals
d. High-dose dexamethasone suppression testing
e. Corticotropin-releasing hormone stimulation and petrosal sinus sampling

Answer: The correct answer is now (d). An elevated ACTH level can be either from the pituitary or from an ectopic focus, which is most often in the lungs. Suppression of ACTH with high-dose dexamethasone indicates a pituitary source.

Let's try the question one more time.

Which of the following would you do first to confirm the etiology of hypercortisolism in a person **with a decreased ACTH level?**

a. Inferior petrosal sinus sampling
b. MRI of the pituitary
c. CT of the adrenals
d. High-dose dexamethasone suppression testing
e. Corticotropin-releasing hormone stimulation and petrosal sinus sampling

Answer: The correct answer is now (c). Hypercortisolism with suppressed ACTH levels is most often either an adenoma or cancer of the adrenals.

> Pituitary ACTH suppresses with dexamethasone. Ectopic ACTH doesn't suppress.

▶ **TIP**

Never start with an imaging study in endocrinology.

High-Dose Dexamethasone Suppression Testing

The cause of hypercortisolism with an elevated ACTH level can be either in the pituitary or from an ectopic site of production, often the lungs. We know that a pituitary adenoma retains enough normal function to still suppress on feedback. Ectopic foci of overproduction of ACTH will not suppress.

High ACTH level with hypercortisolism=pituitary or ectopic focus

Response to High-Dose Dexamethasone	
Pituitary adenoma	**Ectopic production of ACTH**
Suppresses ACTH	Does *not* suppress ACTH

Which of the following would you do first to confirm the etiology of hyper-cortisolism in a person whose ACTH level suppresses in response to high-dose dexamethasone?

a. Inferior petrosal sinus sampling
b. MRI of the pituitary
c. CT of the adrenals
d. CT scan of the chest
e. Corticotropin-releasing hormone stimulation and petrosal sinus sampling

Answer: The correct answer is (b). If the ACTH level suppresses in response to high-dose dexamethasone, we know that the source is in the pituitary. An MRI should be done to confirm this. Never start with an imaging study. Always confirm the site of production of hypercortisolism prior to imaging.

> At least 10% of the population has a pituitary incidentaloma.

Inferior Petrosal Sinus Sampling

Petrosal sinus sampling for ACTH is the most sensitive test you can do to detect a hyperfunctioning pituitary lesion. If the person's biological testing suggests a pituitary source of hypercortisolism (elevated ACTH, suppression with high-dose dexamethasone) and the MRI does **not** show a lesion, the "most appropriate next step in management" is to place a catheter into the inferior petrosal sinus for a sample of ACTH. The MRI can be falsely normal even when the pituitary adenoma is present.

CRH stimulation will increase the release of ACTH from the pituitary in a pituitary adenoma. **The single most accurate test you can do to detect a pituitary adenoma is inferior petrosal sinus sampling for ACTH after giving CRH.** CRH will increase ACTH output from the pituitary with a pituitary adenoma. CRH will not increase output of ACTH if there is an ectopic focus of ACTH production.

> CRH testing distinguishes ectopic from pituitary sources of hypercortisolism.

Response to Corticotropin-Releasing Hormone	
Pituitary adenoma	**Ectopic production of ACTH**
Increases ACTH release	Does not increase ACTH release

▶ **TIP**

Never start with imaging of the adrenals.

Summary of Diagnostic Testing for Hypercortisolism

> At least 4% of the population has an adrenal incidentaloma.

1. The first step is to confirm hypercortisolism with a 24-hour urine cortisol.
   - If the test is equivocal, do 1-mg overnight dexamethasone suppression testing or late-night salivary cortisol.
   - The most common **wrong answer is random cortisol level**.

2. The second step is to confirm the source (location) of the hypercortisolism with an ACTH level.
   - ACTH **low**: CT of the adrenals
   - ACTH **high**: high-dose dexamethasone suppression testing
     - **Yes** suppression: MRI of the pituitary
     - **No** suppression: CT of the chest (look for ectopic focus)

> Diagnosis of Cushing is complex because adrenal and pituitary incidentalomas are so common.

3. If the MRI of the pituitary is unrevealing, do petrosal sinus sampling for ACTH possibly with CRH stimulation. This is the single most sensitive test of an ACTH-producing pituitary adenoma.

TREATMENT

The **treatment** of hyperfunctioning endocrine lesions is a much easier question: **Remove whatever you find**.

Pituitary lesions are removed by a transsphenoidal approach. Adrenal lesions are removed via laparoscopy. Pulmonary lesions are resected. If transsphenoidal surgery does not work for the pituitary lesion, radiation should be done. In the occasional case in which neither surgery nor radiation is effective in controlling a pituitary lesion, medications are used to inhibit the function of the adrenal gland. These are:

- Metyrapone
- Ketoconazole

Addison Disease (Adrenal Insufficiency)

Addison disease is a much easier disease to address in boards questions.

- It has very few causes: **90% of cases are autoimmune** in nature.
- There are very few relevant tests: Cosyntropin stimulation is virtually the only question.
- **Urgent hormone replacement is more important than waiting for test results** in acute adrenergic crisis.

ETIOLOGY

The 10% of Addison disease that is not autoimmune in etiology can be from:

- Infections (e.g., HIV, TB, fungus)
- Cancer metastasizing to the adrenal gland
- Hemorrhage
- Medications such as the ones previously described for treatment of hypercortisolism

PRESENTATION

Adrenal insufficiency from any cause presents with **weakness**, **fatigue**, weight loss, **hypotension**, **hypoglycemia**, nausea, vomiting, and abdominal pain. Weakness can be from electrolyte disturbance. Just as hypercortisolism is a manifestation of exaggerated activity of cortisol, adrenal insufficiency presents with the opposite. Fever is often present.

> Hyperpigmentation is one of the most characteristic features of chronic Addison disease.

▶ TIP

Look for a mention of salt craving in the case, such as "drinking pickle juice."

DIAGNOSTIC TESTS

The most accurate test of adrenal gland hypofunctioning is the cosyntropin stimulation test. Cortisol levels are measured before and after the administration of cosyntropin. Cosyntropin is artificial ACTH. It is a stimulatory diagnostic test. A healthy person's cortisol level should rise in response to cosyntropin.

Metabolic Effects of Adrenal Disorders		
	Cushing syndrome (hypercortisolism)	**Addison disease (hypoadrenalism)**
Potassium	Low	High
Blood pressure	High	Low
Glucose	High	Low
Leukocytosis	Neutrophilia	Eosinophilia
Imbalance	Metabolic alkalosis	Metabolic acidosis

TREATMENT

Treatment should be hormone replacement with prednisone, sometimes combined with fludrocortisone.

The most important point about Addison disease management in acute, severely ill patients is to **start replacement with hydrocortisone and fluids while waiting for the results of diagnostic testing**. When the case is clear:

- Hypotension
- Hyperkalemia
- Metabolic acidosis
- Weakness, hyperpigmentation

You should:

1. Draw a blood **cortisol level**.
2. Start dexamethasone or **hydrocortisone**.
3. Give several liters of normal **saline**.

Long-term Management

For those with permanent adrenal gland destruction, chronic oral treatment is used.

1. **Hydrocortisone**
2. Adding **fludrocortisone**, which has the **highest mineralocorticoid activity of all the steroids**. Mineralocorticoid effect is desirable in the long term in combination with hydrocortisone to simulate the effect of having aldosterone in addition to cortisol.

Pheochromocytoma

PRESENTATION/"WHAT IS THE MOST LIKELY DIAGNOSIS?"

Look for a patient with hypertension that:

- Is episodic
- Is associated with palpitations
- Includes headache, sweating, and tachycardia

Ten percent are **malignant**. Ten percent are **not in the adrenal**. Ten percent are **bilateral**.

DIAGNOSTIC TESTS

The best initial test is **24-hour urine for metanephrines and catecholamines**.

The most **common *wrong* answers** for initial test are:

- Vanillylmandelic acid
- Chromogranin A levels

> Dexamethasone does not interfere with blood testing for cortisol levels.

> There is orthostatic hypotension in between episodes of hypertension.

> Multiple Endocrine Neoplasia
> - Pheochromocytoma
> - Hyperparathyroidism
> - Medullary thyroid carcinoma

Diagnostic Plan

After finding an elevation of the 24-hour urine for metanephrines and catecholamines, the next step is a CT scan of the abdomen to detect the lesion in the adrenal. If no lesion is found in the adrenal, the most appropriate next step is to do an MIBG scan. The MIBG scan detects occult (hidden) non-obvious sources of catecholamine-producing tissue.

TREATMENT

Pretreatment with medication to block the sympathetic nervous system is mandatory prior to removal of lesions from the adrenal gland. The steps are:

1. Alpha-adrenergic blockade with **phenoxybenzamine**
2. **Beta blockade** with propranolol
3. Calcium channel blockers (can be used instead of alpha blockers)
4. **Surgery**

Primary Hyperaldosteronism

ETIOLOGY

The frequency of occurrence is as follows:

Solitary **adenoma: 85%**

Bilateral hyperplasia: 14%

Cancer: 1%

PRESENTATION

Patients present with the effects of **hypokalemia** such as **muscular weakness** and fatigue. Potassium is necessary for normal muscular contraction. Hypertension is most often asymptomatic as it is with most patients.

> Hypertension +
> Hypokalemia =
> Hyperaldosteronism

DIAGNOSTIC TESTS

The presence of **hypertension and hypokalemia** are the clues to obtain renin and aldosterone levels. Metabolic **alkalosis** is present because aldosterone causes an increase in the urinary and colonic excretion of hydrogen ions.

The elevated blood pressure will suppress renin production. The ratio is greater than 20:1 for aldosterone to renin.

The most accurate (or confirmatory) test is the failure of suppression of aldosterone levels in response to salt loading. Patients are given intravenous saline or oral salt. A healthy person should suppress his or her aldosterone levels. This is because the usual stimulant for aldosterone release is either angiotensin or hyperkalemia. Patients with primary hyperaldosteronism will continue to make aldosterone despite the fact that their potassium levels are low, and intravascular volume is expanded with salt or salt and water, which suppresses angiotensin II.

> "Primary" means production is happening without the usual stimuli.

Only after these functional tests are done should you do a CT scan of the adrenal glands. Remember, 4% of the population has an adrenal incidentaloma. You must confirm the presence of primary hyperaldosteronism with functional tests before imaging.

TREATMENT

Solitary adenomas are removed with **surgery**. Bilateral hyperplasia is treated with an aldosterone antagonist such as **spironolactone** or **eplerenone**.

Management of the Asymptomatic Adrenal Incidentaloma

How far do you have to go in the evaluation of an adrenal lesion found by accident?

- Urinary catecholamines and metanephrines
- 1-mg dexamethasone suppression test (the only good use of this test)
- Renin and aldosterone levels in those who are hypertensive

MALE HYPOGONADISM

DEFINITION/ETIOLOGY

> Klinefelter syndrome is the most common cause of primary hypogonadism.

Male hypogonadism is the decreased output of the testes resulting in deficiency of the reproductive hormone testosterone. Primary defects are **Kallmann syndrome** or **Klinefelter syndrome**. Androgen insensitivity syndrome is a lack of adequate receptors to bind testosterone present from conception. This is also known as "testicular feminization." The karyotype in androgen insensitivity is male or XY, but there is no receptor for the testosterone that is produced.

- Prolactinomas and other causes of increased prolactin can decrease gonadal function by prolactin's ability to suppress LH and FSH release.
- Infections such as mumps, echovirus, or flavivirus can cause hypogonadism.
- Medications: Chemotherapy, particularly the combination chemotherapy used for lymphoma, can damage gonadal tissue, leading to infertility. MOPP/ABVD therapy for lymphoma can render up to 95% of patients sterile. Ketoconazole can be so antiandrogenic as to simulate the effects of orchiectomy. Spironolactone, particularly at higher doses, is antiandrogenic and can produce gynecomastia. Heroin-dependent persons are also markedly hypogonadal.

- Testicular injury from trauma or radiation can cause hypogonadism in adults.
- Cryptorchid (undescended) testicles can become nonfunctional.

The gonadotropins (LH and FSH) can be up or down depending on the etiology.

PRESENTATION

All causes of hypogonadism present with:

- Decreased libido *and Potency*
- Erectile dysfunction
- Shrinking of the testicles
- Decreased sperm count and infertility
- Decreased muscle mass

→ Incomplete sexual development
→ Ginecomastia
→ Decreased early morning erections
→ Decreased secondary sexual characteres (ej: decrease shaving frecuency)

Those who were hypogonadal before puberty show:

- Underdeveloped genitals
- Decreased body hair
- Absence of acne at puberty
- Eunuchoid habitus

Small testes (normal adult testes: leng 4-7cm, volomen 20-25mL)

Osteoporosis, Hot flashes

Primary Hypogonadal Disorders

Klinefelter syndrome presents with small testes, eunuchoid appearance, and long limbs. It may go unnoticed until adulthood.

Kallmann syndrome is characterized by anosmia.

Androgen insensitivity gives the external appearance of a female (breasts, vulva, and distal vagina). These patients are socially female. At puberty they fail to menstruate and then are found to be missing a cervix. The testicles are present, but they are undescended or buried in the vulva.

DIAGNOSTIC TESTS

By definition, all have low testosterone levels except for androgen insensitivity syndrome.

Kallmann syndrome has decreased LH and FSH. Klinefelter is hypergonadotrophic (increased LH/FSH).

Prolactin levels may be elevated depending on the cause.

TREATMENT

Testosterone replacement is the most important, and often the only, treatment. Those with **hyperprolactinemia** are managed with **dopamine agonists** such as cabergoline if the cause of the hyperprolactinemia cannot be eliminated.

Androgen insensitivity is managed with removal of the undescended testicles. This is important because of the increased risk of testicular cancer. There is no point in giving testosterone to those with androgen insensitivity because these persons are functionally female and can achieve normal social and sexual development as women, with the exception of infertility because an androgen-insensitive person lacks a cervix, uterus, and ovaries. They naturally make some estrogen because Sertoli cells make estradiol and adipose tissue has aromatase. After the testicles are removed, estrogen replacement is used to maintain development as women.

GASTROENTEROLOGY

by Niket Sonpal, MD

ESOPHAGEAL DISEASE

Esophageal disease is the most common gastrointestinal disorder affecting Americans, with as much as 44% of the population suffering from "heartburn" at least once a month.

A 47-year-old obese male investment banker presents with burning chest pain in duration of 6 months with a frequency of 4 to 6 times per week. He admits to having a sour taste in his mouth and for the remainder of the day he feels like he is "sucking on pennies." He states that the "heartburn" is worse at night and especially when he is lying flat just after eating. He also complains of waking up coughing and feels his voice has been hoarse. Over-the-counter antacids no longer help.

What is the most appropriate next step in the management of the patient?

a. Proton pump inhibitors (PPIs)
b. Esophagogastroduodenoscopy (EGD)
c. 24-hour pH monitoring
d. Barium swallow
e. Nissen fundoplication

Answer: The correct answer is (a). This patient has a prototypic presentation of gastroesophageal reflux disease (GERD) characterized by a metallic and sour taste in his mouth. He also is suffering from nocturnal reflux that causes him to wake up coughing and leaves his voice hoarse from acidic effect on the larynx. His risk factors include obesity and a stressful lifestyle. Starting this patient on PPIs for 4 weeks is both diagnostic and therapeutic in up to 90% of cases. As this patient's symptoms have been going on for less than 6 months, concern of malignant potential is considerably lower. A return visit in 4 weeks should delineate relief of symptoms and improvement in quality of life. EGD is performed only in patients with long-standing symptoms for more than 5 years. Adenocarcinoma develops in 0.5% per year after developing Barrett esophagus. 24-hour pH monitoring will be indicated only if PPI treatment failure occurs and the diagnosis is not clear. It is the most accurate diagnostic test. A barium swallow is indicated if the patient has dysphagia or a possible motility disorder. A Nissen fundoplication is a surgical alternative indicated when all medical options have been exhausted.

Gastroesophageal Reflux Disease

GERD is a condition in which stomach contents leak backward into the esophagus, causing pain and discomfort.

PRESENTATION

- Substernal chest pain without cardiac disease
- Chronic cough
- Belching
- Metallic or sour taste
- Wheezing without reactive airway disease

Helicobacter pylori infection does **not** cause reflux disease.

Risk Factors for GERD	
Risk factor	**Mechanism of increased risk**
Obesity	A BMI above 28 increases the risk of GERD.
Hiatal hernia	Stomach is pulled up through the diaphragm.
Hypercalcemia	Calcium is a second messenger for **gastrin**. Calcium increases acid production.
Zollinger-Ellison syndrome	This gastrinoma massively increases gastric acid output.
Medications	Theophylline, diazepam, prochlorperazine, promethazine, and estrogen replacements all relax the LES.
Motility disorders	Scleroderma, gastroparesis (diabetic neuropathy)
Other	Cigarette smoking, xerostomia, caffeine, chocolate, alcohol, and peppermint

DIAGNOSTIC TESTING

The **best initial test is PPI administration**. It is also therapeutic. If after 4 to 6 weeks treatment failure occurs, the **most accurate test is a 24-hour pH monitoring** and should follow. Endoscopy is indicated when symptoms persist despite maximal therapy. It is also indicated for "alarm symptoms," which are:

24-hour pH is indicated when:

- Asthma begins as an adult in the setting of GERD.
- Hoarseness persists for a prolonged duration.
- Sleep apnea is a comorbid finding.
- Medical treatment has failed.

- Dysphagia (difficulty swallowing)
- Odynophagia (painful swallowing)
- Gastrointestinal bleeding or anemia
- Weight loss

Alarm symptoms in GERD = immediate endoscopic examination

TREATMENT

1. **Lifestyle modification**
   - Elevate the head of the bed.
   - Stop tobacco, caffeine, chocolate, alcohol, and peppermint. These all reduce lower esophageal sphincter (LES) pressure.
   - Don't sleep within 3 hours of a meal, when acid production in the stomach is at a peak.
   - Lose weight.

2. **Medical therapy**
   - **PPIs:** best medical therapy
   - **H2 blockers:** not as effective as PPIs. Only 50 to 70% of patients are controlled with H2 blockers.

3. **Surgical treatment**
   - **Nissen fundoplication** is the answer when PPIs fail.
   - Transoral incisionless fundoplication (TIF) endoscopically rebuilds the LES through the esophagus.

> **Antacids** provide short-term relief in only 20% of cases.

> Carafate is always the wrong answer.

Commonly Tested Points in Dysphagia

A 34-year-old woman presents with difficulty swallowing solids and liquids. She recently returned from Brazil. She states she feels like the food is getting stuck in the middle of her chest and takes many hours to pass. She does not feel nauseated and has not vomited. She has lost 10 pounds in a month. Barium swallow reveals an abnormality at the lower esophageal sphincter.

What is the most likely diagnosis?

a. Achalasia
b. Adenocarcinoma
c. Schatzki ring
d. Zenker diverticulum
e. Esophageal spasm

Answer: The correct answer is (a). The patient is suffering from achalasia secondary to Chagas disease. She just acquired Trypanosoma cruzi from a trip to South America. T cruzi destroys the Auerbach plexus, which is the neural control of esophageal peristalsis. Adenocarcinoma is unlikely in young people. Cancer presents with progressive dysphagia for only solid food at first. Schatzki ring presents with intermittent dysphagia and a midesophageal narrowing on barium swallow. Zenker diverticulum presents with regurgitated food and severe halitosis. Esophageal spasm gives intermittent severe chest pain. The best treatment options for achalasia are pneumatic dilation or surgical myotomy.

A 26-year-old college student comes to the office with bad breath. At times he wakes up with regurgitated foul-smelling food on his pillow. Physical examination reveals foul-smelling breath.

Which of the following is *contraindicated* in this patient?

a. Nasogastric tube placement
b. Barium studies
c. Surgical resection
d. Endoscopic stapling

Answer: The correct answer is (a). The patient has a Zenker diverticulum causing retention of food within the blind pouch in the posterior pharyngeal constrictor muscles. Food rots and causes halitosis. Nasogastric tube placement can cause perforation. The most common location of the diverticulum is at the cervical area of the esophagus. This makes regurgitation of food more likely at night, when the body is supine. Symptomatic patients need surgical repair. Endoscopic stapling allows for repair with faster recovery times.

A 45-year-old woman presents to the ED with severe crushing substernal chest pain that is "knocking the wind out of her." The pain began 30 minutes ago while she was walking to work drinking an iced latte. She is unable to swallow and is drooling. Her pain resolves a few minutes after arriving in the ED. EKG shows no ST segment abnormalities. While awaiting discharge, she has another episode of chest pain that brings her to her knees.

What is the most likely diagnosis?

a. Achalasia
b. Adenocarcinoma
c. Schatzki ring
d. Zenker diverticulum
e. Esophageal spasm

Answer: The correct answer is (e). Sudden chest pain after drinking cold liquids is classic for nutcracker esophagus or esophageal spasm. Spasm can be clinically indistinguishable from an acute coronary syndrome except there is no relationship with exertion. You cannot assess the patient without a normal EKG and often a stress test. The most accurate test is esophageal manometry. Treat with calcium channel blockers. Barium studies will be abnormal only at the time of the spasm, and it is difficult to time the barium study to a spastic event.

Dysphagia

Dysphagia is **difficulty** swallowing while **odynophagia** is **painful** swallowing. Dysphagia in young patients is secondary to a motility disorder. In older patients, stroke is a more common cause.

Odynophagia is typically in the setting of an infectious process and requires biopsy during EGD.

		Causes of Dysphagia			
Disorder	**Type**	**Etiology**	**Best initial test**	**Most accurate test**	**Best therapy**
Achalasia: incomplete LES relaxation with swallowing	Solids and liquids	Idiopathic and Chagas disease	Barium swallow with a "bird's beak" sign and massively dilated esophagus	Esophageal manometry shows high LES pressure with swallowing and aperistalsis	1. Pneumatic dilation 2. LES injections of botulinum toxin type A 3. Heller myotomy
Esophageal cancer: weight loss and heme-positive stools/anemia	Progressive worsening from solids to liquids	Long-standing GERD, alcohol, tobacco	EGD with biopsy and further imaging (CT scan, PET, ultrasound) for staging	EGD (in cancer, tissue biopsy only if definitive)	Surgical resection and 5-fluorouracil therapy +/– radiation
Peptic strictures (rings from acid exposure)	Solids or liquids	Long-standing GERD	Barium study	EGD is diagnostic and therapeutic	Pneumatic dilation
Zenker diverticulum: associated with halitosis	Solids and liquids	Congenital	Barium study	Barium study	Surgical resection or endoscopic stapling
Esophageal spasm	Acute difficulty in swallowing solids and liquids with chest pain	Diffuse, uncoordinated esophageal contractions	Barium study at time of attack showing a "corkscrew" esophagus	Manometry in the setting of clinical symptoms	Calcium channel blockers

Plummer-Vinson syndrome is a stricture that is associated with iron deficiency anemia. It is treated with oral iron supplements and pneumatic dilatation.

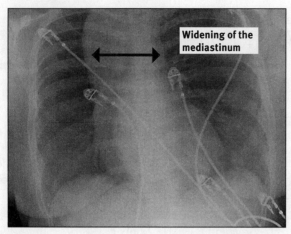

Figure 6.1: Achalasia x-ray. Widening of the mediastinum to the right of the spine from a dilated esophagus.

Source: Juliet Azie, MD

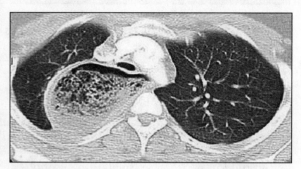

Figure 6.2: Achalasia CT. Food within the obstructed esophagus.

Source: Juliet Azie, MD

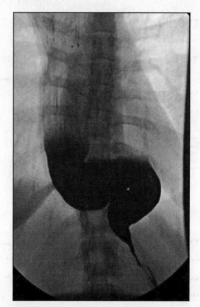

Figure 6.3: Barium esosphagram. Dilated esophagus coming to a point from loss of the ability to relax the lower esophageal sphincter.

Source: Juliet Azie, MD

Esophagitis

Esophagitis is inflammation of the esophagus causing **pain upon swallowing** (odynophagia). The pain occurs due to the food bolus irritating the inflamed area of the mucosa.

The most common cause of esophagitis is GERD, also known as reflux esophagitis. Endoscopy is done to monitor reflux esophagitis for Barrett esophagus.

A 52-year-old man with HIV presents with odynophagia. He has recently been noncompliant with his antiretroviral medications. Oral examination is normal. CD4 count shows 50 cells. He has had no previous opportunistic infections.

Which of the following is the most appropriate next step in the management of this patient?

a. Fluconazole
b. EGD with biopsy
c. Foscarnet
d. Acyclovir
e. Do nothing

Answer: The correct answer is (a). In patients with immunocompromise from HIV who have fewer than 100 CD4 cells, the first step is to start antifungal therapy since 95% of odynophagia is from esophageal candidiasis. A patient can have esophageal candidiasis without oral lesions. EGD is the answer if the patient's symptoms do not improve with 5 to 7 days of treatment with fluconazole. CMV and herpes can cause esophagitis in AIDS, but are far less common than candidiasis. Foscarnet is incorrect because it is for CMV. Acyclovir is for HSV esophagitis.

A 72-year-old woman presents with severe substernal chest pain that is burning in nature. The pain has been intermittent for several weeks and is sometimes worsened with food. She has a history of osteoporosis. Physical examination reveals a diaphoretic, distressed woman with no crepitus around the clavicles. The patient had one episode of hematemesis prior to admission.

What is the most likely diagnosis?

a. Myocardial infarction
b. Pill esophagitis
c. Mallory-Weiss tear
d. GERD

Answer: The correct answer is (b). This patient presents with odynophagia from esophagitis. Given her history of osteoporosis, she must be taking bisphosphonates such as alendronate. Pill esophagitis can also occur from doxycycline, NSAIDs, and potassium. The pill has eroded through the mucosa and caused an upper GI bleed. Endoscopy is the most accurate test. Although surgical intervention may sometimes be needed, most cases resolve with stopping the medication. To prevent it, patients are instructed to drink copious amounts of water with the pill and sit upright for 30 minutes after having taken the pill. Crepitus is found in full thickness perforation, which is rare in pill esophagitis.

A 17-year-old adolescent presents with difficult, painful swallowing for the last 6 months. He has exercise-induced asthma for which he uses an albuterol inhaler. Barium swallow is normal including a normal transit time of contrast. Upper endoscopy with biopsy is done and shows a furrowed-appearing esophagus with concentric grooves.

What will biopsies demonstrate on microscopic examination?

a. Eosinophils
b. Viral inclusion bodies
c. Auer rods
d. Neutrophils

Answer: The correct answer is (a). Eosinophilic esophagitis is found in young patients with odynophagia. Endoscopy typically shows a furrowed mucosa. Biopsies will show many eosinophils. Steroids are the best initial therapy. Allergen skin testing can sometimes reveal the cause. Viral bodies are seen with ulcerations secondary to cytomegalovirus (CMV) or herpes simplex virus (HSV). Auer rods are a finding in acute myelocytic leukemia. Neutrophils would be a nonspecific finding.

Causes of Esophagitis				
Disease	**Signs and symptoms**	**Endoscopic findings**	**Diagnostic test**	**Therapy**
Candidiasis	Dysphagia and odynophagia	Diffuse raised white plaques, easily removed	Treat patients with AIDS who have <100 CD4 cells with fluconazole	Fluconazole
CMV	Dysphagia and odynophagia in an immunocompromised patient	Large deep ulceration	EGD with biopsy with viral cultures	Ganciclovir or foscarnet
HSV	Dysphagia and odynophagia in an immunocompromised patient	Multiple small ulcerations that can coalesce and look like "black esophagus"	EGD with biopsy with viral cultures	Acyclovir, valacyclovir, and famciclovir
Pill esophagitis	New-onset dysphagia and odynophagia in a patient on bisphosphonates or doxycycline	Large deep crater with pill remnants or "kissing ulcer"	EGD to rule out other causes	Prevention with copious water with pills and sitting up 3 hours postingestion
Eosinophilic esophagitis	Dysphagia and odynophagia in a young patient with atopy and normal motility	Furrowed appearance with concentric grooves	EGD with biopsy followed by allergen testing to identify causative agent	Pneumatic dilatation and oral corticosteroid therapy

> Viral cultures must be taken from the ulcer margin in CMV and HSV esophagitis; otherwise you may get a false negative.

Barrett Esophagus

Barrett esophagus is a precancerous lesion that is found on endoscopic exam usually at the gastroesophageal junction.

ETIOLOGY

The normal squamous epithelium lining the esophagus is replaced by **metaplastic columnar epithelium from GERD** after prolonged disease lasting many years. This tissue is similar to gastric or colonic tissue and is marked by the presence of goblet cells. In patients with colonic-type mucosa, the risk of malignant transformation is increased.

DIAGNOSTIC TESTS

Upper **endoscopy** is the only way to visualize and biopsy the lesions.

TREATMENT

Biopsies are categorized into 4 levels of findings:

1. Non-dysplastic or Barrett esophagus: Give PPIs and repeat EGD in 3 years.
2. Low-grade dysplasia: Give PPIs and repeat EGD in 3 to 6 months.
3. High-grade dysplasia: Perform surgical resection.
4. Carcinoma: Perform surgical resection.

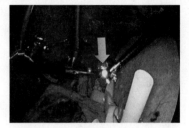

Intraoperative endoscopy showing Boerhaave's defect in the esophagus
Source: Niket Sonpal

A 58-year-old known alcoholic man presents to the ED with chest pain that began shortly after vomiting. Physical examination reveals a diaphoretic patient clutching his chest with a crunching, rasping sound, synchronous with the heartbeat heard over the precordium. EKG and troponin are normal.

What is the most likely diagnosis?

a. Boerhaave syndrome
b. Mallory-Weiss tear
c. Myocardial infarction
d. Food bolus impaction

Answer: The correct answer is (a). Boerhaave syndrome is a **full thickness tear** of the esophagus secondary to retching. The patient will have a history of severe incessant vomiting, often due to alcoholism. Mallory-Weiss tears do not have subcutaneous air, and an MI would have elevated troponins and an abnormal EKG. Food bolus impaction also would not have subcutaneous air, and would not have chest pain as severe as with perforation.

Esophageal Perforation

Esophageal perforation is caused by a sudden increase in intraluminal esophageal pressure with negative intrathoracic pressure caused by vomiting that leads to a full thickness tear.

Perforation of the esophagus can present with:

- **Severe retrosternal chest pain** that begins shortly after vomiting
- **Odynophagia** and hematemesis
- Crunching, rasping sound, synchronous with the heartbeat from subcutaneous emphysema
- Radiation of the pain to the left shoulder

DIAGNOSTIC TESTS/TREATMENT

The most accurate test is a **gastrografin esophogram** that will reveal extravasation of contrast outside of the esophageal lumen. **Closure of the perforation is done surgically** with debridement of the mediastinum. Endoscopic stents can be placed to close the perforation in patients not amenable to surgery.

Mallory-Weiss Syndrome

ETIOLOGY/PRESENTATION

This is a **mucosal** tear due to vomiting that occurs most commonly at the gastroesophageal junction. It presents with **chest pain and hematemesis**, but will **not have subcutaneous air**. It commonly occurs in alcoholics and bulimics.

DIAGNOSTIC TEST/TREATMENT

Upper endoscopy is both diagnostic and therapeutic. It will reveal a laceration-like lesion, and endoscopic **closure of the mucosal defect** is the treatment.

> Mallory-Weiss tears usually occur just below the gastroesophageal junction on the lesser curvature of the stomach.

A 53-year-old obese man presents with abdominal pain that is worse with food for the last 8 months. He describes the pain as a deep stabbing sensation. He has dark stools that are foul smelling. He says lately he is afraid of eating, feels full quickly, and has lost 10 pounds in the last month. The patient has a full bottle of esomeprazole in his pocket. He takes ibuprofen for knee pain. His hemoglobin is 9.3 g/dL (normal range is 14 to 17).

What is the most likely diagnosis?

a. Peptic ulcer disease
b. Pancreatitis
c. Cholecystitis
d. Non-ulcer dyspepsia
e. Esophagitis

Answer: The correct answer is (a). The patient has peptic ulcer disease. He has all 3 of the warning signs: weight loss, anemia, and early satiety. The patient's bottle filled with PPIs demonstrates he is noncompliant with his medication. Abdominal pain that is worse with eating is typical of gastric ulcer, while pain that is better with eating is more common with duodenal ulcers. He also has a history of NSAID use, which is a risk factor for ulcer development. He should discontinue NSAIDs immediately and start a PPI daily. He will also need an upper endoscopy. Pancreatitis presents with abdominal pain that radiates to the back, while cholecystitis is right upper quadrant pain. There is no bleeding with non-ulcer dyspepsia, which is a diagnosis of exclusion.

> Barium or gastrografin studies are always the wrong answer in Mallory-Weiss tears.

Peptic Ulcer Disease

ETIOLOGY

Risk factors for peptic ulcer disease (PUD) include:

1. *Helicobacter pylori* infection
2. NSAID use: 20% prevalence of having an ulcer with NSAID use and 5% incidence of symptoms in the course of one year
3. Burns: Curling ulcers
4. Head injury: Cushing ulcers
5. Inflammatory bowel disease: Crohn disease

> Alcohol and smoking prevent ulcer healing but do not directly **cause** ulcers.

6. Cancer: the tumor itself becomes ulcerated
7. Mechanical ventilation: stress gastritis

PRESENTATION

The patient often presents with **gnawing abdominal pain** localized to **epigastrum**. Severe ulcers may also have gastric outlet obstruction causing early satiety and bleeding leading to anemia and heme-positive stools. The most common cause of epigastric pain is non-ulcer dyspepsia. There is no way to be certain of the etiology of epigastric pain without endoscopy. There is no unique physical finding to answer the "most likely diagnosis" question.

> All vented patients must be on PPIs to prevent stress ulcers.

> Gastric ulcer has a 4% risk of cancer.

DIAGNOSTIC TESTS

Upper endoscopy is the mainstay of diagnosis in patients with suspected PUD. It is necessary to directly visualize the stomach for ulcers. Biopsies are necessary with gastric ulcer to exclude cancer. Duodenal ulcers do not have malignant potential.

Zollinger-Ellison syndrome (ZES), a state of hypersecretion of acid, must be considered if there are **multiple large ulcers**, especially if they occur on the distal duodenum and recur after treatment for *H pylori*.

Diagnosis of Helicobacter pylori

If endoscopy and biopsy are performed, no further testing for *H pylori* is needed. If endoscopy is not performed, the other tests are:

Serology: This test is **very sensitive**. A negative result means the patient has not previously been infected with the organism. **Serology is not accurate** in distinguishing old from new infections (ie, not useful for testing for disease eradication).

> The best test for a cured *Helicobacter* infection is urea breath test or stool antigen testing.

Breath testing and stool antigen: Both of these methods are highly specific only for active infection. **Neither of them is routine** for the initial diagnosis. They are useful as a test of cure after treatment, unless there is recurrence of symptoms. The sensitivity of both tests is affected by treatment with PPI, bismuth, and antibiotics.

TREATMENT

1. **Discontinue NSAIDs.**
2. Treat *Helicobacter pylori* with triple therapy (PPI, clarithromycin, and amoxicillin).
3. Recurrent/persistent symptoms are likely due to either noncompliance or resistance. In these cases, treatment with a bismuth-based quadruple therapy containing metronidazole (rather than clarithromycin) is indicated.
4. Repeat endoscopy may be warranted if symptoms do not resolve.
5. Gastric ulcer must be re-scoped to ensure resolution of the ulcer. This is the only 100% accurate way to exclude cancer even if the biopsy is normal.

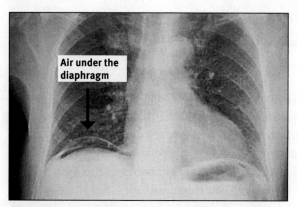

Figure 6.4: Perforation. Air under the diaphragm is always seen best on an upright chest x-ray. Abdominal x-ray does not always show the diaphragm.

Source: Derek DeSa and Anuraag Sahai, MD

Zollinger Ellison Syndrome

ETIOLOGY/PRESENTATION

ZES is a syndrome of increased gastrin production and increased levels of acid production in the stomach from a gastrinoma (a type of pancreatic neuroendocrine tumor).

Patients will present with:

- Severe abdominal pain
- Anemia
- Watery diarrhea and weight loss (acid inactivates lipase)
- Anorexia

Diagnostic Tests

Pursue a diagnosis of ZES in those with PUD if the patient is found to have:

- **Multiple large** ulcerations greater than 1 cm in size
- Ulcerations **beyond** the **first part of the duodenum**
- Symptoms **after** recurrent HP treatment

Increased gastrin level + increased acid output = ZES

Secretin in healthy patients should decrease gastrin levels and acid output; however, in patients with ZES, no change will be seen. Best initial test is a secretin stimulation test.

The most accurate tests are **endoscopic ultrasound (EUS) and nuclear somatostatin scan**. EUS has the advantage of being able to directly gain tissue samples and endoscopically tattoo the lesion with ink for future surgical resection.

TREATMENT

Localized: surgical resection. **Metastatic disease:** lifelong PPI + chemotherapy, tumor embolization (if hepatic), octreotide

A 46-year-old woman presents with long-standing abdominal pain that is persistent. The pain has recently become unbearable. She also has heartburn 3 to 4 times per week. An EGD demonstrates active inflammation but without ulcers, and severe edema in the antrum. Biopsies reveal numerous colonies of *H pylori* and a region of mucosa-associated lymphoid tissue (MALT) lymphoma.

What is the most appropriate next step in the therapy of this patient?

a. Immediate surgical gastrectomy
b. Repeat EGD in 6 months
c. PPI therapy alone
d. PPI therapy with clarithromycin and amoxicillin

Answer: The correct answer is (d). This patient is found to have H pylori and MALT lymphoma (MALToma), which has a very strong association with this infection. This patient will require antibiotic treatment for 10 to 14 days and repeat EGD to evaluate for eradication. EUS is necessary to stage and investigate if this MALToma has invaded other tissue layers. 75% of MALTomas are found to regress after therapy for H pylori. A repeat EGD is warranted, but not as the first step. PPI alone will not cure the infectious process in a symptomatic patient.

> Don't let negative antigen fool you. Over years *H pylori* antigen levels fade in patients with MALTomas, but the infection is still present. You must initially always treat for *H pylori* in patients with MALToma.

Helicobacter pylori

PRESENTATION/ETIOLOGY

Gastritis is inflammation of the stomach wall lining that can be caused by *H pylori*, pernicious anemia, and alcohol.

More than 50% of patients harbor *H pylori* in their GI tracts. *H pylori* infection is associated with a 1% to 2% lifetime risk of stomach cancer and a less than 1% risk of gastric MALT lymphoma. *H pylori* is associated with 80% of MALT lymphomas of the stomach. It is one of the few cancers that can be eradicated by treating an infectious agent.

> If initial treatment fails, re-treat with:
> - tetracycline
> - metronidazole
> - bismuth sulfate
> - PPI

DIAGNOSTIC TESTS

There are 4 major methods of testing for *H pylori*.

1. Stool antigen testing is used to evaluate for disease eradication.
2. Urease breath testing is used to evaluate for disease eradication.
3. Serology is highly sensitive, but cannot distinguish between previous infection and active infection.
4. EGD with biopsy and Giemsa staining is the **most accurate test**.

TREATMENT

Treat *H pylori* with a PPI, clarithromycin, and amoxicillin for 14 days. If the patient is penicillin allergic, replace amoxicillin with metronidazole.

A 19-year-old woman presents with a 3-month history of crampy abdominal pain not related to eating. She also has bloody diarrhea, is fatigued, and has lost 5 pounds. She **has both constipation and diarrhea.** She has tender red sores on the anterior aspects of her lower extremities and decreased range of motion at the lumbar spine. She has anemia with a hemoglobin of 10.8 g/dL.

Which of the following is the most likely diagnosis?

a. Inflammatory bowel disease
b. Infectious colitis
c. Irritable bowel disease
d. Diverticulitis
e. Anal fissure

Answer: The correct answer is (a). This is a typical presentation of inflammatory bowel disease, specifically ulcerative colitis. Infectious colitis and diverticulitis would not last 3 months. Irritable bowel disease would not have bloody diarrhea. Anal fissure has extremely painful defecation.

Inflammatory Bowel Disease (IBD)		
	Crohn	**Ulcerative colitis**
Presentation	Weight loss, abdominal pain, and diarrhea	Weight loss, bloody diarrhea, tenesmus
Antibody	Antineutrophil cytoplasmic antibodies (ANCA) negative; anti-saccharomyces cerevisiae antibody (ASCA) positive	ANCA positive; ASCA negative
Areas involved	Most commonly ileal involvement, though can affect any portion of the GI tract; rectal sparing	Starts in rectum but ileum spared; may involve entire colon
Depth of involvement	Transmural	Mucosal involvement only
Appearance	Cobblestone appearance to mucosa Granulomas Aphthous ulcers	Pseudopolyps = 2 ulcers close together pushing up normal tissue to form a polyp Crypt abscesses
Ulcer spread	Skip lesions	Continuous

(continued)

Inflammatory Bowel Disease (IBD) *(continued)*		
	Crohn	**Ulcerative colitis**
Extraintestinal manifestations	Arthritis Erythema nodosum Uveitis, episcleritis	Arthritis Pyoderma gangrenosum Sclerosing cholangitis Uveitis
Complications	Fistulas Strictures Colorectal cancer Osteopenia, osteoporosis, fractures Vitamin deficiencies	Toxic megacolon Colorectal cancer Cholangitis, cholangiocarcinoma (secondary to increased incidence of PSC) Osteopenia, osteoporosis, fractures
Cancer risk	3% risk	10% risk for colon cancer starting at 10 years postdiagnosis
Diagnosis	Colonoscopy with biopsy	Colonoscopy with biopsy
Treatment	Aminosalicylates Topical steroids (budesonide) Oral steroids (for short-term use) Immunomodulators (6-mercaptoprine, methotrexate, azathioprine) Anti-tumor necrosis factor-alpha biologic agents (infliximab, adalimumab) Surgery is not curative	Aminosalicylates Topical steroids (budesonide) Oral steroids (short-term use only) Immunomodulators (6-mercaptoprine or azathioprine) Cyclosporine Infliximab Hemi- to total colectomy for severe disease is curative

Extraintestinal Manifestations of IBD
Iritis and uveitis
Erythema nodosum
Primary sclerosing cholangitis
Ankylosing spondylitis

Fistulas
- Enteroenteral → bowel to bowel (**most common**)
- Enterocutaneous → bowel to skin
- Enterovesicular → bowel to bladder
- Enterovaginal → bowel to vagina
- Enteromuscular → bowel to muscle, leading to abscesses
- Enteroaortic → bowel to aorta (**most fatal**)

Screening for colon cancer in ulcerative colitis (UC) begins 8 to 10 years after diagnosis. Repeat colonoscopy every 1 to 2 years with multiple biopsies.

Every patient who starts infliximab must have a PPD to detect latent tuberculosis.

A 27-year-old ambitious male resident on call at work develops nausea, vomiting, and severe diarrhea and a fever of 103°F. He denies any travel history, but does admit to blood in the diarrhea. Prior to symptoms he had a salad at the hospital cafeteria. He insists he can continue working; however, his blood pressure is 100/84 while sitting and 84/72 while standing and he is tachycardic. His skin shows signs of tenting and he is extremely lethargic. Laboratory findings show a WBC of 15,600 cells, elevated BUN and creatinine, and elevated hematocrit.

Which of the following is the most appropriate next step in management of this patient?

a. CT of the abdomen and pelvis
b. Discharge home
c. Fluid resuscitation
d. Stool ova and parasite (O&P) analysis
e. Fluid resuscitation and empiric antibiotic delivery

Answer: The correct answer is (e). This resident will require aggressive fluid resuscitation and antibiotics as he also has orthostatic hypotension and tachycardia and blood in his diarrhea. Fluid resuscitation alone is insufficient. Radiological imaging and stool studies are all less important than the resuscitation of the patient. Antibiotics have shown to decrease mortality in patients with severe dysentery. Discharging this patient could be fatal without both treatments.

Diarrhea

PRESENTATION

Mild disease is self-limiting. Severe disease is defined as having:

- Fever
- Abdominal pain
- Hypotension
- Tachycardia
- **Blood** in the stool (**most important diagnostic criteria**)

DIAGNOSTIC TESTS

The **best initial test** is fecal leukocytes and the **most accurate test** is stool culture.

TREATMENT

Fluid resuscitation antibiotics (fluoroquinolones or rifaximin) are useful for acute traveler's diarrhea and for severe disease.

> Loperamide is always the wrong answer if the patient is not on antibiotics and has bloody diarrhea.

Causes of Bloody Diarrhea

Name	Cause	Illness
Campylobacter jejuni	Fecal-oral transmission or from raw meat	Most common cause of gastroenteritis Febrile illness Associated with Guillan-Barré and reactive arthritis Left lower quadrant mimicking diverticulitis. Usually self-limited after 1 week; treatment with macrolides (resistant to fluoroquinolones).
Escherichia coli	Undercooked beef Fresh produce Unpasteurized dairy products Petting zoos	Three forms: 1. 0157:H7: associated with hemolytic uremic syndrome—never give antibiotics. Usually outbreaks. Afebrile. 2. Enterotoxigenic: traveler's diarrhea 3. Enterohemorrhagic
Salmonella	Chicken and eggs	Usually self-limited
Shigella	Shiga toxin: most severe	Associated with reactive arthritis and daycare settings
Yersinia	Rodent urine or feces and old creamy pastries	Right lower quadrant mimicking appendicitis
Giardia	Drinking fresh water Detected with 3 O&P studies or 1 ELISA antigen Treat with metronidazole	Can simulate fat malabsorption
Entamoeba histolytica	Travelers in endemic areas	Abdominal pain, bloody diarrhea

> Do not give antibiotics with 0157:H7.

Causes of Non-bloody Diarrhea		
Name	**Cause**	**Illness**
Viral gastroenteritis	Rotavirus: Daycare setting Norwalk (Noro) virus: cruise ship gastroenteritis	Gastroenteritis that is self-limiting
Staphylococcus aureus	Creamy foods such as mayonnaise	Vomiting and diarrhea within 6–8 hours of ingestion due to toxin
Tropheryma whippelii	Unknown reservoir	EGD biopsy shows PAS-positive macrophages Treatment with antibiotics for 1 year or more
Strongyloides	Ascends through the skin of the foot to the lung, and then is swallowed	Diarrhea, epigastric pain, anemia, and eosinophilia Treat with ivermectin or thiobendazole
Bacillus cereus	Refried rice	Nausea and vomiting within 2 hours of ingestion
Scombroid food poisoning	Tuna, mackerel, and mahi-mahi	Diarrhea within 10 minutes of ingestion Treat with antihistamines
Cryptosporidiosis	Fecal-oral	HIV-positive patient with fewer than 100 CD4 cells
VIPoma/ glucagonoma and Zollinger-Ellison syndrome	Neuroendocrine origin	Profuse watery diarrhea Positive skin rash with glucagonoma and severe ulcerations with ZES
Vibrio parahemolytics	Undercooked seafood, usually oysters	Look for oysters eaten in warm weather environments
Vibrio vulnificus	Eating raw seafood such as sushi	Associated with skin blisters and liver lesions

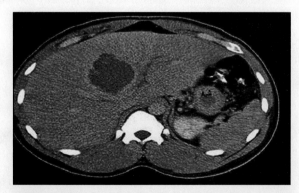

Figure 6.5: Liver abscess before drainage. Many liver abscesses arise from colonic flora.

Source: Akash Ferdaus, MD

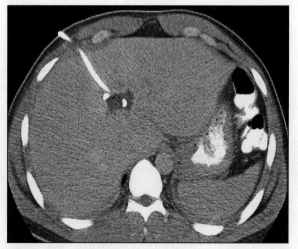

Figure 6.6: Liver abscess after drainage. Repeating the CT shows a smaller lesion after drainage.

Source: Akash Ferdaus, MD

C. difficile–associated Diarrhea

PRESENTATION

The most common presentation is **after extended antibiotic use** of any kind. Hospital stays of longer than 4 weeks have a 50% incidence of *C. difficile*–associated diarrhea. Symptoms include:

- Profuse mucous and foul-smelling watery diarrhea
- Cramps and tenesmus
- Increased bowel sounds and tenderness over the left lower quadrant

Complications include toxic megacolon, perforation, and sepsis.

> BI/NAP1 is the strain most associated with toxic megacolon.

DIAGNOSTIC TESTS

The best initial test is the **stool toxin ELISA**, which has a sensitivity of 75% to 85%. Several stool determinations are needed. The most accurate test is biopsy during colonoscopy showing active infection.

> In severe *C. difficile* infections (high WBC counts and renal failure), patients should be on combination therapy of vancomycin and metronidazole.

TREATMENT

Discontinue antibiotics. Once the diagnosis of *C. difficile* diarrhea is confirmed, **the best initial therapy is with oral metronidazole**. Vancomycin is for the patient who has failed or is allergic to therapy with metronidazole. If the patient's diarrhea resolves and then recurs, the answer is to re-treat with metronidazole.

Vancomycin is to be used if that patient has a third occurrence or relapses after second treatment with metronidazole. Combination treatment is when the disease is very severe.

Fidaxomicin, a narrow spectrum macrocyclic, eradicates illness with the smallest chance of recurrence.

Chronic Diarrhea

When assessing patients with chronic diarrhea, the best initial tests are stool weight for 24 hours, stool osmolality and stool for quantitative fat:

1. If the patient has a **normal osmotic gap** and **normal stool weight**, the most likely diagnosis is irritable bowel syndrome.
2. If the patient has **normal osmotic gap** but with **increased stool weight**, the patient is abusing laxatives.
3. If patient has an **increased osmotic gap** and **normal fecal fat**, the most likely diagnosis is lactose intolerance.
4. If the patient has an **increased osmotic gap** and **increased fecal fat**, the most likely diagnosis is either pancreatic insufficiency or bacterial overgrowth.

Causes of Chronic Diarrhea			
Cause	**Signs and symptoms**	**Diagnosis**	**Treatment**
Lactose intolerance	Bloating Cramps Flatulence Diarrhea	Removing milk products is both diagnostic and therapeutic. Hydrogen breath test is the most accurate test.	No milk products Lactase supplements
Carcinoid syndrome	Flushing Wheezing Watery diarrhea	5-HIAA urinary level	Octreotide

A 44-year-old alcoholic man presents to the ED with constant abdominal pain. He frequently comes to the ED with abdominal pain and diarrhea. Tonight he says his stools smell very bad and they won't flush no matter how hard he tries. He has bruises on his arms. His INR is 1.9, and abdominal x-ray reveals punctate calcifications over the epigastrum.

Which of the following is the most accurate test to diagnose his condition?

a. CT scan of the abdomen without contrast
b. Endoscopic ultrasound
c. Secretin stimulation test
d. Serum amylase and lipase levels

Answer: The correct answer is (c). This patient presents with chronic pancreatitis, a condition resulting from chronic alcohol use. The most accurate test is a secretin stimulation test. In normal individuals, secretin will cause a large outflow of bicarbonate from the pancreas into the duodenal bulb; however, in patients without adequate pancreatic tissue, bicarbonate levels will be severely reduced. CT scan, EUS, and MRI are not as accurate as the secretin stimulation test. Serum amylase and lipase levels are usually normal by the time the pancreas is "burnt out" enough to cause a fat malabsorption. This is analogous to finding normal AST/ALT levels in cirrhosis.

Acute Pancreatitis

ETIOLOGY/PRESENTATION

Causes of pancreatitis include:

- Alcohol: most common
- Gallstone obstruction of the duct: second most common
- Autoimmune
- Trauma, most likely with blunt abdominal impact
- Scorpion stings
- Hypertriglyceridemia >1,000

- Post-endoscopic retrograde cholangiopancreatography (ERCP)
- Drugs: azathioprine, didanosine, valproic acid, mercaptopurine

Patients will present with fever, severe midabdominal pain radiating to the back, nausea and vomiting, abdominal distension, and sometimes an ileus.

DIAGNOSTIC TESTS

The best initial tests are amylase level, which is sensitive, and lipase level, which is more specific to the pancreas. **Levels of amylase and lipase do not correlate with disease severity.** CT scan is the most accurate test to assess both the presence of acute pancreatitis and as its severity. The greater the degree of pancreatic necrosis, the worse the disease. ERCP can be used to clear stones and stent strictures.

> Levels of amylase and lipase do not correlate with disease severity.

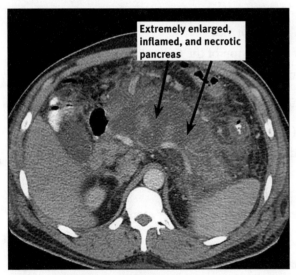

Figure 6.7: Necrotic pancreatitis. The dark areas are necrosis. >30% necrosis is an indication for antibiotics and a biopsy.

Source: Eduardo Andre, MD and Eduardo Lopez, MD

TREATMENT

Aggressive IV fluids and NPO until symptoms resolve.

There is no evidence for **starting imipenem** prophylactically unless there is more than **30% necrosis on the CT scan**. If there is necrosis on the CT, a biopsy must be done for culture and antibiotic therapy must be started. The best initial antibiotic is imipenem. If the necrotic pancreas is infected, debridement must be performed.

Pancreatic enzyme inhibitors and octreotide have **not** been shown to improve outcome. They are the wrong answer.

> The Ranson criteria were developed to guide operative debridement.

Assessing Severity of Pancreatitis (Ranson Criteria)	
On admission	**At 48 hours**
Age >55 years	Calcium (<8.0 mg/dL)
White blood cell count >16,000	Hematocrit fall >10%
Blood glucose (>200 mg/dL)	Oxygen: PO$_2$ <60 mm Hg)
Serum AST >250 IU/L	BUN increased by 1.8 or more after IV fluid hydration
Serum LDH >350 IU/L	Base deficit >4 mEq/L
	Sequestration of fluids >6 L

Malabsorption

Chronic diarrhea with fat malabsorption typically presents with:

- **Weight loss**
- Oily greasy stools known as steatorrhea
- **Foul-smelling** stools that float on top of the toilet water
- Abdominal pain, cramping, and bloating

All forms of fat malabsorption are associated with:

> Pancreatic enzymes are not necessary to absorb iron.

- **Vitamin B12 deficiency** (pancreatic enzymes are necessary for absorption)
- Vitamin K deficiency leading to easy bruising, elevated prothrombin time, or INR
- **Hypocalcemia** from vitamin D deficiency
- Oxalate overabsorption leading to oxalate kidney stones
- **Osteoporosis**

The best initial test for fat malabsorption is a Sudan black stain of the stool. The most sensitive test to determine the presence of fat malabsorption is a 72-hour fecal fat collection.

Malabsorption			
Disease	**Etiology and presentation**	**Diagnostic testing**	**Treatment**
Chronic pancreatitis	History of alcoholism with pancreatitis causing "burnout" of the pancreas Sphincter of Oddi dysfunction Chronic abdominal pain localized to the epigastrum radiating to the back	Normal amylase and lipase levels Best initial test: Abdominal x-ray shows calcifications: 60% sensitive. CT scan is 85% sensitive. Endoscopic ultrasound: sensitivity 85%–90% Most accurate test: Secretin stimulation with a lack of bicarbonate release (95% sensitive)	Oral pancreatic enzyme replacement Insulin occasionally in severe cases Pain control/analgesics
Celiac sprue or gluten-sensitive enteropathy	Gluten sensitivity causing reaction to small bowel tissue and villi destruction Vitamin deficiencies (A, D, E, and K) Dermatitis herpetiformis Concomitant IgA deficiency has been seen with anaphylaxis to blood transfusions.	Best initial test: Antigliadin, antiendomyseal, and anti-tissue transglutaminase antibodies Most accurate test: Small bowel biopsy with loss of villus architecture Biopsy excludes enteropathy-associated T cell lymphoma. D-xylose testing is abnormal.	Lifelong gluten-free diet; no wheat, rye, or barley can be consumed
Tropic sprue	Similar presentation to celiac disease with travel to a tropical region	Most accurate test is small bowel biopsy showing microorganisms.	Treat with doxycycline or sulfamethoxazole/trimethoprim for 6 months
Bacterial overgrowth	Excessive colonic bacteria in the small intestine; caused by intestine dysmotility or hypochlorhydria	Vitamin deficiency (including B12); elevated folate	Tetracycline, amoxicillin-clavulanate, or rifaximin

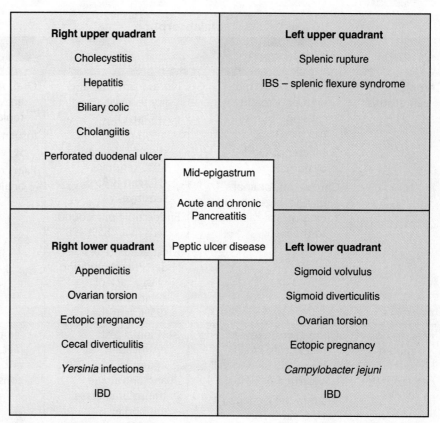

Figure 6.8: Abdominal pain chart.
Source: Niket Sonpal, MD

A 25-year-old woman presents with abdominal pain in the left upper quadrant most acutely after eating, as well as constipation. Her symptoms have been persistent for 6 months except while she was in Aruba with her boyfriend. She states she feels better after defecation but does not feel fully evacuated and at times has tenesmus. She has diarrhea at other times and there is no blood in the stool. Physical exam reveals left upper quadrant tenderness.

What is the most likely diagnosis?

a. Irritable bowel syndrome (IBS)
b. Inflammatory bowel disease
c. Chronic pancreatitis
d. Infectious diarrhea

Answer: The correct answer is (a). Abdominal pain with alternating bouts of constipation and diarrhea is consistent with IBS. Symptoms of IBS are also described as resolving on weekends or vacation. Colonoscopy and stool studies are needed to exclude other diseases. IBD would have a history of bloody diarrhea, while infectious diarrhea would not last 6 months. Chronic pancreatitis has constant, dull pain that is localized to the epigastrum and is not relieved by defecation.

Irritable Bowel Syndrome (IBS)

ETIOLOGY/PRESENTATION

IBS presents with abdominal pain or discomfort in association with frequent changes in bowel movements. It is more common in women and in those with a history of depression.

- Symptoms must be present for **at least 3 days** a week over the **previous 3 months**.
- The abdominal pain must be **relieved by a bowel movement, decrease** at **night** and on the **weekends**, and may have **constipation alternating with diarrhea**.
- The pain will be described as in the **left upper quadrant** and is known as splenic flexure syndrome. It is caused by viscous distension from gas buildup in the splenic flexure.

IBS can be classified into 4 major categories:

1. Diarrhea-predominant
2. Constipation-predominant
3. IBS with alternating stool pattern

DIAGNOSTIC TESTS

No diagnostic test proves a person has IBS. It is a diagnosis of exclusion. Patients must have negative:

- Stool guiac and cultures
- O&P (3 negative)
- Colonoscopy
- Serologies for celiac disease (if diarrhea present)

TREATMENT

The best initial therapy is with **stool-bulking agents** such as fiber supplements. The next best therapy is to add **antispasmodic agents** such as hyoscyamine or dicyclomine. **Tricyclic antidepressants** are used if there is no response.

Lubiprostone is a gastrointestinal agent used for the treatment of constipation-predominant IBS.

Linaclotide is an experimental peptide agonist of guanylate cyclase 2C used for constipation predominant IBS.

> Opioid-induced constipation is treated by subcutaneous methylnaltrexone bromide.

Fecal Incontinence

Fecal incontinence is continuous or recurrent uncontrolled passage of fecal material for at least one month in an individual older than 3 years of age.

Clinical history and flexible sigmoidoscopy or anoscopy is the best initial test. The most accurate test is anorectal manometry.

There are 3 forms of treatment for fecal incontinence: Medical therapy, biofeedback, and surgery. Medical therapy includes bulking agents such as fiber. Biofeedback includes control exercises and muscle strengthening exercises. Prior to surgical intervention injection of dextranomer/hyaluronic acid has been shown to decrease incontinence episodes by 50 percent. If this fails colorectal surgery is needed.

Diverticulitis

ETIOLOGY/PRESENTATION

Diverticulitis most **commonly** occurs in **elderly** patients whose diets are **low in fiber** and high in fat. It is a complication of long-standing diverticulosis. The most common location is in the sigmoid region. It presents with:

- Lower left quadrant pain
- Tenderness
- Fever
- Leukocytosis

DIAGNOSTIC TESTS/TREATMENT

The most accurate test is a CT scan of the abdomen. Treatment is with ciprofloxacin and metronidazole. Surgical intervention may be necessary if recurrent bouts of diverticulitis occur.

Barium enema and colonoscopy are contraindicated in diverticulitis due to the risk of perforation.

Hepatobiliary Disorders

Acute hepatitis can be caused by:

- Viruses
- Drug- or alcohol-induced
- Ischemia
- Autoimmune or fat deposition

They each present in similar ways on physical examination and can all cause cirrhosis. Each patient will present with:

- Severe right upper quadrant pain
- Jaundiced appearance

- Dark urine from bilirubin
- Elevated transaminases

  - AST and GGT are elevated in drug- and alcohol-induced hepatitis.
  - AST is generally elevated in a 2:1 ratio with ALT in alcohol-induced hepatitis.
  - ALT is greater than AST with viral hepatitis. AST is greater than ALT with drug- and alcohol-induced hepatitis.
  - AST and ALT are classically elevated greater than 1,000 in ischemic, acute viral, and medication-overdose (classically acetaminophen) hepatitis.

Hepatitis			
Type	**Etiology**	**Diagnostic testing**	**Treatment**
Viral hepatitis	AST/ALT ratio 1:2. Hepatitis A is from contaminated food, water, or via sexual transmission. Hepatitis B is associated with polyarteritis nodosa. Hepatitis C is associated with mixed cryoglobulinemia. Genotypes 2 and 3 have better response to therapy than genotype 1. Hepatitis D is a superimposed infection with hepatitis B. Hepatitis E in pregnant women.	Serologic testing for A: anti-HAV IgM B: anti-HBc IgM, HBsAg C: anti-HCV IgM, HCV RNA are the best initial tests. The most accurate tests are viral PCR.	A: Self-resolving B: Treat chronic disease (HBeAg+) with lamivudine, entecavir, adefovir, or interferon C: Ribavirin and interferon
Drug- or alcohol-induced hepatitis	Post "alcoholic binge"	AST/ALT ratio of 2:1	Severe illness is treated with steroids.
Ischemic hepatitis	Decreased perfusion of the liver from any form of shock	AST and ALT greater than 1,000 U/L	Self-resolving.
Autoimmune hepatitis	An immune response against the patient's own liver. Concomitant autoimmune diseases such as ITP are also seen.	Positive ANA, LKM-1, or positive antibodies against soluble liver antigen	Glucocorticoids or azathioprine. Can lead to cirrhosis.
Alpha 1-antitrypsin deficiency (A1AT)	Look for COPD/emphysema.	Best initial test: Low A1AT level. The most accurate test is liver biopsy.	Lung disease is treated with enzyme replacement. Severe cases require liver transplant. Can lead to cirrhosis.
Nonalcoholic steatohepatitis (NASH)	Fatty infiltration common in obese diabetics.	Liver biopsy: Most accurate test. Resembles alcohol-induced hepatitis on histology.	Weight loss. Manage underlying diabetes.

LKM = liver kidney microsomal antibody

Acute Hepatitis B				
	Surface antigen	e-Antigen	Core antibody	Surface antibody
Acute disease	Present	Present	Present	Not present
Window period	Not present	Not present	Present	Not present
Vaccinated	Not present	Not present	Not present	Present
Recovered	Not present	Not present	Present	Present
Chronic hepatitis	Positive	Positive	Positive	Negative

A 36-year-old man presents to his doctor's office saying that he looks more tan than usual. His joints also hurt every morning. In addition, he feels like he has to urinate more frequently and is drinking a lot more water than usual. His wife also mentions they have been trying to have a baby for the last 3 years. Physical exam reveals darkening of the skin around the eyes and trunk. Finger stick reveals a blood sugar of 275 mg/dL (normal range is 80 to 115).

What would be the most likely cause of death in this patient?

a. Cardiac ischemia
b. Cardiogenic shock
c. Arrhythmia
d. Cirrhosis
e. Hepatoma

Answer: The correct answer is (d). This patient has a presentation of hereditary hemochromatosis manifested by infertility, darkening of the skin, and diabetes all secondary to iron deposition in various tissues of the body. The most common cause of death in these patients is complications of cirrhosis. Restrictive cardiomyopathy is not the most common cause of death. It develops in only 15%.

Cirrhosis

DEFINITION/PRESENTATION

Cirrhosis is a result of long-standing liver infection or inflammation leading to fibrosis. Patients with cirrhosis present with:

- **Gynecomastia and hypogonadism:** increased circulating estrogen
- **Hepatosplenomegaly**
- **Ascites:** due to hypoalbuminemia—treat with sodium restriction and diuretics; if refractory, large-volume paracentesis is used.
- **Thrombocytopenia:** secondary to hypersplenism
- **Caput medusa:** abdominal venous congestion
- **Fetor hepaticus:** bad breath from dimethyl sulfide
- **Jaundice**
- **Asterixis:** wrist flapping on extension due to encephalopathy
- Spider angiomata and palmar erythema

Complications of cirrhosis include:

- **Esophageal varices:** Prevent bleeding with a non-selective beta blocker such as propanolol; if bleeding occurs, treat with endoscopic banding.
- **Encephalopathy presents with altered mental status to coma;** treat with lactulose.
- **Hepatic encephalopathy (HE)** presents with altered mental status to coma; The best initial treatment is with lactulose. The best treatment to reduce recurrent episodes of HE is with rifaximin.
- **Hepatorenal syndrome leading to renal failure: Transplant is the only true cure.**
- **Hepatopulmonary syndrome** presents with "orthodeoxia" or desaturation on sitting up.
- **Hepatocellular carcinoma:** Screen with ultrasound and alpha-fetoprotein levels in patients with advanced liver disease; transplant is indicated for patients with limited disease. Treatments when transplant is not possible are: chemoembolization, ethanol ablation, radiofrequency ablation, and chemotherapy.

> Rifaximin is superior to neomycin as an adjunctive agent for hepatic encephalopathy.

Ascites

Patients with cirrhosis and new-onset ascites or ascites in the presence of **pain, fever, or abdominal tenderness** must undergo a diagnostic paracentesis. The fluid must be sent for albumin level, Gram stain, and cytology. If the serum ascites to albumin gradient (**SAAG**) is **less** than 1.1, then portal hypertension is not present. A SAAG greater than 1.1 is indicative of portal hypertension as the cause of the ascites.

Spontaneous bacterial peritonitis (SBP): Defined as an ascitic neutrophil count greater than 250 per mm^3, it is treated with cefotaxime or ceftriaxone for 5 to 7 days. After recovery, prophylactic antibiotics such as ciprofloxacin or norfloxacin must be continued.

Causes of Cirrhosis			
Type	**Etiology and presentation**	**Diagnostic tests**	**Treatment**
Alcoholic cirrhosis	Drinking for longer than a decade AST/ALT ratio 2:1 Diagnosis of exclusion	Best test: Liver biopsy with macrosteatosis and Mallory bodies	Supportive treatment and in severe cases liver transplant
Primary biliary cirrhosis (PBC)	Middle-aged woman with pruritus, fatigue, and xanthalasmas History of other autoimmune disorders (thyroid, vitiligo, Addison)	Best initial test: Alkaline phosphatase level and antimitochondrial antibodies Most accurate test: Liver biopsy	Ursodeoxycholic acid; liver transplant for advanced cases

(continued)

Causes of Cirrhosis *(continued)*			
Type	**Etiology and presentation**	**Diagnostic tests**	**Treatment**
Primary sclerosing cholangiitis	Ulcerative colitis (80% of cases) and pruritus Elevated bilirubin and serum alkaline phosphatase Increased risk of cholangiocarcinoma	Most accurate test: ERCP showing *beading* (strictures and dilatation) of the common bile duct	Ursodeoxycholic acid and cholestyramine are used for symptomatic relief. Transplant is the only cure.
Wilson disease (autosomal recessive)	Choreiform movements Psychiatric abnormalities, tremor Pathologic accumulation of copper in various organs	Best initial test: Kayser-Fleischer rings on slit lamp eye examination Elevated serum copper; low ceruloplasmin level in 80%–95% of cases Most accurate test: Liver biopsy	Penicillamine for copper chelation. Trientine HCl as a chelator and zinc to further prevent absorption of copper. Liver transplantation is curative.
Hemochromatosis	Over-absorption of iron in tissues leads to skin hyperpigmentation ("bronze appearance"). Pseudogout Restrictive cardiomyopathy Infertility Panhypopituitarism	Best initial test: Iron studies. Fasting transferrin saturation of >60% and ferritin >300 ng/mL Most accurate test: Liver biopsy for Prussian blue staining Genetic test: mutations in HFE gene	Serial phlebotomy weekly until normalization of iron levels. If phlebotomy is not tolerated, deferoxamine (an iron chelator) by subcutaneous injection. 15%–20% will develop hepatocellular carcinoma if untreated.

Ascending Cholangiitis

ETIOLOGY/PRESENTATION

Ascending cholangiitis is an infection that rises up the common bile duct (CBD) due to an obstruction by gallstones.

It most commonly occurs in obese patients and is characterized by:

- RUQ abdominal pain
- Jaundice
- Fever
- Septic shock: hypotension and tachycardia
- Mental confusion

The most common bacteria linked to ascending cholangiitis are *Escherichia coli*, *Klebsiella*, and *Enterobacter*. This is similar to pyelonephritis.

> Charcot's triad = jaundice + fever + right upper quadrant abdominal pain

> Reynolds pentad = Charcot's triad + shock + altered mental status

Diagnostic Tests/Treatment

ERCP with clearance of the bile duct stone is the most accurate diagnostic test and treatment with biliary decompression.

Colon Cancer Screening

Diagnostic Tests

Colon cancer screening should follow the following guidelines:

General population:

- Begin at age 50.

If one family member has colon cancer:

- Begin at age 40, or 10 years before the age of onset in the family member who had cancer.

Hereditary non-polyposis colon cancer: Three family members over the course of 2 generations and one premature (less than 50 years of age):

- Colonoscopy should begin at age 25 and continue every 1 to 2 years thereafter.

Methods of Screening

- **Colonoscopy:** most sensitive and specific, the most accurate test
- **Flexible sigmoidoscopy:** performed every 5 years in conjunction with occult blood testing for patients not tolerating colonoscopy
- **Stool occult blood testing:** if positive, must lead to endoscopy; performed annually
- **Double contrast barium enema:** if abnormal, endoscopy must be performed
- **Virtual colonoscopy:** always the wrong answer
- **CEA level: never used for screening;** used only to monitor progression of known colon cancer after therapy

Post-colonoscopy Findings

- **Tubular adenoma:** repeat colonoscopy in 3 years
- **Hamartomas:** benign findings
- **Hyperplastic polyp:** benign finding
- **Dysplastic polyp (malignant):** repeat colonoscopy every 3 to 5 years
- **Ulcerative colitis:** Start 8 to 10 years after the original diagnosis. Repeat colonoscopy every 1 to 2 years with biopsies every 10 cm in 4 quadrants.

Colon Cancer Syndrome		
	Description	**Screening**
Familal adenomatous polyposis	100% risk of colon cancer by age 40–50	Screening sigmoidoscopy at age 10–12 and total colectomy when polyps are found
Gardner syndrome	Osteomas and thyroid cancer	Same as general population
Peutz-Jegher syndrome	6%–10% lifetime risk of cancer Hamartomatous polyps can lead to obstruction and intussusception Melanotic spots on lips and gingival surfaces	Same as general population

A 67-year-old man with a history of CAD with two stents placed presents with multiple dark black bowel movements over the course of 1 week. The patient's ejection fraction on recent echocardiography is 55%. He denies abdominal pain and during physical examination has an episode of coffee ground emesis. His blood pressure is 123/67 mm Hg and pulse is 87 per minute. Hemoglobin is found to be 7.1 g/dL.

What is the most appropriate next step?

a. IV fluid bolus and packed red blood cells for ongoing anemia
b. Capsule endoscopy
c. IV proton pump inhibitor
d. CT scan of the abdomen

Answer: The correct answer is (a). This patient likely has an upper GI bleed from long-standing gastritis in the setting of aspirin and clopidogrel. This patient will require IV fluids to maintain his pressure, even though he is not in shock yet, and will require packed red blood cells for a hemoglobin goal of greater than 9 given his history of CAD. Neither IV PPIs nor a CT scan of the abdomen is critical at this time. Capsule endoscopy is a means of diagnosing small bowel bleeding if the upper and lower endoscopies do not show the cause of bleeding.

GI Bleeding

ETIOLOGY/PRESENTATION

Upper GI bleeding presents with dark black stool and is defined as a bleed occurring proximal to the ligament of Treitz.

- Tarlike stool or **melena** requires 100 to 125 cc of blood loss.
- Coffee ground emesis is usually from a gastric, esophageal, or duodenal bleeds and requires only 10 cc of blood.

Causes include:

- Peptic ulcer disease: long-standing ulcer from NSAIDs or *H pylori*
- Esophagitis: secondary to GERD
- Hemorrhagic gastritis: consider *H pylori*
- Mallory-Weiss tear
- Cancer

TREATMENT

Variceal bleeding occurs in cirrhotic patients. Treatment is with IV fluids, endoscopic banding, and octreotide. In refractory bleeding from varices, a transjugular intrahepatic portosystemic shunt (TIPS) is performed.

> The most common cause of death in GI bleeding is cardiac ischemia.

▶ TIP

Lower GI bleeding usually presents with bright red blood per rectum or hematochezia, blood mixed with stool.

Causes include:

- Arteriovenous malformation (AVMs): most common cause; also known as angiodysplasia
- Diverticular bleed: painless bright red blood from the rectum; most commonly from the right colon (as opposed to left-sided diverticulitis)
- IBD: associated with abdominal pain and flares; most common cause of flares is NSAID use
- Hemorrhoids: self-resolving and described as blood in toilet and tissue paper
- Ischemic colitis: secondary to hypovolemic state affecting the "watershed" areas of the bowel; treat with volume resuscitation and pain control
- Cancer

DIAGNOSTIC TESTS

1. Endoscopy: Upper and lower endoscopy are the mainstays of treatment, as they are both diagnostic and therapeutic.
   i. Injection with epinephrine
   ii. Sclerotherapy for varices that cannot be treated with banding
   iii. Argon plasma electrocoagulation for actively bleeding ulcers
   iv. Vascular clipping
   v. Biopsy to establish a diagnosis of cancer or *Helicobacter pylori*

2. If endoscopic therapy cannot find an active bleeding source, technetium bleeding scan is the next best step.

> Upper GI: Bleeding from mouth and the upper part of the small intestine
> Lower GI: Bleeding from upper part of the small intestine to the anus

3. Angiography can also be selected if the location of the bleeding is known, as it can identify and embolize the right vessel. Angiography is most useful to guide surgical resection.

4. Capsule endoscopy is an outpatient evaluation for chronic anemia and is the answer for evaluating portions of the small bowel not reachable by endoscopy.

5. Small bowel enteroscopy has been essentially replaced with capsule endoscopy.

TREATMENT

The best initial therapy is hemodynamic maintenance with IV fluid resuscitation.

- Packed red blood cells are given for hematocrit less than 20 (below 30 in patients with coronary artery disease).
- Transfuse platelets if they are below 50,000 with active bleeding.
- Fresh frozen plasma (FFP) is given for elevated INR/PT. Vitamin K will be the wrong answer because it is too slow.

Both intervention for diagnostic purposes and therapy are antecedent to the previous steps.

- IV proton pump inhibitor for upper GI bleeds

Management of Esophageal Varices

The best initial step is fluid resuscitation including FFP, platelets, and packed red cells as needed. This part is the same in all forms of bleeding. The best initial therapy specific for variceal bleeding is:

1. Octreotide (vasoconstrictor) to decrease portal pressure
2. Upper endoscopy for banding. Sclerotherapy and banding have equal efficacy in stopping bleeding, but sclerotherapy has a greater risk of strictures and ulceration after controlling the bleeding.
3. If bleeding continues, perform an urgent portosystemic shunt with a catheter (TIPS).
4. A nonselective beta blocker such as propranolol or nadolol is used to prevent recurrences of bleeding.

Propranolol has no benefit in acute bleeding.

GERIATRICS

7

DELIRIUM

Delirium is a waxing and waning "altered level of sensorium." This is relatively common in elderly patients, those with advanced dementia, and hospitalized patients. Delirium specifically means that patients do not appear awake and alert. They do not register your presence and they may appear too sleepy and confused to comply with a mini-mental state exam.

Causes of Delirium

Delirium has numerous etiologies:

1. • Metabolic (alterations in sodium, glucose, oxygen, calcium)
2. • Infectious (meningitis, UTI, pneumonia)
3. • Intoxication or withdrawal of medications
4. • Toxin accumulation (such as from liver and kidney failure)
5. • Vascular (stroke, vasculitis)

▶ **TIP**

When severe, the causes of delirium are the same as the causes of seizures.

DEMENTIA

DEFINITION

Dementia is loss of memory. It is also associated with a persistent decline in cognitive functions such as language, problem-solving, and eventually attention span. The level of consciousness is intact until the disease is very far advanced.

> Dementia is specifically not lethargy, obtundation, stupor, coma, or sleepiness.

PRESENTATION/"WHAT IS THE MOST LIKELY DIAGNOSIS?"

The diagnosis of dementia is based on the results of the mini-mental state exam.

- What is the date: month, day, year
- Location: state, city
- Name three objects after 5 minutes.
- "Draw a clock face set at 10 after 11."
- Serial 7s ("Count back from 100 by 7.")
- **Test of agnosia:** Name several objects (e.g., pen, watch, book).
- **Test of executive function:** "Take a piece of paper. Fold it. Place it on the floor."
- **Test of apraxia:** "Show me how you comb your hair, or tie your tie."
- **Test of aphasia:** Repeat "No ifs, ands, or buts" or write a sentence on a blank piece of paper.

Diagnostic Criteria for Dementia

These disturbances must be persistent and severe enough to interfere with work, social activities, or relationships. These disturbances cannot occur only during episodes of delirium to be defined as dementia.

- Cortical dementia (as with Alzheimer dementia) is characterized by deficits in language (**aphasia**), movement (**apraxia**), and recognition (**agnosia**).
- Subcortical dementia (progressive supranuclear palsy, Parkinson dementia, and Huntington disease) is characterized by psychomotor slowing and extrapyramidal signs.

DIAGNOSTIC TESTS

Dementia rarely has a single diagnostic test. This is particularly true for Alzheimer dementia (AD). The biggest issue is how far to go in testing.

Routine tests are:

- Thyroid function
- Vitamin B12
- Head CT or MRI

Under appropriate circumstances only, syphilis testing, lumbar puncture, cerebral angiography, and EEG may be considered. These tests are not routine.

TREATMENT

Only Alzheimer dementia, and Lewy body dementia have routine therapy with the anticholinesterase medications (donepezil, rivastigmine, galantamine). Normal pressure hydrocephalus is treated with shunting. Most of the others have no therapy.

► **TIP**

The most frequently asked dementia question is: What is the diagnosis of each dementia syndrome?

Alzheimer Dementia

ETIOLOGY

AD has no clear cause, occurs exclusively in older persons, and cannot be explained by other disorders.

The questions can be:

- What is the most common risk factor?
- What is commonly found on brain pathologic specimens?
- Which of the following is the most effective preventive method?

The most important risk factor for AD is age.

AD is almost universally present in patients with **Down syndrome** in advanced age.

Neuritic amyloid plaques and neurofibrillary tangles are classically found on brain pathology specimens in patients with AD. The extent of distribution of these findings correlates well with disease severity.

The best methods to prevent AD are:

- Physical activity
- High IQ/intellectual achievement

It is perhaps a matter of semantics to determine whether intellectual achievement is itself "protective"—or whether, when dementia occurs, it is less noticeable because there is simply more IQ and cognitive function to lose. Either way, the answer to the question is either increased levels of physical activity or high level of intellectual achievement.

TREATMENT

1. Anticholinesterases (**donepezil, rivastigmine, galantamine**)
2. **Memantine** (an N-methyl-D-aspartate receptor antagonist): used as a neuroprotective agent in those not controlled with anticholinesterase medications

► **TIP**

Cholinesterase inhibitors **treat the symptoms of** dementia, but generally **do not prevent it, reverse its symptoms, or halt its progression.**

> Treatments that don't prevent dementia are:
> - Vitamin E
> - Gingko biloba
> - B vitamin supplementation
> - Estrogen

Lewy Body Dementia

Lewy body dementia (LBD) is characterized by the features of dementia previously described as well as:

- Features of **Parkinson disease**
- Prominent **visual hallucinations**
- Marked **fluctuation in cognitive function**

LBD is irreversible, and is treated with the same medications as Alzheimer dementia.

> LBD, not vascular dementia, is the second most common cause of dementia.

Progressive Supranuclear Palsy

Progressive supranuclear palsy (PSP) is characterized by dementia in association with:

- Vertical gaze palsies
- **Parkinsonism** with its postural **instability**, **bradykinesia**, and **rigidity**

Because of the gait and postural problems combined with the inability to look down, PSP often presents with frequent falls in the patient. There is no therapy besides treating the parkinsonism.

Frontotemporal Dementia (Pick Disease)

Frontotemporal dementia has all the features of dementia with:

- **Loss of social appropriateness** first
- Loss of control of emotions
- Aphasia

> In frontotemporal dementia, behavior and personality problems precede memory loss.

Loss of social appropriateness most commonly manifest as defects in personal hygiene and grooming. Language and executive function are more markedly impaired than in AD. The "most accurate test" is CT or MR imaging showing involvement of the frontal and temporal lobes out of proportion to the other parts of the brain. This is why frontotemporal dementia is sometimes called "lobar atrophy." There is **no specific effective therapy for frontotemporal dementia**.

Vascular Dementia

Vascular dementia is the answer when the question describes a "stepwise decrease in cognitive ability." This is because each stroke, no matter how small, decreases cognitive function. A stroke affects the brain in the same way that a myocardial infarction can lead to congestive heart failure: Just as myocardial infarction destroys tissue and weakens the output of the heart, so strokes destroy brain tissue and decrease the output of the brain. The output of the brain is thoughts and the creation of new memories.

Look for standard risk factors for vascular disease such as hypertension, diabetes, smoking, and hyperlipidemia.

The most accurate test is CT or MRI of the brain. There is no specific therapy to reverse vascular dementia. Anticholinesterase medication or memantine are wrong answers when they are in the choices.

Normal Pressure Hydrocephalus

Normal pressure hydrocephalus (NPH) has a triad of:

- **Dementia**
- Gait **ataxia** (described as shuffling)
- Urinary **incontinence**

Although CT scan of the brain that shows enlarged ventricles strongly supports the diagnosis, it is not always seen and, therefore, is not required for the diagnosis. The most accurate test is a lumbar puncture. Although the pressure will be normal, the most accurate feature of NPH is an improvement in symptoms with removing CSF. Long-term **treatment** is with **ventriculoperitoneal shunt** placement.

▶ **TIP**

When asked the "most accurate test for NPH," the answer is to remove CSF with a lumbar puncture.

Creutzfeld-Jakob Disease

Creutzfeld-Jakob disease (CJD) is caused by proteinacious particles called prions. A prion is not a virus and its precise nature is unknown. We do know that prions are transmissible. Patients have contracted CJD from:

- Pooled growth hormone from pituitary glands
- Improperly cleaned stereotactic brain biopsy needles
- Dural grafts
- Corneal transplants

CJD is the reason dementia excludes a person from being a cornea donor.

PRESENTATION/"WHAT IS THE MOST LIKELY DIAGNOSIS?"

Look for a person too young to have AD with:

- **Rapidly progressive dementia**
- Healthy person progressing to death in 6 months
- **Myoclonic jerks**

DIAGNOSTIC TESTS/TREATMENT

Rapidly progressive dementia + myoclonus = CJD

The best initial test is head CT/MRI. Lumbar puncture can show a special **14-3-3 protein on CSF.** The most accurate diagnostic test is a brain biopsy showing spongiform encephalopathy. There is no effective therapy; the disease is fatal in 100% of sufferers.

Huntington Disease

Huntington disease (HD) is an autosomal dominant disorder that presents, most commonly in the fourth and fifth decades, with progressive:

- **Dementia**
- **Choreiform movement disorder**
- **Emotional and behavior problems**

Tetrabenazine is a drug unique to Huntington for movement problems.

The diagnostic test is CAG trinucleotide repeat sequences found on genetic testing. Treatment of HD with antipsychotic medications does not reverse or slow down disease progression, but is used to simply control behavioral disturbance. Use quetiapine or risperidone. Tetrabenazine is used to control choreiform movements.

Mild Cognitive Impairment

Mild cognitive impairment is a problem with poor memory function, apraxia, agnosia, or aphasia that **does not interfere with the activities of daily living.** All test results will be normal. Do not treat with anticholinesterase medications.

▶ **TIP**

The most common wrong answer for mild cognitive impairment is to treat with anticholinesterase medications.

Up to 12% per year of patients with mild cognitive impairment will progress to Alzheimer's disease.

Summary of Treatment for Dementia Syndromes	
Disease	**Treatment**
Alzheimer dementia	Anticholinesterase medications first, memantine if no response
Lewy body dementia	Same as above
Normal pressure hydrocephalus	Fluid removal with lumbar puncture; ventriculoperitoneal shunt
Frontotemporal	None
Creutzfeld-Jakob disease	None
Vascular dementia	None
Progressive supranuclear palsy	None beyond treating parkinsonism

URINARY INCONTINENCE

Stress Incontinence

PRESENTATION/"WHAT IS THE MOST LIKELY DIAGNOSIS?"

All incontinence implies the inability to control the flow of urine, with urinary leakage. "Stress" incontinence specifically means the loss or leakage of a small volume of urine with coughing, sneezing, standing, laughing, lifting heavy objects, or anything that increases intraabdominal pressure. There is **no pain** with stress incontinence. Stress incontinence occurs almost exclusively in:

- Older women
- Men after a radical prostatectomy

DIAGNOSTIC TESTS

There are no specific diagnostic tests to prove that a person has stress incontinence. The first important step is to rule out any potential reversible causes (DIAPERS = **D**rugs, **I**nfections, **A**trophic vaginitis, **P**sychiatric or neurologic, **E**ndocrine/metabolic, **R**estriction of mobility, **S**tool impaction). When the case describes the symptoms of "urinary leakage with coughing" the "most appropriate next step in management" is:

1. The patient is asked to stand up.
2. The patient is instructed to cough.
3. The examiner bends over to inspect the perineal area for urine.

Urinalysis should be done to exclude infection. Do not get a urine culture unless there are white blood cells in the urine. If there is still a large volume of urine in the bladder after voiding, the diagnosis is not stress incontinence. A large "post-voiding residual" implies an obstruction to the flow of urine such

> Stress incontinence is like erectile dysfunction. You must ask; patients will often not volunteer the information.

> Post-void residual is a test of urinary obstruction.

as benign prostatic hypertrophy in a man, tumors in the bladder or cervix, or bladder neck obstruction. **You can test for the presence of post-void residual only by the placement of a urinary catheter or ultrasound.**

TREATMENT

The best initial therapy for stress incontinence in women is pelvic floor muscle exercises, also known as Kegel exercises. The patient must:

1. Contract the circumvaginal muscles as if she is stopping urination mid-flow.
2. Hold the contraction for 10 seconds and repeat 10 times. Do this 3 to 4 times a day.
3. If properly done, an examiner's finger will be "drawn in" to the vagina.

If Kegel exercises cannot be performed accurately, biofeedback methods are added to increase accuracy. When the question says that a patient still has stress incontinence "after several weeks of attempts at pelvic floor muscle exercises," the "most appropriate next step in management" is surgical correction. Estrogen cream has been used in the past to increase the growth of the epithelium of the distal third of the urethra. The efficacy of estrogens, both topically and orally, is marginal at best.

▶ **TIP**
The most common wrong answer is estrogen cream.

> Only 30% of women can perform Kegel exercises effectively enough to provide clinical benefit.

Urge Incontinence (Detrusor Overactivity)

Urge incontinence is characterized by pain in the bladder followed by an intense urge to urinate a large volume of urine. The most accurate test is a urodynamic study. In urodynamic studies, a pressure transducer is placed into a half-full bladder to measure pressures. The best initial therapy is bladder training exercises. In bladder training, the patient tries to gradually increase the amount of time between urinations by 15 to 30 minutes. If this is unsuccessful, the "most appropriate next step in management" is the use of anticholinergic medications such as:

- Oxybutynin
- Tolterodine
- Trospium
- Darifenacin
- Solifenacin

All of these medications are approximately the same in terms of mechanism, efficacy, and adverse effects. They are muscarinic receptor antagonists that have their action predominantly at the receptors in the bladder. The most common adverse effects are anticholinergic symptoms such as dry mouth and constipation.

PRESSURE ULCERS

DEFINITION/ETIOLOGY

Pressure (decubitus) ulcers are common in patients with a stroke or advanced dementia leading to profound immobility. As the ulcer progresses, the skin breaks down and may become infected, potentially spreading into the surrounding bone and causing osteomyelitis.

Which of the following is the most effective method of preventing ulcers?

a. Rotating the patient every 2 hours
b. Assisting the patient to a chair twice a day
c. Nutritional support
d. Mental status improvement
e. Prevention of wetness
f. Air or foam mattresses
g. Sheepskin overlay on the bed

Answer: The correct answer is (a). Although placing the patient in a chair twice a day is helpful, it is not frequent enough to be as helpful as rotating the patient every several hours. All of the choices listed will help prevent ulcers, but the one that helps the most in preventing the development of the local tissue hypoxia that leads to a pressure ulcer is very frequent rotation of the patient.

> Do not place urinary (Foley) catheters to prevent pressure ulcers.

Diagnosis

The most important element in diagnosing pressure ulcers is to **inspect the skin daily**. Wrong choices about diagnosis are:

• X-ray or CT
• Swab or superficial wound cultures

▶ TIP

Culturing the surface of any ulcer is always a wrong choice.

TREATMENT

Besides preventing and relieving pressure, the most important management is to avoid cytotoxic solutions like hydrogen peroxide, iodine solutions, or Dakin solution. They are toxic to tissue. Debridement of superficial necrotic tissue should be done on the ulcer. Antibiotics are generally to be avoided unless there is very clear purulent infection as evidenced by fever, leukocytosis, or draining purulent material. You cannot sterilize damaged tissue in which the skin has broken down. That is why it is always wrong to attempt to treat with antibiotics until the ulcer resolves.

FALLS

Falls are far more common in the older adults than many people realize.

- 30% of those over 65 will fall at some point in their lifetime.
- 50% of those over 80 will fall.

Which of the following is the most likely cause of increased falls in older people?

a. Musculoskeletal weakness
b. Visual impairment
c. Hearing impairment
d. Proprioception
e. Medications
f. Postural hypotension

Answer: The correct answer is (a). Though mechanical falls (e.g., tripping on a rug or furniture) are the most common cause of falls in older adults, generalized musculo-skeletal weakness is the most common risk factor for falls and fractures among those listed. However, all of the answers listed contribute to falls in the older population.

Environmental Factors

Don't forget to correct "environmental factors." These are responsible for about a third of falls in older patients. Environmental factors means:

- Lighting
- Loose rugs
- Electrical cords
- Anything else a person can trip over

Which of the following is most likely to prevent falls in older adults?

a. Resistive exercise
b. Wrist restraints
c. Hip protector
d. Levodopa/carbidopa
e. Tai chi or yoga

Answer: The correct answer is (a). It is resistive exercise, not simple physical activity, that decreases the risk of falls and the fractures that result. Tai chi and yoga increase general well-being but they do not specifically decrease the risk of falls. Hip protectors were a nice idea but did not prove to be effective. Levodopa/carbidopa is excellent for treating Parkinson disease, but does not specifically prevent falls.

> Muscle weakness is far more common than Parkinson disease as a risk of falls.

PREVENTIVE MEDICINE IN OLDER ADULTS

All of the following should be done routinely in the general population as they age:

- Pneumococcal vaccine at age 65
- Abdominal aortic aneurysm (AAA) screening:
  - In men who have ever smoked in the past
  - With an ultrasound at age 65
  - One screening ultrasound only
- DEXA bone desitometry starting at age 65 in women
- Varicella vaccine at age 60 to prevent shingles
- Influenza vaccine yearly. Use the injected inactivated vaccine.

> There is no benefit to repeating the screening for AAA if the results are normal.

HEMATOLOGY

8

Hematology is a specialty with few distinct physical findings. The questions, therefore, center on diagnostic tests and treatment. In the entirety of hematology, the most common physical findings are bleeding, petechiae, purpura, and splenomegaly.

ANEMIA

All forms of anemia have, at the root of the case stem, the same history of fatigue, tiredness, and, when more severe, shortness of breath (dyspnea) and lightheadedness. This includes every disease in which anemia is present, not just specific anemias such as iron deficiency. As the anemia becomes more severe, patients will become confused with severe dyspnea on exertion.

▶ TIP

You cannot answer the "most likely diagnosis" question based only on the symptoms or the presentation of anemia.

PRESENTATION

Anemia presents with symptoms of decreased oxygen carrying capacity. The body cannot distinguish between anemia, hypoxia, carbon monoxide poisoning, or methemoglobinemia. The cells perceive all of these as a decrease in oxygen carrying capacity and a decrease in oxygen delivery. More than any other disease, the symptoms of anemia are based on the underlying functional status of the patient. For example, young, healthy pregnant women routinely have hematocrits between 25 and 30% in the later months of pregnancy with virtually no symptoms, while an older patient or one with vascular disease may have a fatal event with a hematocrit of 25%.

Which of the following is the most common cause of death in a person with anemia?

a. Respiratory failure

b. Stroke

c. Congestive heart failure

d. Myocardial infarction

e. Embolic events

Answer: The correct answer is (d). Ultimately, a low hematocrit will decrease the oxygen carrying capacity to the point where the myocardium will become ischemic. Although many of the symptoms of anemia, such as shortness of breath, are related to the respiratory system, there is nothing intrinsically wrong with the lungs and they do not fail. Although severe anemia makes it difficult to think clearly, stroke is rare. Even in the event of stroke, it is less likely than a myocardial infarction to result in death. Ultimately, the myocardium cannot distinguish between ischemia and anemia. Both are identical physiologically in impairing oxygen delivery.

> For the left ventricle, anemia is the same as coronary disease. Both produce ischemia.

Correlation of Levels of Anemia with Symptoms	
Hematocrit (Normal ranges are 39%–49% in men, 35%–45% in women)	**Symptoms**
30–35	Generally asymptomatic
25–30	Fatigue, tiredness
20–25	Dyspnea, especially on exertion, some will be lightheaded
<20–25	Lightheadedness, confusion, incapacitating fatigue and dyspnea

The ranges in the preceding table are approximate because the symptoms of anemia are extraordinarily variable based on the underlying condition of the patient, the rapidity with which the hematocrit falls, and at what hematocrit the patient typically lives. The decision to transfuse should be based on these factors, and not strictly on the hematocrit. There is no benefit in transfusing a healthy person until the hematocrit is below 20. The heart is healthy enough to withstand the decreased oxygen carrying capacity until the reticulocytes are high enough to raise the hematocrit. Older patients, particularly those with coronary artery disease, can wait for transfusion until the hematocrit is below 30%.

DIAGNOSTIC TESTS

The best initial test after the hemoglobin and/or hematocrit reveals an anemia is the mean corpuscular volume (MCV). The MCV classifies the anemia as microcytic, normocytic, or macrocytic and is the first method of determining the etiology of the anemia. Although a reticulocyte count should be done, this test does not offer as much clarity in terms of establishing a diagnosis since virtually all forms of production problems have a low reticulocyte count.

All microcytic and macrocytic anemias will have a low reticulocyte count, with one exception.

The peripheral smear should also be done, but all forms of anemia with a low MCV will potentially have the same smear, which is hypochromic small cells.

Which of the following is associated with an increased reticulocyte count?

a. Iron deficiency
b. Alpha thalassemia with 3 genes deleted (HgH)
c. Alpha thalassemia with 2 genes deleted
d. Beta thalassemia trait
e. Beta thalassemia
f. B12 deficiency
g. Folate deficiency
h. Anemia of chronic disease

Answer: The correct answer is (b). All of the other forms of anemia have a low reticulocyte count. With the exception of the very specific circumstance of 3 gene-deleted alpha thalassemia, all production problems in the bone marrow have a low reticulocyte count.

Microcytic Anemia

ETIOLOGY/PRESENTATION

Microcytic anemia is defined as having a low MCV (normal level is between 80 and 100). The most common causes of microcytic anemia are:

- Iron deficiency
- Anemia of chronic disease
- Sideroblastic anemia
- Thalassemia

The anemia of chronic disease is sometimes called "inflammatory anemia" because it can be secondary to chronic inflammatory conditions (such as rheumatoid arthritis). The anemia of chronic disease can have a low or normal MCV. Sideroblastic anemia is also variable in its presentation, as it can also be macrocytic.

You cannot distinguish the nature of the anemia from the symptoms. Symptoms are based on the severity of the drop in hematocrit, not on the underlying cause. There are some features in the history that can suggest the diagnosis.

"WHAT IS THE MOST LIKELY DIAGNOSIS?"

Although there is nothing on physical examination to allow you to answer the "most likely diagnosis" question, there are some features in the history that will help.

> Nothing on physical examination can help you answer the "most likely diagnosis" question for the specific cause of the anemia.

Answering the "Most Likely Diagnosis" Question	
Feature in history	**Most likely diagnosis**
• Blood loss • Pica (craving ice) • Celiac disease • Malabsorption	Iron deficiency
Rheumatoid arthritis, cancer, end-stage renal disease	Anemia of chronic disease
Alcohol, lead, isoniazid	Sideroblastic anemia
Asymptomatic with profound microcytosis, <60	Thalassemia

DIAGNOSTIC TESTS

After the CBC is done, the "most appropriate next step in management" for microcytic anemia is the iron studies. Although the peripheral smear should be done, there is nothing specific on smear to allow you to answer the "most likely diagnosis" question. All the microcytic anemias can give target cells. The only one that has an elevated red cell distribution width is iron deficiency (RDW). This is because the cells are different sizes. As time goes on, the cells become more iron deficient, resulting in smaller cells being made. The older cells are larger because they have more hemoglobin content.

> Only iron deficiency has an elevated RDW. In all the others, the cells are all the same size.

> Very high RDW implies a "dimorphic" pattern with both microcytic and macrocytic anemia.

Findings on Iron Studies with Microcytic Anemia				
	Iron deficiency	**Chronic disease**	**Sideroblastic**	**Thalassemia**
Iron level	Low	Low	**High**	Normal
Iron binding capacity	High	**Low**	Normal	Normal
Ferritin	**Low**	Normal	Normal	Normal

> Ferritin is an acute phase reactant and is falsely normal in 30% of cases of iron deficiency anemia.

Unique Diagnostic Features of Each Disorder			
Iron deficiency	**Chronic disease**	**Sideroblastic**	**Thalassemia**
Low ferritin = iron deficiency RDW elevated Platelets elevated One-third with iron deficiency have a normal ferritin	Decreased iron binding capacity	Only anemia with high circulating iron level	Microcytic anemia with normal iron studies Most likely to have target cells

Answering "What Is the Most Accurate Diagnostic Test?"

There is a considerable difference between the "most appropriate next step in management," which in microcytic anemia means iron studies, and the "most accurate diagnostic test."

Iron deficiency: bone marrow biopsy for stainable iron

Sideroblastic: bone marrow biopsy with Prussian blue stain reveals iron accumulated in mitochondria in the red blood cells

Thalassemia: hemoglobin electrophoresis, which is routinely done when there is a microcytic anemia with normal iron studies

Beta thalassemia shows:

- Decreased hemoglobin A
- Increased hemoglobin A2 (fetal hemoglobin is sometimes elevated)

Alpha thalassemia shows:

- One gene deleted: no clinical or laboratory abnormalities
- Two genes deleted: normal electrophoresis with mild microcytic anemia
- Three genes deleted: hemoglobin H (beta-4 tetrads) with high mortality secondary to heart failure

> Alpha thalassemia with a single gene deletion does not come to medical attention. These patients are in normal health.

> Four gene deletion (hydrops fetalis) causes fetal death in utero.

TREATMENT

The least efficient way to replace iron is with oral ferrous sulfate. Only 1% to 2% of the oral dose is absorbed. This is why it turns the stool black. Despite the black stool, however, elemental iron will not make the stool guaiac (heme) positive. Blood causes diarrhea. Profound anemia of chronic disease can be treated with erythropoietin only in those with end-stage renal disease or who have a documented low erythropoietin level. There is no evidence that increasing the hemoglobin to greater than 10 has any clinical benefit. Occasional persons with sideroblastic anemia will respond to vitamin B6 replacement, but not the ones who had their disease caused by alcohol or lead poisoning. There is no treatment for thalassemia trait.

> Ferrous sulfate is constipating; blood causes diarrhea.

After iron replacement, which of the following will increase first?

a. Hematocrit
b. Reticulocyte count
c. Mean corpuscular volume
d. Mean corpuscular hemoglobin concentration (MCHC)
e. Red cell distribution of width

Answer: The correct answer is (b). Reticulocytes are the newest cells to be released from the bone marrow. They will increase first with iron replacement. They are a sign of new cells being formed. The other parameters go up based on the release of reticulocytes. You can't raise the MCV or MCHC without new cells.

Macrocytic Anemia

ETIOLOGY

An elevated MCV (above 100 fL) can be caused by:

> Macrocytic means the MCV is elevated. Megaloblastic means hypersegmented neutrophils.

- Vitamin B12 (cobalamin) and folate deficiency
- Liver disease
- Alcohol effect on the bone marrow
- Drug effects such as sulfa medication, zidovudine, methotrexate, or phenytoin
- Hypothyroidism

Causes of B12 and Folate Deficiency

B12 deficiency can be caused by:

- Pernicious anemia
- Chronic pancreatitis (pancreatic enzymes are needed to detach B12 from R-proteins)
- Celiac disease, Whipple disease, tropic sprue, or anything else that affects the terminal ileum, leading to malabsorption
- Nutritional deficiency

Folate deficiency is caused by:

> Everyone with sickle cell disease and all pregnant women need folic acid supplementation.

- Nutritional deficiency, particularly in alcoholics or anyone who does not eat green leafy vegetables or overcooks their vegetables
- Pregnancy
- Hemolysis, psoriasis, or any other disease with high cell production and turnover
- Phenytoin, which accelerates folate metabolism and contributes to deficiency

PRESENTATION

> Isolated folate deficiency is not associated with neurological abnormalities.

You cannot determine the etiology of macrocytic anemia solely by symptoms related to anemia. Fatigue and dyspnea are too nonspecific. The presence of neurological abnormalities tells you that it cannot be folate deficiency alone as the cause of the macrocytic anemia.

The most common neurological abnormality in B12 deficiency is peripheral neuropathy. The least common is dementia. B12 deficiency can present with *any* neurological abnormality.

Other features of vitamin B12 deficiency are:

- Glossitis (smooth tongue)
- Weight loss
- Pale, yellow skin

An MCV > 110 FL strongly suggests B12 or folate deficiency.

DIAGNOSTIC TESTS

The best initial test for B12 and folate deficiency is a peripheral blood smear. This is because only B12 and folate deficiency have hypersegmented neutrophils. If the serum folate level is low, you do not need to do any further tests to diagnose folic acid deficiency. If the serum folate level is normal, then the answer is one of the following:

- Red cell folate level
- Homocysteine level (increased in B12 and folate deficiencies)
- Methylmalonic acid (increased in B12 deficiency and normal in folate deficiency)

B12: MMA elevated, homocysteine elevated

Folate: MMA normal, homocysteine elevated

If the B12 level is decreased, no further tests are needed to diagnose the presence of B12 deficiency. If the level is low normal, the next step in establishing a diagnosis is an elevated level of methylmalonic acid (MMA). Once a diagnosis of B12 deficiency is established, the "most appropriate next step in management" is to determine the etiology or cause of the B12 deficiency. The "best initial test" to establish pernicious anemia as the cause of B12 deficiency is:

- Anti-intrinsic factor antibodies (70% sensitive, 100% specific)

▶ TIP

In B12 deficiency, be careful to answer the precise question asked: initial diagnosis or cause.

Smear: Hypersegmented neutrophils mean megaloblastic anemia (B12 or folate)

B12 or folate level: Establishes the presence of deficiency but not the reason for the deficiency

MMA or red cell folate: Use if the initial folate and B12 levels are normal.

Schilling test is always a wrong answer.

Additional Lab Abnormalities in B12 Deficiency

- Macro-ovalocytes
- Increased indirect bilirubin and increased LDH from early cell death just after release from the marrow
- Homocysteine is elevated in both B12 and folate deficiency
- Low reticulocyte count
- Hypercellular marrow

B12 deficiency can give low WBC count and low platelet count.

TREATMENT

Oral replacement can be used for either B12 or folate deficiency. Hypokalemia can occur as a complication of treatment with B12 or folic acid. The cells start to be made so rapidly that they use up all the potassium.

Hemolysis

PRESENTATION

All forms of hemolysis classically present with:

- Rapid onset of anemia from destruction of cells
- Increase in reticulocytes
- Increase in LDH, uric acid, and indirect bilirubin level
- Decreased haptoglobin level

Intravascular hemolysis (DIC, TTP, HUS, HELLP syndrome, ABO blood group incompatibility) will also give:

- Abnormal blood smear with microangiopathic hemolytic anemia (schistocytes, helmet cells, fragmented red cells)
- Hemoglobin in the urine

> No form of hemolysis gives bilirubin in the urine since only direct bilirubin can get into the urine.

Sickle Cell Disease: The Questions You Are Asked

1. What is the **best initial diagnostic test? Peripheral smear**. The smear can tell the difference between sickle cell disease and sickle cell trait. Trait produces normal smear results.
2. What is the **most accurate test? Hemoglobin electrophoresis**. This is the answer for both sickle cell disease (the homozygote or SS disease) and the sickle cell trait (the heterozygote or AS disease).
3. What is the **best initial therapy? Oxygen, hydration, analgesics**. Do **not** use meperidine as the analgesic since the metabolite can cause seizures.
4. When are **antibiotics** the answer? Ceftriaxone, levofloxacin, or moxifloxacin is the answer when there is an obvious infection or just **for "fever" in the history**. Because adults with sickle cell disease have no functional spleen, fever alone is a dramatic emergency that can indicate a rapid decline into sepsis. The other time to answer "antibiotics" is when there is a marked **increase in the WBC count**. Patients with sickle cell disease often have an elevated WBC count from stress to the marrow. The indication for antibiotics must specifically describe a WBC count that has jumped up.
5. When is **exchange transfusion** the answer? Life-threatening sickle-cell crises with critical infarctions of organs such as:
   - **Eye** (visual disturbance secondary to retinal infarction)
   - **Lung** (acute chest syndrome)
   - **Penis** (priapism)
   - **Brain** (stroke)

6. When is **hydroxyurea** the answer? When the patient has **four or more crises per year** and the case says "the patient is going home" or "**best long-term therapy.**" Hydroxyurea decreases the frequency of sickle cell crises by increasing the production of fetal hemoglobin and decreasing the WBC count.

7. When is **folic acid replacement** and *Pneumococcus, Haemophilus*, and *Meningococcus* vaccine the answer? They are indicated for everyone.

Additional Sickle Cell Questions in the Homozygote		
Question	**Answer**	**Reason**
What physical finding is most likely to be found?	Icterus	Chronic hemolysis
Right upper quadrant pain and tenderness	Bilirubin gallstones	Chronic increase in indirect bilirubin
What is the most common cause of osteomyelitis?	*Salmonella*	Published reports describe *Salmonella* (even if you think it is *Staphylococcus*)
What is the most common chronic lung disease?	Pulmonary hypertension	Repeated episodes of acute chest syndrome

Parvovirus B19

1. When is **Parvovirus B19** is the "**most likely diagnosis**"? Look for a description of a "**drop in hematocrit over 2 to 3 days.**" Interestingly, sickle cell crisis does not usually decrease the hematocrit rapidly during a crisis. Usually, the crisis will give a change in shape of the cells and pain, but not a decrease in hematocrit.

2. What is the "**best initial diagnostic test**" for parvovirus? **Reticulocyte count.** Sickle cell disease is a chronic, compensated hemolytic anemia. That means red cells have a shortened lifespan and the only way to maintain the hematocrit at a steady level is to have a markedly elevated reticulocyte count all the time. Parvovirus "freezes" the growth of the marrow. This is first detected by a drop in reticulocyte count from the usual level of 10% to 20% in sickle cell down to 2% to 3%.

3. What is the "**most accurate test**"? Parvovirus **PCR for DNA**.

4. What is the "**best initial therapy**"? Intravenous immunoglobulin (IVIG).

> Parvovirus in sickle cell often lacks the rash and joint pain found when it infects otherwise normal persons.

> A normal reticulocyte count in sickle cell is a life-threatening abnormality. Anemia will rapidly develop.

Frequent Most Common Wrong Answers in Sickle Cell Disease

- Answering "splenic sequestration" when the hematocrit suddenly drops. You cannot sequester into a spleen that has autoinfarcted.

- Thinking that the smear **can't** show the difference between sickle cell disease and trait. It can.

- Answering "parvovirus IgM or IgG" as the "most accurate test" for parvovirus. PCR-DNA is far more specific.

Sickle Cell Trait (Heterozygous or AS)

Sickle trait has only one significant manifestation despite the fact that 50% of the hemoglobin in the heterozygote is sickle hemoglobin. Sickle trait presents with renal involvement such as:

- Proteinuria (25%)
- Hematuria
- Renal concentrating defect ("isosthenuria")
- Urinary infection

There is no treatment for sickle trait. The patient will develop an acute sickle cell crisis only under conditions of extreme hypoxia such as high-altitude parachute drops or mountain climbing.

Hemoglobin SC Disease

The patient is heterozygous for sickle cell disease but the other half of the hemoglobin is HgC instead of HgA. Manifestations are:

> The most frequent manifestation of SC disease is vision problems.

- More sickle crises than the usual sickle trait (or AS disease)
- Fewer crises than homozygous sickle disease (or SS disease)
- Increased frequency of retinopathy and orthopedic complications

Autoimmune Hemolysis

> As much as 50% of autoimmune hemolysis has no identified etiology.

> Smear in autoimmune hemolysis can show microspherocytes.

1. When is autoimmune hemolysis the **"most likely diagnosis"**? When **the case describes another autoimmune disease in the history** such as **SLE, rheumatoid arthritis**, or a **lymphocytic malignancy** such as chronic lymphocytic leukemia **(CLL)** or **lymphoma**.
2. What is the **most accurate test? Coombs test.** The direct and indirect Coombs tests tell basically the same information. Antibodies are made against red blood cells.
3. What is the **best initial therapy?** Prednisone or other glucocorticoids.
4. When is **splenectomy** the right answer? **Recurrent episodes** or a failure to control the disease with prednisone.
5. When is **intravenous immunoglobulin** the right answer? The answer is IVIG when the hemolysis is **extremely severe, rapid, and not responsive to prednisone.**

Cold Agglutinin Disease

1. When is cold agglutinin disease the **"most likely diagnosis"**? When the case describes *Mycoplasma* or **Epstein-Barr virus** in association with hemolysis under cold temperatures. Look for **"clumping of red cells"** on the smear or a falsely elevated MCV and MCHC.
2. What is the **"best initial therapy"**? **Stay warm.** If **rituximab** is in the choices, then it is the answer. Cold agglutinin disease does not respond to steroids or splenectomy. Other choices that can be correct as treatment are cyclophosphamide or mephalan.

Hereditary Spherocytosis

1. When is hereditary spherocytosis the **"most likely diagnosis"**? When the case describes:
   - Recurrent episodes of lifelong hemolysis
   - Family history of hemolysis
   - Splenomegaly (time and recurrences are necessary to enlarge the spleen)
   - Bilirubin gallstones
2. What is the **best initial diagnostic test**? Peripheral smear or elevated mean corpuscular hemoglobin concentration (MCHC).
3. What is the **most accurate diagnostic test**? Osmotic fragility.
4. What is the **most effective therapy**? Splenectomy.

> Everyone with chronic hemolysis should be on folic acid supplementation.

Paroxysmal Nocturnal Hemoglobinuria

1. When is paroxysmal nocturnal hemoglobinuria (PNH) the **"most likely diagnosis"**? When the case describes:
   - Dark morning urine
   - Pancytopenia
   - Large vessel thromboses (mesenteric artery or vein, hepatic vein)

PNH can transform into acute leukemia.

2. What is the **"most accurate diagnostic test"**? The defect in PNH is the inability to remove complement from the red cell before its destruction. An abnormal covering of platelets with complement results in abnormal platelet activation and large vessel thrombosis. This factor that removes complement is known as decay accelerating factor, which is tested for with **CD55 and CD59**. There is also a defect in the anchoring protein that binds CD55 and CD59 so they cannot remove complement. **Flow cytometry** is the test that detects the specific CD55/59 cells.
3. What is the **best initial therapy**? **Steroids** are the best initial therapy during acute events. Steroids inhibit the activation of complement and inhibit all the defects in the system. **Eculizumab** is the monoclonal antibody that gets rid of abnormal complement.

> PIG-A is the gene that codes for the protein that anchors CD55 and CD59 to the cell to remove complement.

> PNH is associated with aplastic anemia, myelodysplasia, and acute myelogenous leukemia.

Most Common Wrong Answers in PNH

Choices that are always wrong in PNH are:

- Sugar water (sucrose hemolysis) test
- Ham test (acidifying medium)

Both of these test are older "functional" tests of PNH. In the first test, sucrose was used to provoke hemolysis. In the second (Ham test), the media was acidified to provoke hemolysis. Neither should be used any longer. They may be in the choices and they are always wrong. Transplant is curative.

> PNH can change into AML.

▶ **TIP**

A frequent question in PNH is "what is the most common cause of death?" The answer is thrombosis.

Glucose-6-Phosphate Dehydrogenase Deficiency

1. When is glucose-6-phosphate dehydrogenase (G6PD) deficiency the **"most likely diagnosis"**? Sudden onset of hemolysis after the use of certain oxidizing substances (sulfa drugs, primiquine, dapsone, fava bean) or acute events (infections) in a male patient.

2. What is the **"best initial diagnostic test"**? Peripheral smear revealing **Heinz bodies and bite cells.** Acute oxidant stress produces precipitants of hemoglobin in the red cell membrane known as Heinz bodies, which are removed from the cell by the spleen, producing a bite cell. Heinz bodies are not visible on a normal smear. They need a special "supravital stain" such as brilliant cresyl blue.

3. What is the **"most accurate diagnostic test"**? Obtain a **level of G6PD after waiting 2 months.** Immediately after an episode of hemolysis, the G6PD level will be normal. This is because the most deficient cells are destroyed. The cells left behind are those with normal G6PD levels.

4. What is the **"best initial therapy"**? **No specific therapy.** Nothing can reverse the hemolysis. Avoid oxidant stress in the future and use folic acid routinely.

> G6PD deficiency is X-linked and occurs almost exclusively in men.

APLASTIC ANEMIA

DEFINITION/ETIOLOGY

Aplastic anemia literally means a marrow "without growth." There are many causes of a pancytopenia, which is the decrease in all three cell lines (white, red, and platelet). Aplastic anemia does not have a specific diagnostic test. You must exclude all the other causes of pancytopenia and then, by exclusion, the patient has aplastic anemia. Although the presumed mechanism is a T cell that begins to attack its own marrow, there is no identified cause found in aplastic anemia. In fact, if there is a clear cause, it is by definition not aplastic anemia.

> Heinz bodies are not seen on routine stain. Use cresyl blue.

▶ **TIP**

The answer is aplastic anemia only if all other causes of pancytopenia have been excluded.

Causes of Pancytopenia

The answer to all the "best initial treatment" and "most effective treatment" questions is based on the cause. Pancytopenia is most often caused by diseases that invade or infiltrate the marrow and shut off production of cells. Sometimes there is increased destruction such as SLE or splenic sequestration.

Causes of Decreased Marrow Production

- Infection infiltrating the marrow (tuberculosis, fungus, bacterial)
- Infection damaging production (HIV, CMV, hepatitis)
- Cancer, either metastatic or leukemia
- Myelodysplasia
- Myelofibrosis
- Drugs, alcohol, or radiation
- B12 or folate deficiency
- Paroxysmal nocturnal hemoglobinuria
- Congenital aplastic anemia (Fanconi anemia)

PRESENTATION

Pancytopenia can present with bleeding (thrombocytopenia), fatigue (anemia), or infection (leucopenia). This is the same no matter what the etiology.

▶ **TIP**

Symptoms alone cannot help you answer aplastic anemia for the "most likely diagnosis" question.

DIAGNOSTIC TESTS

The best initial test is a CBC showing pancytopenia. The most accurate test is a bone marrow biopsy. The diagnosis is confirmed by excluding cancer and infection infiltrating the bone marrow.

A CT of the chest is often done because detection, and subsequent removal, of a thymoma can be curative.

> There is no blood test to detect myelofibrosis, metastatic cancer, and many of the other causes of pancytopenia without bone marrow biopsy.

TREATMENT

The "best initial management" is always to correct the underlying cause of the pancytopenia. There is no cause identified for aplastic anemia in most patients. Treat with immunosuppressives and transplant in those with moderate to severe disease.

▶ **TIP**

When is bone marrow transplant (BMT) the answer? Age younger than 50 with a suitable match (about 30% of patients).

If the patient is too old to be transplanted or does not have a suitable matched donor, long-term treatment is with immunosuppressive medications. Since the presumed mechanism is an aberrant T cell, treatment is based on eliminating T cells with:

> Aplastic anemia must have an allogeneic BMT; you cannot do an autologous transplant from someone with no marrow.

> In aplastic anemia, it is as if the body's own T cells are rejecting it as foreign. That is why drugs that prevent organ transplant rejection are effective.

- Prednisone
- Cyclosporine (or tacrolimus)
- Antithymocyte globulin

There is an excellent response to these medications. 60% to 80% of patients will see recovery of marrow function.

▶ **TIP**

Growth factors are not the answer for aplastic anemia. Controlling T cells is the answer with BMT or drugs.

MYELODYSPLASTIC SYNDROME

DEFINITION/PRESENTATION

> There is no specific physical finding characteristic of MDS.

Myelodysplastic syndrome (MDS) is a preleukemic disorder with a cytopenia in the peripheral blood. Although certain cytogenetic abnormalities (e.g., 5q deletion) are characteristic of MDS, its cause is unknown. Patients are often above age 60 with infection, fatigue, bleedings, or splenomegaly.

DIAGNOSTIC TESTS

The best initial test is a CBC, which shows cytopenia which is sometimes a pancytopenia with an increased MCV. This is why it is essential for the question to give you the information that there are no B12 or folate deficiencies and there is no alcohol use. Bone marrow biopsy is then done to determine the percentage of blasts, which, in addition to the aggressiveness of the anemia, is the main determinant of survival. Finally, chromosome analysis is done as a predictor of response to therapy.

> The marrow is variable in MDS. It can be hypercellular or hypocellular.

Which of the following is most specific to MDS?

a. Macro-ovalocytes
b. Bilobed nucleus of neutrophil (Pelger-Huët cell)
c. Ringed sideroblasts on Prussian blue stain
d. Blasts
e. Teardrop-shaped cells

Answer: The correct answer is (b). The Pelger-Huët cell is the most characteristic of MDS. Macro-ovalocytes are seen in MDS, but they are common in B12 deficiency as well. Ringed sideroblasts are seen in lead poisoning and with alcohol effect on the development of red cells as well as MDS. Blasts are definitely seen in MDS, just in smaller percentages (5% to 19%) than would be seen in acute leukemia (more than 20%). Teardrop-shaped cells are found in myelofibrosis.

5q Deletion

Isolated partial deletion of chromosome 5 (5q deletion) is characteristic of certain groups of patients with MDS. 5q deletion is critically important because this subset of patients is responsive to more medications than other patients with MDS. 5q deletion is most responsive to therapy with lenalidomide.

TREATMENT

Besides supportive therapy with blood transfusion, erythropoietin, and treating infections as they arise, MDS is treated with:

1. **Erythropoietin** and **G-CSF**
2. Azacitidine and decitabine
3. **Lenalidomide** (for 5q deletion syndrome)
4. **Allogeneic BMT** in the occasional person who presents below age 50
5. Chelation therapy (may be required for patients with iron overload secondary to chronic transfusions)

> Bone marrow transplant (BMT) is the only cure for myelodysplasia.

What is the most common cause of death in MDS?

a. Infection and bleeding
b. Transformation into acute myelocytic leukemia
c. Transformation into acute lymphocytic leukemia
d. Adverse effects of medications

Answer: The correct answer is (a). The majority of patients with MDS do not live long enough for the disease to transform into acute leukemia. Most dwindle away with infection and bleeding.

ACUTE LEUKEMIA

DEFINITION/PRESENTATION

By definition, acute leukemia has more than 20% blasts on bone marrow. Although radiation and toxins such as benzene or toluene are associated with the development of acute leukemia, this is not a useful part of the history to answer the "most likely diagnosis" question. Look for signs of pancytopenia with infection, bleeding, easy bruising, and fatigue. This is true even if the WBC count is elevated. Leukemic blasts do not "work": They are not functional.

▶ **TIP**

There is no physical finding unique to acute leukemia. Of note, in contrast to patients with acute lymphocytic leukemia (ALL), patients with acute myelogenous leukemia (AML) do **not** have lymphadenopathy or hepato-splenomegaly.

DIAGNOSTIC TESTS/TREATMENT

The best initial diagnostic test is blasts on peripheral smear. If the WBC count has more than 20% blasts, the diagnosis of acute leukemia is established. When there is less than 20% blasts on peripheral blood, the bone marrow is examined for blasts. There is often leukocytosis with accompanying anemia and thrombocytopenia.

Serum electrolytes (e.g., calcium, phosphorous, uric acid, potassium) and LDH must be measured before and during chemotherapy to monitor for tumor lysis syndrome. Because CNS involvement is common in ALL, lumbar puncture should be performed prior to initiation of therapy.

The most accurate diagnostic test is flow cytometry. This is the "sorting" of cells by specific CD type. This is how to distinguish AML from ALL as well as to distinguish subtypes. For example, CD10 is also known as the "common ALL antigen."

Comparison of AML and ALL Testing and Treatment		
	AML	**ALL**
Lab finding	Auer rods (eosinophilic inclusions)	Common ALL antigen
Specific enzyme abnormality	Myeloperoxidase	Periodic acid Schiff (PAS)
Initial therapy	Daunorubicin (or idarubicin) and cytarabine; also, allopurinol and fluids	Daunorubicin, prednisone, vincristine, asparaginase, cytarabine; also, allopurinol and fluids
Additional therapy	Add all-trans-retinoic acid with or without arsenic trioxide for M3 promyelocytic leukemia	Intrathecal methotrexate to prevent recurrences. Monoclonal antibody therapy: imatinib for Philadelphia chromosome [t(9:22)]; rituximab for CD20 positive

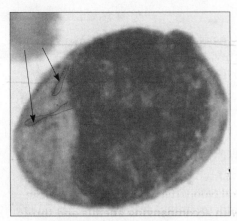

Figure 8.1: Auer rods. Auer rods are found in acute myelogenous leukemia.
Source: Farouk Talakshi, MD

Prognosis and When to Transplant

Although the combination chemotherapy previously listed can produce remission in the majority of patients, relapse will also occur. Relapsed acute leukemia is harder to control, so the question becomes: Who do I transplant in first remission **before** they relapse? The answer is based on cytogenetics, which indicates the risk of relapse. Cytogenetics means the types of genetic defects found in the patient. For example, in AML, monosomy of chromosome 5 or 7 gives a bad prognosis; patients with translocations between chromosomes 15 and 17 and between 8 and 21 have a favorable prognosis. In ALL, older age, presence of Philadelphia chromosome, and, generally, B cell rather than T cell predominance are poor prognostic factors. If BMT kills 10% to 20% of those who undergo the procedure, you would do it only if the patient's risk of relapse was higher than that. This is what we use cytogenetics to determine.

▶ **TIP**

When you are asked "what is the most important factor in prognosis?" the answer is cytogenetics.

MYELOPROLIFERATIVE DISORDERS

Polycythemia Vera

DEFINITION

Polycythemia vera (p. vera) is the overproduction of all three cell lines, but predominantly red blood cells. It is, essentially, red blood cell cancer. The cells grow in the absence of erythropoietin.

Hot showers make people with p. vera itch because of histamine release from basophils.

PRESENTATION

When the hematocrit goes above 55%, blood viscosity increases, leading to:

- Headache, dizziness, and blurry vision sometimes leading to TIAs and stroke
- Epistaxis from **engorged mucosal vessels**
- Thrombosis, especially after surgery (DVT, Budd-Chiari syndrome)
- Splenomegaly (palpable in 75%, detectible by imaging in all patients)

Diagnostic Tests

Besides a marked elevation of the hematocrit, unique features of p. vera are the elevation in WBC and platelet count. Extremely rapid red cell production uses up all the iron, making the RBCs small and eliminating iron stores. Patients often have iron deficiency and a hypercellular bone marrow.

Elevated hematocrit – hypoxia = primary polycythemia vera

The "most accurate test" is JAK2 mutation. JAK2 is found in 95%. If it is missing, you should look for another diagnosis.

No medication can simulate the presentation of p. vera. Testosterone and erythropoietin use can raise the red cell count, but they do not raise the WBC count, elevate platelets, or enlarge the spleen.

Microcytic erythrocytosis (low MCV + high RBC count)

- P. vera
- Thalassemia
- Hypoxia

Additional Lab Abnormalities in p. vera
- Elevated B12 level from increase in transcobalamin
- Hyperuricemia
- Increase in eosinophil and basophil count
- Iron deficiency

Smear is normal. The red blood cells may look normal or slightly hypochromic and microcytic (from iron deficiency); there are just too many of them.

TREATMENT

The best initial therapy is phlebotomy. Everyone who is not bleeding (e.g., epistaxis) should get aspirin. P. vera has an abnormally increased amount of platelet activation, which contributes to stroke, TIAs, and hepatic vein thrombosis (Budd-Chiari syndrome).

If the case says "the patient's symptoms and blood count are not controlled by phlebotomy and aspirin," the "most appropriate next step in management" is interferon or hydroxyurea.

Essential Thrombocythemia

DEFINITION/PRESENTATION

Essential thrombocythemia (ET) is **cancer of platelets**. Patients present with thrombosis or bleeding. ET and p. vera are the two most common causes of "erythromelalgia" which is painful, red hands thought to be from small vessel thrombosis. As with p. vera, ET can lead to large vessel **thrombosis** at unusual sites such as the renal vein or hepatic vein (Budd-Chiari). **Visual disturbance is common.**

DIAGNOSTIC TESTS

The platelet count in ET is always above 600,000/μL and usually over 1,000,000. Oddly, extremely high platelet counts are associated with a greater risk of bleeding. About half of patients will have the **JAK2 mutation**. You must rule out other causes of thrombocytosis (reactive, iron deficiency, malignancy, inflammatory). Bone marrow shows hypercellularity with abnormal megakaryocytes.

> When is JAK2 the cause of thrombocythemia?
> - P. vera 95–97%
> - Myelofibrosis 50%
> - Essential thrombocythemia 50–75%

TREATMENT

Platelet apheresis with high-dose **hydroxyurea** is indicated for life-threatening conditions. Low-dose hydroxyurea is the next best initial therapy. Those who are not bleeding should get aspirin to prevent thrombosis. Alternatives to hydroxyurea are **anagrelide** and interferon. They are not as effective as hydroxyurea.

Myelofibrosis

PRESENTATION/"WHAT IS THE MOST LIKELY DIAGNOSIS?"

Myelofibrosis is an idiopathic disorder in which the bone marrow is "choked off" by reticulin fibers developing within the bone marrow. Although patients are anemic at every stage, the presentation is variable because the production of which blood cells and platelets is variable. If there is pancytopenia, patients may present with **infection**, **fatigue**, and **bleeding** as they would in any person with pancytopenia of any cause. Because progenitor cells (stem cells) leave the marrow and set up residence in the spleen and liver (extramedullary hematopoiesis), **hepatic and splenic enlargement can be quite massive.**

DIAGNOSTIC TESTS

In advanced stages, myelofibrosis will present with pancytopenia. Early on, the WBC count can be elevated as the stressed marrow increases its output and marrow production expands because blood production begins in the spleen and liver. This stress causes release of giant, bizarre-looking platelets.

> Bone marrow aspirate may be "dry" and the biopsy shows fibers.

Blood smear: Teardrop-shaped cells and nucleated RBCs are the most characteristic finding of myelofibrosis.

TREATMENT

The best initial therapy is "supportive" with blood transfusions. The "most effective therapy" is lenalidomide, a variant of thalidomide. Thalidomide has proven to have enormous benefit in hematological malignancies such as myeloma, myelofibrosis, and myelodysplasia. Ruxolitinib is a JAK2 inhibitor.

If the case describes the WBC count as high, hydroxyurea can be a choice as best initial therapy. Hydroxyurea is used to control overproduction of cells such as ET, leukostasis reactions, and p. vera.

In younger (under 50 to 60) and healthier patients, allogenic bone marrow transplant has been used with benefit.

Bone Marrow Transplant with Stem Cells

Stem cell transplant is useful in myelofibrosis and myeloma in the person young enough to undergo the procedure. Autologous stem cell transplantation can be done up to 60 to 70 years of age. There is no rejection or graft versus host disease in an autologous stem cell transplant, so it can be tolerated in patients between 50 and 70 years of age. Stem cells are "partially grown" compared to transplanting the bone marrow in general. Monoclonal antibodies are used to pick out the stem cells, so it is only those cells that are transplanted. This shortens the duration of neutropenia because the blood count comes back faster.

Chronic Myelogenous Leukemia

DEFINITION/PRESENTATION

Chronic myelogenous leukemia (CML) is the proliferation of normal-appearing neutrophils and WBC precursors that are diminished in function, but are far more functional than the blast cells of acute leukemia. Patients often present **without symptoms**, having a **markedly elevated WBC count** found on a CBC done for other purposes. Some patients with advanced disease have **fatigue, fever, night sweats,** and **left upper quadrant pain** from **splenomegaly**.

DIAGNOSTIC TESTS

The "best initial" and "most accurate" diagnostic test is the BCR/ABL gene mutation known as the Philadelphia chromosome. This is the translocation of chromosomes 9 and 22. The **leukocyte alkaline phosphatase (LAP) score is an old test that is abnormally low in CML.** Normal neutrophils have alkaline phosphatase. CML cells have less alkaline phosphatase, so in CML, the WBC count is elevated but the LAP score is low. CML is also associated with increased basophils and a markedly hypercellular bone marrow. Patients

---

JAK2 in 50% with myelofibrosis

Lenalidomide can allow a person with myelofibrosis to become independent of transfusions.

The shorter the period of neutropenia, the smaller the chance of a fatal infection.

Ruxolitinib is a JAK2 inhibitor useful in myelofibrosis.

CML does not bleed, as would happen in an acute leukemia.

typically have a small number of blasts (less than 5%), but, as the disease progresses, blast crisis may occur if/when the blasts surpass 20%.

PCR or fluorescent in-situ hybridization (FISH) for the BCR/ABL oncogene can be done on peripheral blood. Score is always a wrong answer.

> ► **TIP**
>
> If BCR/ABL is in the answer choices, then it is the answer to both the "best initial" and the "most accurate" test.

TREATMENT

The best initial therapy is a tyrosine kinase inhibitor such as imatinib. Nilotinib and dasatinib are alternatives to imatinib. There is an excellent hematologic response in more than 95%, and survival at 5 years is greater than 80%. The only way to cure CML, however, is bone marrow transplantation.

> ► **TIP**
>
> Untreated with imatinib, CML has the highest risk of transformation to acute leukemia of all the hematologic malignancies.

Leukostasis Reactions

Some patients with extremely high WBC counts above 100,000 to 200,000/μL develop signs of "sludging," decreasing perfusion of the lungs, brain, and eyes. This is a leukostasis reaction that comes from WBCs blocking tissue perfusion. Patients will have:

- **Dyspnea**
- **Blurry vision**
- **Confusion, dizziness, and lightheadedness**

Treatment is with leukapheresis to remove WBCs from circulation with a centrifuge and relieve the impairment of flow. Hydroxyurea is added to treatment to help bring down the WBC count a little faster.

CHRONIC LYMPHOCYTIC LEUKEMIA

DEFINITION/PRESENTATION

Chronic lymphocytic leukemia (CLL) is the massive proliferation of normal-appearing lymphocytes in patients at an average age of 70. CLL is most often found on routine CBC in an asymptomatic patient. Some patients present with fatigue, infection, or painful lymph nodes or left upper quadrant pain from splenomegaly. A small number will be in an advanced stage with anemia

---

Sidebar notes:

In CML, the peripheral blood looks like the bone marrow.

Diagnose CML with PCR or FISH for BCR/ABL.

Leukostasis happens with AML and CML because neutrophils and blasts are larger than other cells.

or thrombocytopenia. CLL is different from CML in that the hematocrit and platelet count can be low on an autoimmune basis (ie, hemolytic anemia).

In the setting of CLL, which of the following has the worst prognosis?

a. Low platelets from marrow infiltration with CLL cells
b. Anemia from marrow infiltration with CLL cells
c. Autoimmune thrombocytopenia
d. Autoimmune hemolysis
e. Splenomegaly
f. Frequent pulmonary infections

Answer: The correct answer is (a). Low platelets from infiltration of the marrow with leukemic cells represents stage IV, the most advanced form of disease. Autoimmune thrombocytopenia and anemia are very common in CLL and easily treatable with prednisone. Infections occur because the lymphocytes are, after all, leukemic. They do not produce normal antibodies to defend the body from infection. On average, survival with stage IV CLL is 1 to 2 years.

DIAGNOSTIC TESTS

The best initial test is a CBC with a markedly elevated WBC count that is predominantly normal-appearing lymphocytes. This is extraordinarily specific for CLL in an older person. More specific (accurate) tests are:

- Flow cytometry with increased CD5 and CD20
- Fluorescent in situ hybridization (FISH)

> A smudge cell is a laboratory artifact of a damaged CLL cell. It is not a usual diagnostic finding.

▶ TIP

You should avoid any book or course that tries to make you learn too many CD numbers or genetic defect specifics in CLL. You don't need them to answer the questions.

Staging

Stage 0: Elevated WBC alone

Stage I: Lymphadenopathy

Stage II: Splenomegaly or hepatomegaly

Stage III: Anemia from marrow infiltration/replacement with CLL

Stage IV: Thrombocytopenia from marrow infiltration/replacement with CLL

> Anemia is defined as a hemoglobin less than 11 gm/DL.

▶ TIP

Remember: Autoimmune thrombocytopenia and hemolysis (usually warm agglutinin) do not count as advanced stage CLL or serve as negative prognostic signs.

TREATMENT

The best initial therapy is based on staging.

Stages 0 and I: No therapy is given, especially in an older person; median survival is 10 to 15 years.

Stage II, III, IV, or anyone with B symptoms, discomfort from hepatic or splenic enlargement, or worsening cytopenias: Treat with fludarabine and rituximab, which increase survival.

Autoimmune hemolysis or thrombocytopenia: Glucocorticoids are the best initial therapy. Severe recurrences are treated with splenectomy. Acute, severe hemolysis not responding to steroids gets intravenous immunoglobulins. Alemtuzumab (anti-52) is used for relapsed disease. Chlorambucil is used only to lower WBC in frail, elderly patients.

> Cyclophosphamide adds efficacy and increased toxicity to initial therapy. It is definitely right if the patient does not respond to fludarabine and rituximab.

> Stage II disease (splenomegaly) is treated if symptomatic.

PLASMA CELL DISORDERS

Multiple Myeloma

PRESENTATION/"WHAT IS THE MOST LIKELY DIAGNOSIS?"

The most common presentation of myeloma is with a pathologic bone fracture in an older patient. Patients will also present with symptoms related to hypercalcemia or neuropathy from the effect of paraproteins on the nerves.

DIAGNOSTIC TESTS

The single most specific test for myeloma is the marked elevation in plasma cells on bone marrow biopsy above 30%. The other abnormalities can occur in other conditions such as:

> Blood smear shows rouleaux (stacks of red cells), but this finding has no prognostic, therapeutic, or diagnostic importance.

- Lytic bone lesions
- Bence-Jones proteinuria
- Anemia
- High total protein with a monoclonal spike in the IgG or IgA region
- Hyperuricemia from increased turnover of cells with nuclei
- Amyloid
- Renal insufficiency

Which of the following is the most common cause of death in myeloma?

a. Accelerated atherosclerosis
b. Infection
c. Renal failure
d. Anemia
e. Bleeding

Answer: The correct answer is (b). Normal immunoglobulins are suppressed in myeloma. As the plasma cells increase their production of useless IgG or IgA, they decrease the production of immunoglobulins that might be useful in protecting the body against infection. All of the issues in the answers occur, but infection is the one most likely to prove fatal.

Beta-2 Microglobulin

The beta-2 microglobulin level is useful to stage myeloma: The higher the level, the less the chances of survival. Beta-2 microglobulin decreases in response to treatment and is a good single numerical measure of response to therapy.

▶ **TIP**

When the question says "what is the single most **specific test** in myeloma?" the answer is **percentage of plasma cells** in bone marrow.

▶ **TIP**

When the question asks "what **single test** is most accurate in **determining prognosis**" or "**response to therapy**" the answer is beta-2 microglobulin.

Although plasma cells and the height of the monoclonal (or "M") spike are very good in establishing the initial diagnosis, they are not as good in determining prognosis. That is because they can rapidly disappear with treatment, but they may return rapidly as well.

TREATMENT

Myeloma is not a curable disease. Treatment methods include a combination of:

- Autologous stem cell transplantation in those under age 70
- Thalidomide (or lenalidomide)
- Melphalan and prednisone
- Bortezomib (proteosome inhibitor)
- Vincristine, adriamycin, dexamethasone (VAD) in preparation for transplantation

> Autologous stem cell transplantation should be first for myeloma.

> The precise order or combination of these therapies is not clear at this time.

Monoclonal Gammopathy of Unknown Significance

Monoclonal gammopathy of unknown significance (MGUS) is an elevated spike in IgG or IgA on a serum protein electrophoresis (SPEP). No treatment is required beyond routine monitoring for multiple myeloma or another plasma cell disease.

Look for:

- Older patient (70 or above)
- High total protein
- Asymptomatic, found on routine testing

By definition, MGUS has no abnormalities of the bone, kidney, calcium level, or immune system. Even laboratory criteria for myeloma should be absent. Plasma cell levels should be under 10% and the beta-2 microglobulin level should be low.

Waldenström Macroglobulinemia

DEFINITION/PRESENTATION

Waldenström macroglobulinemia is similar to myeloma in that there is an abnormal immunoglobulin made by plasmacytoid lymphocytes. Unlike myeloma, there are no bone, kidney, or calcium problems. Because Waldenström is caused by an IgM monoclonal gammopathy instead of the much smaller IgG, most of the symptoms are from **hyperviscosity**. Patients present with:

- **Blurred vision**
- Fatigue
- Headache and confusion
- Mucosal bleeding
- Dyspnea and heart failure

> Most of the symptoms in Waldenström relate directly to thickened plasma that blocks the delivery of oxygen to tissues.

▶ **TIP**

Don't confuse the hyperviscosity of Waldenström with leukostasis of blast crisis. The symptoms are the same, but the WBC count is normal.

> Rituximab first for Waldenström

TREATMENT

The "best initial step in management" is unquestionably **plasmapheresis** to eliminate the hyperviscosity.

Long-term management is to use chemotherapeutic agents to get rid of the abnormal plasma cells that make the immunoglobulin. These include:

Best initial therapy is rituximab. For severe disease, add cyclophosphamide. Alternatives are fludarabine, chlorambucil, and cladribine.

> Waldenström therapy looks like a collection of miscellaneous agents because there is no clear answer.

Hairy Cell Leukemia

Look for a middle-aged patient with:

- **Pancytopenia**
- **Massive splenomegaly** without lymphadenopathy
- No teardrop-shaped cells (distinguishes it from myelofibrosis)

> 90% will have hairy cells on blood or marrow smear.

If they want to hand you the diagnosis and ask you treatment, the stem of the question will describe "projections" on the cells. These are the "hairs" of the hairy cell leukemia. Hairy cells are found on both blood and marrow.

DIAGNOSTIC TESTS

> "Dry tap" + no teardrop-shaped cells = hairy cell leukemia

Most specific test is CD antigens on bone marrow. Tartrate resistant acid phosphatase (TRAP) is outdated and wrong.

The "best initial therapy" is **cladribine**, also known as 2-CDA.

LYMPHOMA

PRESENTATION

> Diagnose hairy cell by flow cytometry immunotyping, not TRAP.

Both Hodgkin disease (HD) and non-Hodgkin lymphoma (NHL) present with painless, non-tender enlargement of lymph nodes. Warmth, redness, and tenderness should make you answer infection to the "most likely diagnosis" question. The major difference between HD and NHL lies in their histology, and consequently their treatment. Also, HD is far more likely to be local to the neck with 80% to 90% in stage I or II. NHL is more likely to be widespread with 80% to 90% with stage III or IV. Hence, you rarely radiate NHL.

B Symptoms

The B symptoms are **fever**, **weight loss**, and drenching **night sweats**. They are indicative of more severe, widespread disease. Weight loss is defined as more than 10% loss of body weight.

DIAGNOSTIC TESTS

> Local lymphoma needs cycles of chemotherapy.

The best initial test for lymphoma is an excisional biopsy of the lymph nodes, rather than a fine-needle aspiration. It is necessary to see the entire architecture of the node to establish a diagnosis. This is because individual lymphocytes in lymphoma appear normal. This is like CLL and CML, in which the cells look normal on smear.

Once the diagnosis of lymphoma is made based on lymph node biopsy, flow cytometry, and FISH/cytogenetics, the next best step is to determine therapy. Localized Hodgkin disease (stages I and II) is treated with local radiation and ABVD chemotherapy. Advanced disease (stage III or IV, or any with B symptoms) is treated with ABVD or a more intensive chemotherapy regimen, possibly followed by hematopoietic stem cell transplant. Staging of lymphoma is indispensible to determine therapy.

▶ **TIP**

If the case describes widespread nodal involvement, staging tests are of no value.

Ann Arbor Staging System

Stage I: one lymph node group

Stage II: two lymph node groups on the same side of the diaphragm

Stage III: lymph nodes on both sides of the diaphragm

State IV: diffuse, widespread disease (e.g., bone marrow involvement)

If a patient has lymph node involvement in the neck, the staging evaluation would be to do CT scans of the chest, abdomen, and pelvis to see if there is a second group, particularly on the other side of the diaphragm. If the case describes lymph nodes in the pelvis, then staging is to scan the abdomen and chest. If all the CT and PET scans are normal, you must go as far as a bone marrow biopsy to detect occult disease.

> If you radiate the neck and there are nodes with lymphoma hidden in the abdomen or pelvis, the patient will die.

> Combination chemotherapy has a 1% per year risk of aplastic anemia and AML.

Adverse Effects of Common Chemotherapeutic Medications		
Medication	**Adverse effect**	**Method of assessment**
Adriamycin	Cardiotoxic	MUGA scan (nuclear ventriculogram)
Bleomycin	Pulmonary fibrosis	PFTs, diffusion of carbon monoxide
Vincristine, vinblastine	Peripheral neuropathy	Nerve conduction studies
Cyclophosphamide	Hemorrhagic cystitis	Cystoscopy

▶ **TIP**

Exploratory laparotomy and lymphangiogram are always wrong.

TREATMENT

The standard of care is ABVD for HD and CHOP for NHL. If the CD20 is positive in NHL, it is standard to add rituximab, the anti-CD20 antibody.

ABVD: adriamycin, bleomycin, vinblastine, dacarbazine

CHOP: cyclophosphamide, hydroxydaunorubicin, vincristine (Oncovin), prednisone

COAGULATION DISORDERS

Immune Thrombocytopenic Purpura

PRESENTATION

Immune thrombocytopenic purpura (ITP) can be classified as acute (generally occurring in childhood and self-resolving) or chronic (more common in adulthood). ITP can present with new episodes of bleeding (from mild gingival bleeding and epistaxis to life-threatening GI bleeds and intracranial hemorrhage), petechiae, and ecchymosis; or it can present as an incidental finding on a CBC.

▶ TIP

Always start with the type of bleeding when assessing a bleeding disorder. Don't start with the lab tests. If you start with lab tests, you will not get the correct answer.

DIAGNOSTIC TESTS

Antiplatelet antibodies are too nonspecific to be useful in the assessment of an acute episode of bleeding. Too many people in the general population have circulating antiplatelet antibodies to make them a useful test. They do not have the same specificity for ITP as a Coombs test does for hemolytic anemia. Anti-GPIIb/IIIa antibodies, on the other hand, are more specific; this test for ITP is far more similar to a Coombs test for hemolytic anemia.

Increased megakaryocytes in ITP are similar in significance to increased reticulocytes in anemia. Because megakaryocytes are found only in the bone marrow, this makes testing for an increased level of megakaryocytes accurate, but inconvenient. This is why when a patient presents with bleeding, the answer for "best initial step" or "what would you do first" is never megakaryocyte level.

Splenic enlargement is one of the few things that can decrease the platelet count without affecting the other cell lines. In the evaluation of thrombocytopenia, it is important to assess spleen size to see if that is the cause of the low platelets. A patient with ITP has a normal spleen size even though the spleen is the site of the destruction of the platelets.

Isolated low platelet count – splenomegaly = ITP

TREATMENT

The best initial therapy of ITP is based on the severity of the disease.

Mild bleeding, platelet count below 50,000/µL: prednisone

Bleeding repeatedly recurring after stopping steroids:

- Splenectomy leads to improvement in 70%
- Rituximab (anti-CD20 antibodies)

Dangerous/severe bleeding, platelet count below 10,000 to 20,000/μL:
IVIG or RHO(D) immune globulin (human) (RhoGAM). This is the fastest way to inhibit the destruction of platelets; both agents are both far more effective than giving a platelet transfusion in raising platelet counts.

Recurrent thrombocytopenia despite splenectomy:

- Rituximab (anti-CD20 antibodies)
- Eltrombopag and romiplostim: These are thrombopoietin receptor agonists that increase platelet counts when the ITP does not respond to steroids or to splenectomy. Recombinant human thrombopoietin has not been effective.
- Danazol is an anabolic steroid that has some benefit in raising the platelet count when the other therapies fail. Cyclophosphamide and azathioprine are also used in refractory cases.

> Eltrombopag and romiplostim stimulate platelet production directly from the megakaryocyte.

▶ **TIP**

Plasmapheresis does not help ITP. It is always a wrong answer in ITP.

Heparin-induced Thrombocytopenia

Heparin-induced thrombocytopenia (HIT) occurs with the use of any amount of heparin. It is an idiosyncratic allergic reaction and can occur equally with full-dose intravenous heparin or as small an amount as a heparin-coated catheter or a heparin flush. Low molecular weight heparin has a much lower risk of HIT compared with IV unfractionated heparin.

Which of the following is the most common manifestation of HIT?

a. Venous thrombosis
b. Arterial thrombosis
c. Mucosal bleeding
d. CNS bleeding
e. Gastrointestinal bleeding

Answer: The correct answer is (a). HIT leads to thrombosis, not bleeding. Although arterial clots can occur, venous thromboses are 3 to 4 times more common than arterial clots.

PRESENTATION

HIT presents with a drop in the platelet count several days after starting heparin. HIT causes venous thromboses such as DVT and pulmonary emboli. The platelets "clump," causing clots.

A 64-year-old woman is admitted with a pulmonary embolus secondary to intravenous unfractionated heparin.

What is the most appropriate management of this patient?

a. Switch to low molecular weight heparin
b. Decrease the dose
c. Transfuse platelets
d. Start warfarin
e. Switch heparin to argatroban

Answer: The correct answer is (e). If the patient has thrombocytopenia with IV unfractionated heparin, you cannot just switch to low molecular weight heparin, even though this agent gives less of a risk of thrombocytopenia than unfractionated heparin. You cannot effectively treat the clot by just switching to warfarin. Patients with HIT who must continue heparin should be treated with a direct-acting thrombin inhibitor such lepirudin, bivalirudin, or argatroban. If you transfuse platelets, you will make the clot worse.

> Fondaparinux has an extremely small risk of HIT.

DIAGNOSTIC TESTS

The best initial test is simply to look for a decrease in the number of platelets (below 150,000). Since the platelet count can start from very high, a drop in platelet count by 50% is consistent with HIT even though the platelet level is still normal.

The most accurate test is the **antiplatelet factor IV antibody** or the **serotonin release assay**.

TREATMENT

1. Stop all heparins including low molecular weight heparin.
2. If acute anticoagulation must be given, switch to a direct-acting thrombin inhibitor such as **lepirudin** or **argatroban**.
3. Delay the use of warfarin until the platelet count has recovered to above 100,000/μL.
4. Use thrombin inhibitors to **prevent** thrombosis in those in whom it has not yet developed.

> Avoid heparin permanently after an episode of HIT.

Thromboses may develop in as much as 20% to 50% of those with HIT who do not get treated with an anticoagulant. This is another excellent reason not to use heparin routinely in atrial fibrillation while waiting to achieve a therapeutic INR. Not only does the bolus of heparin put the patient at risk of bleeding, there is also the risk of thrombosis from HIT.

Von Willebrand Disease

PRESENTATION

Von Willebrand disease (VWD) presents with signs of bleeding related to platelets such as epistaxis, petechiae, menorrhagia, or gingival bleeding. Look for the phrase "worse after using aspirin." VWD has an enormous range of presentation because the deficiency of von Willebrand factor (VWF) is variable. Many patients have a borderline normal level that becomes abnormal only with the use of aspirin.

DIAGNOSTIC TESTS

CBC shows a normal platelet count. The bleeding time is prolonged, but this is a test with limited accuracy. The bleeding time is a functional test looking at platelet function in those with a normal platelet count. If VWF multimers or factor VIII levels are in the answer choices, they are the right answer.

The most specific tests are:

- VWF level
- Ristocetin cofactor assay (an in-vitro test of platelet function)

> The aPTT is elevated in 50% of patients because VWF and factor VIII coagulant (hemophilia factor) are bound to each other.

> Platelet type of bleeding plus a normal platelet count = von Willebrand disease

TREATMENT

The best initial therapy is desmopressin, which releases subendothelial stores of VWF and factor VIII. If there is no response to desmopressin, the "most appropriate next step in management" is to give factor VIII concentrate replacement, which contains VWF as well. Cryoprecipitate contains high levels of VWF.

▶ **TIP**

Cryoprecipitate is never the "best initial therapy" for anything.

Uremia-induced Platelet Dysfunction

Uremia causes a disorder of the release of the granules inside of platelets. The platelet number is normal but they do not degranulate. This is a direct result of the effect of uremia on the platelets. The best initial therapy is with desmopressin, which improves platelet activity.

Factor XI Deficiency

Factor XI deficiency causes an elevation of the aPTT but the prothrombin time (PT) stays normal. Under normal conditions there is no bleeding. Bleeding occurs in factor XI deficiency only under conditions of stress such as trauma or surgery. The best initial test to evaluate any type of bleeding seemingly related to clotting factor deficiency with an elevated PT or aPTT is a mixing study.

When the mixing study corrects to normal, the next best step is to measure the level of the specific clotting factor. When bleeding does occur, the "best initial therapy" is fresh frozen plasma.

Mixing Study

A mixing study is used to determine if the patient has a deficiency of a clotting factor. If the aPTT is elevated from a clotting factor deficiency, the test result will correct to normal when the patient's plasma is mixed 50:50 with a sample of normal plasma. This is based on the fact that the aPTT will not begin to elevate until the level of the factor decreases to less than 20% to 30% of normal.

Factor XII Deficiency

Factor XII deficiency is always detected by the accidental finding of an elevated aPTT on testing done for other reasons (incidental finding) or as part of pre-operative screening. **Patients with factor XII deficiency do not bleed. No treatment is needed.**

Factor XIII Deficiency

Factor XIII deficiency presents with **delayed bleeding after trauma**, surgery, or other injury. Factor XIII normally functions to cross-link clotting factors that have already been involved in forming a clot. Factor XIII functions as a stabilizer of clots. Factor XIII, however, is not part of the normal clotting cascade that begins at factor XII. When treatment is needed, **fresh frozen plasma** is the best initial step. Test with urea clot lysis time. A normal clot should be stable in 5M urea.

Liver Disease and Vitamin K Deficiency

All of the clotting factors are made in the liver with the exception of factor VIII and von Willebrand factor. Since vitamin K is responsible for the production of factors II, VII, IX, and X, the clinical presentation is nearly identical with an initial increase in PT followed by a prolonged aPTT. Liver disease will also be associated with a decrease in albumin, an elevated d-dimer (from decreased clearance), and thrombocytopenia from splenic sequestration. Treatment is with vitamin K orally, or fresh frozen plasma in the acute setting.

Disseminated Intravascular Coagulation

Disseminated intravascular coagulation (DIC) will not occur in a healthy person. DIC occurs in patients with severe, often overwhelming illness such as sepsis, amniotic fluid embolus, snake bites, burns, or crush injury. Besides elevation of both the PT and the aPTT, there will be low platelets, low serum fibrinogen, and evidence of hemolysis on the smear and in the labs. The most accurate test for the presence of DIC is elevation of the level of fibrin split products and d-dimers. The treatment of DIC is to correct the underlying cause and to replace both the clotting factors and the platelets.

THROMBOPHILIA OR HYPERCOAGULABLE STATES

All forms of thrombophilia present with abnormal clotting in people without the usual risk factors of immobility, trauma, surgery, pregnancy, or malignancy. Investigation should also occur when a stroke occurs in a young person (less than 45 years old).

Thrombophilia Questions

- **What is the most common cause of thrombophilia?** Factor V Leiden mutation. This disorder results in factor V becoming unresponsive to the usual inhibitory effects of protein C.
- **When do I answer an antithrombin deficiency?** When the case describes a patient who is placed on heparin but on whom it has no effect. Heparin works through potentiating the effects of antithrombin. If you give a bolus of heparin and there is no effect, the "most likely diagnosis" is antithrombin deficiency.
- **When do I answer protein C deficiency?** When the patient is placed on warfarin and the patient develops skin necrosis as an effect of the warfarin.
- **When do I answer lupus anticoagulant?** When the patient clots with an elevation of the aPTT and a normal PT.
- **When do I answer anticardiolipin antibody or antiphospholipid syndrome?** Look for a female patient with multiple first-trimester spontaneous abortions or one second-trimester spontaneous abortion.

A patient comes to the hospital with a pulmonary embolus developing after a long transatlantic flight.

What is the most appropriate action in the management of this patient?

a. Evaluate for thrombophilia
b. Evaluate for thrombophilia if there is a recurrence
c. No evaluation for thrombophilia
d. Evaluate for thrombophilia only if the clot recurs on warfarin

Answer: The correct answer is (a). Healthy people do not clot on long plane rides. The people who clot on long plane rides have a thrombophilia that is "unmasked" or produces clinical symptoms brought on by the extended period of immobility. This does not mean to do the tests immediately. You must wait for the person to be completed with 6 months of warfarin to get an accurate assessment for thrombophilia with the exception of factor V mutation and prothrombin-20210 mutation.

> The only thrombophilia with an elevated aPTT is the lupus anticoagulant.

DIAGNOSTIC TESTS

Most diagnostic tests for the etiology of thrombophilia are not accurate at the time of the acute thrombosis. This is because protein C and protein S are vitamin K–dependent anticoagulations. In addition, antithrombin and lupus anticoagulant testing is not accurate during the use of heparin.

The only tests that are accurate during the time of the acute thrombosis are:

- Factor V mutation
- Prothrombin 20210 mutation

The "most accurate test" for the cause of thrombophilia is to wait 6 months until the end of anticoagulation. Perform the evaluation one month after stopping warfarin.

TREATMENT

The intensity and duration of anticoagulation in a person with thrombophilia is:

- Target INR 2 to 3
- Duration 6 months

There is no conclusive proof that lifelong anticoagulation should be given. **The strongest potential indication for lifelong anticoagulation is with the antiphospholipid syndromes.**

TRANSFUSION REACTIONS

Major Blood Group (ABO) Incompatibility

Look for the sudden onset of back pain, hypotension, shortness of breath, confusion, tachycardia, and dark urine specifically described as occurring "during the transfusion." Renal failure can occur from the toxic effect of hemoglobin on the kidney tubule. The "best initial step" is to stop the transfusion. The most common cause is administrative error in which the wrong person's blood is administered to the patient. Treatment is with:

- Hydration, mannitol, and oxygen
- Epinephrine for anaphylaxis
- Dopamine or norepinephrine as needed to maintain blood pressure

Minor Blood Group Reaction (Delayed Hemolytic Reaction)

Reactions between the numerous minor blood groups (e.g., rH, Kell, Duffy, Lewis, Kidd) present with fever and jaundice 7 to 14 days after the transfusion. There will also be a failure of the expected rise in hematocrit with lab studies consistent with hemolysis. There is no specific therapy. It will resolve on its own without fatality, renal failure, or hyperkalemia.

> TRALI is fatal in 5% to 10%. The rest recover.

Transfusion-related Acute Lung Injury

This reaction is also called a "leukoagglutination reaction." Transfusion-related acute lung injury (TRALI) is from antibodies in the donor plasma attacking and agglutinating neutrophils in the recipient. This causes the precipitation of WBC in the microcirculation of the lung. This results in modest but transient shortness of breath in less than 6 hours following transfusion. TRALI can mimic ARDS and volume overload. Therapy is supportive care, as with mechanical ventilation. Resolution should occur in 3 to 4 days.

Febrile Nonhemolytic Transfusion Reaction

This mild elevation in temperature of about 1°C is the most common transfusion reaction. The reaction is of recipient antibodies against donor WBC antigens. No therapy is needed for the acute event except to give antipyretics. Leukocyte reduction filters are done to prevent recurrences.

> Blood donations should be routinely WBC depleted.

Urticarial Reactions

Wheals and urticaria can occur from the reaction of recipient antibodies against donor plasma proteins. Bronchospasm may occur. The acute reaction is managed with antihistamines. Subsequent reactions are prevented by transfusing washed red cells. If you wash the plasma proteins off the donor blood, the reaction will not occur.

Transfusion Reactions	
Type of reaction	**Mechanism**
Minor blood group reaction	Recipient antibodies against donor minor blood groups
TRALI	Donor antibody against recipient WBCs
Febrile nonhemolytic reaction	Recipient antibody against donor WBCs
Urticarial reaction	Recipient antibody against donor plasma proteins

INFECTIOUS DISEASES   9

CENTRAL NERVOUS SYSTEM INFECTIONS

"WHAT IS THE MOST LIKELY DIAGNOSIS?"

All of the infections of the central nervous system (CNS) present with **fever** and **headache**. In addition, any of them can also have:

- Nausea and vomiting
- Seizures

There is considerable overlap in the additional findings of:

- Focal neurological abnormalities
- Confusion and altered mental status
- Neck stiffness or nuchal rigidity

If the question describes more than one of these findings (**stiff neck, focal abnormalities, confusion**) you cannot answer the "most likely diagnosis" question without additional information. These patients **will need a head CT or a lumbar puncture** to establish a diagnosis. If the question describes only one of them, you can answer the question.

Answering the "Most Likely Diagnosis" Question	
Presentation	**Most likely diagnosis**
Stiff neck (nuchal rigidity)	Meningitis
Confusion	Encephalitis
Focal neurological abnormalities	Abscess

▶ TIP

The advantage of a board examination is that the questions say "What is the most likely diagnosis?" not "What is the diagnosis?" If they want you to know the answer, they have to tell you something.

219

Meningitis

PRESENTATION

Meningitis does not always give all of the manifestations of fever, headache, nuchal rigidity, and photophobia at the same time. However, if you are expected to be able to answer the question about diagnosis, then most will have to be shown.

> At least one-third of patients with meningitis have focal neurological deficits and/or altered mental status.

> Hearing loss is the most common neurological complication of meningitis.

▶ **TIP**

Answer **meningococcus** when shown:

- **Young adult**
- **Petechial** rash
- Thousands of neutrophils on cerebrospinal fluid (CSF) culture

DIAGNOSTIC TESTS

The **most accurate test** for bacterial meningitis is a **culture of the cerebrospinal fluid**. The best initial test is the CSF cell count. Culture is never available at the time of initial presentation. Hence, in infectious diseases, with rare exception, all treatment is initiated empirically—that is, without a culture to guide you.

Accuracy of Diagnostic Testing in Bacterial Meningitis			
Test of CSF	**Sensitivity**	**Specificity**	**Bottom line**
Culture	90%–95%	Almost 100%	Culture is great, but never available at the time you are starting treatment.
Gram stain	60%–70%	>95%	If the stain is positive, it is extremely specific. A negative Gram stain is useless.
Protein	Very high	Very low	**Any kind of meningitis can elevate the protein.** A normal protein excludes bacterial meningitis.
Glucose	Poor	Poor	Severe bacterial meningitis sometimes has a CSF glucose of less than 60% of serum.
Bacterial antigen detection	60%–90%	Almost 100%	Bacterial antigen testing is useful in those given antibiotics before a culture is obtained. It is close to Gram stain in accuracy.
Cell count	>95%–98%	Modest	Very high neutrophil count is fairly specific for bacterial meningitis.

Protein levels are extremely nonspecific. Not only can every type of infection raise the CSF protein level, but trauma, dementia, and autoimmune disorders such as Guillain-Barré syndrome also raise the protein level.

Cell Count

The CSF cell count is the most important initial step in determining if there is meningitis. In addition, the differential on the cell count is the best you can do to distinguish acute bacterial meningitis from the many causes of an elevated lymphocyte count. You cannot distinguish the specific bacterial pathogen without a CSF culture.

Who Has to Get a Head CT before a Lumbar Puncture?

CT before lumbar puncture (LP) is the answer when there is:

- **Papilledema**
- **Focal neurological deficits**
- **Seizure or severe confusion**

CT is also "strongly considered" for any immunocompromised patient. Although it is possible to still have a small mass lesion without these findings, it is not clinically relevant. If the lesion is too small to cause focal findings or papilledema, then it is too small to cause cerebral herniation. You cannot adequately perform a neurological examination on an uncooperative or confused patient.

▶ **TIP**

If a CT is needed before an LP, the answer is "first give antibiotics." Don't send patients off to the CT scan to let their brain "fry" from an infection without giving antibiotics.

Etiology of Bacterial Meningitis

Pneumococcus is the most common cause of bacterial meningitis in adults. The environmental reservoir of pneumococcus has never been identified. *Listeria* should be suspected if the patient is immunocompromised or pregnant. By definition, elderly patients (older than 70) and neonates are immunocompromised. Suspicion for *Listeria* from the history is indispensable because you must **add ampicillin to treatment.** *Listeria* is **resistant to cephalosporins** and vancomycin.

Summary of Bacterial Meningitis	
Organism	**Associations**
Pneumococcus (most common, 60%–70%)	Reservoir unknown, trauma, CSF leak
Neisseria meninigitidis	Young, healthy, military, college students
Haemophilus influenzae	Rare since introduction of group B vaccine
Listeria monocytogenes	Immunocompromised
Staphylococcus aureus	Neurosurgery, penetrating trauma, skin damage

---

Normal CSF protein excludes bacterial meningitis.

Without culture, the CSF characteristics (cell count, protein, glucose, color) **cannot** distinguish between:
1. Pneumococcus
2. Neisseria
3. Listeria
4. Staphylococcus
5. Haemophilus

Thousands of neutrophils = acute bacterial meningitis

You can't detect a focal neurological abnormality without an accurate neurological examination.

Better to have a false negative CSF culture than an accurate test with brain damage.

Add ampicillin for:
- Elderly
- Pregnant
- Immunocompromised

Treatment of Bacterial Meningitis

Initial treatment is started without knowing the results of culture. When the CSF cell count shows thousands of neutrophils, the "next best step in management" is to start:

- Ceftriaxone + vancomycin + glucocorticoids (usually dexamethasone)

If **immunocompromised** (risk of *Listeria*):

- **Add ampicillin** to ceftriaxone/vancomycin/dexamethasone.

Eliminating the Nasopharyngeal Carrier State for Meningococcus

The close contacts of patients with *Neisseria meningitidis* should receive either rifampin or ciprofloxacin to prevent nasopharyngeal colonization and a "carrier" state. Ceftriaxone and azithromycin are considered alternatives. Prophylaxis should be given within 24 hours of identification of the source case.

Preventing/eliminating the carrier state of meningococcus is the entire reason that meningitis patients are placed on respiratory isolation (droplet precautions).

The hardest issue is **who is considered a "close contact" for meningococcus.** These are:

- **Household** contacts
- Anyone with possible **salivary** contact (kissing, eating utensils)
- Healthcare workers only if in direct contact with oral or respiratory secretions with mouth-to-mouth resuscitation.

Who is not considered a "close contact" for meningococcus?

- Routine school and work contacts
- Routine contact with healthcare workers

Meningococcal prophylaxis is not needed if a respiratory mask is used for ventilation.

▶ **TIP**

The most common question brings a "routine" school or work contact to your office requesting prophylaxis for meningococcus. The answer is "reassurance" only.

Listeria monocytogenes

Special considerations for *Listeria* are:

- Occurs in pregnant, elderly, or immunocompromised patients
- Must add ampicillin or penicillin to empiric therapy
- Use trimethoprim/sulfamethoxazole in the penicillin allergic.

Neisseria meningitidis

Special consideration for meningococcus are:

- Respiratory isolation is indicated.
- Give rifampin or ciprofloxacin for close contacts.

- Look for a **young adult** in the **military** or a dormitory with **petechial rash** and neutrophils in CSF.
- When recurrent episodes occur, test for terminal complement (C5–C9) deficiency.
- Don't give prophylaxis to medical students or nurses unless intubation or respiratory secretion contact is specifically described.

A patient comes to the emergency department with fever, headache, stiff neck, and photophobia for the last 6 hours. On physical examination he has a gaze palsy and weakness of his left arm.

What is the next best step in the management of this patient?

a. Head CT
b. Lumbar puncture
c. Ceftriaxone
d. Ceftriaxone and dexamethasone
e. Ceftriaxone, vancomycin, and dexamethasone

Answer: The correct answer is (e). When a patient has a presentation consistent with acute bacterial meningitis and there is a contraindication to doing an immediate lumbar puncture, the most important step is to give antibiotics. In questions like this one, the contraindication to the lumbar puncture is most often recognized. The major mistake is to send the patient for a CT scan instead of starting treatment. The patient does need a head CT, but he needs to start treatment even more.

Nonbacterial Meningitis (CSF Lymphocytosis)

There are numerous causes of an elevated CSF lymphocyte count. In the past this was referred to as "aseptic" meningitis. Aseptic simply means nonbacterial.

- All can elevate the protein.
- None is visible on Gram stain.
- None grows on bacterial culture media.
- They are indistinguishable without other features in the history or lab testing.

Meningitis characterized by an increased CSF lymphocyte count is caused by:

- *Cryptococcus*
- Tuberculosis
- Rocky mountain spotted fever (Rickettsia)
- Lyme
- Viruses

Cryptococcal Meningitis

HIV/AIDS is the most common risk for cryptococcal meningitis. Without AIDS in the history, there is no specific CSF finding that would compel you to answer "India ink" or "cryptococcal antigen" as the diagnostic tests.

Cryptococcus does not form a spore at room temperature, but it is inhaled. The precise source is not clear in most patients.

Cryptococcus acts like the dimorphic fungi (the causes of histoplasmosis, blastomycosis, and coccidioidomycosis) that exist as spores in the environment and then germinate into a growing yeast in the warm 98.6°F environment of the body. **All of these:**

> The dimorphic fungi (spore in the environment, yeast in the body) do not need antifungal treatment in immunocompetent hosts without dissemination.

- Enter through the respiratory system
- Occur more frequently, but not exclusively, in AIDS
- Disseminate to the brain, bone, skin, and prostate
- Are self-limited in immunocompetent hosts and feel like a transient "viral syndrome"
- Do not need treatment unless disseminated

Cryptococcal meningitis differs from bacterial meningitis in that it:

- Is slower in onset
- Does **not** usually have fever, headache, stiff neck, and photophobia all present at the same time
- May have a normal CSF WBC count

DIAGNOSTIC TESTS

India ink: The "best initial test" of CSF. India ink is like a Gram stain. It is 60% to 70% sensitive, but nearly 100% specific when it is positive.

> Serum and CSF antigen testing seem to have equal accuracy.

Cryptococcal antigen: The antigen is more than 95% sensitive and specific.

Fungal culture: The only test more specific than an antigen test. The culture needs more time than an antigen detection method.

TREATMENT

The **best initial therapy** is **amphotericin and flucytosine**. After several weeks, this is followed by fluconazole. If the CD4 count goes up above 100/µl, then fluconazole can be stopped. If the CD4 stays low, then lifelong fluconazole is needed. Caspofungin and the other echinocandins will not treat cryptococcosis. Liposomal amphotericin is used only if there is renal insufficiency. The greatest predictor of mortality is:

- Low CSF cell count (<20 HPF)
- High opening pressure of CSF (>250 mm H_2O)
- High antigen titer (>1:1024)

> Adding flucytosine to amphotericin sterilizes the CSF faster than using amphotericin alone.

Antiretroviral therapy should not be started at the same time as the initial treatment of cryptococcal meningitis or any other opportunistic infection. Immune reconstitution syndrome is a rare, idiosyncratic worsening of AIDS just after initiating antiretroviral therapy.

Daily lumbar puncture is indicated in signs of increased intracranial pressure to maintain CSF pressure < 200 mm H_2O.

▶ **TIP**

The worst mortality from *Cryptococcus* is in those with the lowest CSF cell counts.

A man with AIDS comes to the office for routine evaluation. He is asymptomatic and has recently found he is HIV positive. His CD4 count is 18/μl and his viral load is 450,000 copies.

What would you recommend?

a. Trimethoprim/sulfamethoxazole (TMP-SMX), azithromycin, and fluconazole
b. TMP-SMX, azithromycin, and antiretrovirals
c. TMP-SMX, azithromycin, fluconazole, and antiretrovirals
d. TMP-SMX, azithromycin, fluconazole, antiretrovirals, and ganciclovir
e. TMP-SMX, azithromycin, antiretrovirals, and ganciclovir

Answer: The correct answer is (b). There is no routine antifungal prophylaxis with fluconazole for Cryptococcus. Antiretroviral medications should be started under 500 CD4 cells, pneumocystis pneumonia prophylaxis under 200, and atypical mycobacterial prophylaxis under 50 CD4/μl. Routine cytomegalovirus prophylaxis is not indicated either.

Tuberculous Meningitis

Tuberculous meningitis is extremely rare, occurring in less than 1% of those with tuberculosis (TB). Look for meningitis when you see:

- Lung lesions
- A recent immigrant
- Extremely high CSF protein level

The sensitivity of a single acid-fast (AFB) smear is less than 10%. The "most accurate test" is:

- Take three high-volume CSF samples for culture.
- Centrifuge the samples to concentrate the organisms.

> PCR is only 60% sensitive for CSF TB infection.

TREATMENT

TB meningitis is treated in the same way as pulmonary tuberculosis, except:

- Add dexamethasone to decrease neurologic complications
- Extend the length of treatment

Rocky Mountain Spotted Fever

Rocky Mountain spotted fever (RMSF) is caused by *Rickettsia rickettsii* in the geographic distribution of its tick vector. RMSF is the answer when the case describes:

> Of patients with RMSF, 60% will recall a tick bite.

- Petechial rash moving from the wrists and ankles inwards toward the body (centripetal pattern)
- Camping or hiking
- Many nonspecific symptoms such as arthralgias, myalgias, headache, and fever

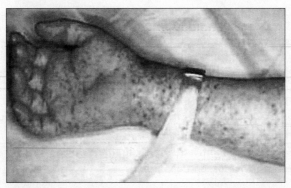

Figure 9.1: Rocky Mountain spotted fever. The rash of RMSF starts at the wrists and ankles and moves toward the trunk.

Source: Conrad Fischer, MD

DIAGNOSTIC TESTS/TREATMENT

RMSF is detected with serologic testing in 95% of cases, but the indirect fluorescent antibody test will take as long as 2 to 3 weeks to become positive. Skin biopsy is more difficult to obtain, but can give a definite diagnosis immediately. Doxycycline is the best initial therapy, even for children.

Lyme

Lyme is geographically localized to the northeastern United States in Connecticut, Massachusetts, New Jersey, and New York. **Only 20% of patients will recall a tick bite** because the tick is so small. Because there is nothing specific on CSF in terms of cell count, stain, or protein level, you will answer Lyme as the diagnosis when there is:

PCR has poor sensitivity in detecting CNS Lyme.	

- History of hiking/camping in endemic area
- Previous "target-shaped" rash
- Joint pain, AV block, or facial palsy

The most accurate test is the ELISA or Western blot of the CSF. Treatment is with intravenous ceftriaxone, cefotaxime, or penicillin. Lyme titers are higher in CSF than serum.

Do not perform serologic testing on asymptomatic tick bites.	

▶ **TIP**

There is no such disease as "chronic Lyme disease." A prolonged (months-long) course of antibiotics for Lyme is never the right answer.

Permanent pacemaker is usually not needed in Lyme.	

Viral Meningitis

Although viral meningitis is the most common cause of "aseptic" meningitis, there is no routine testing performed to confirm the etiology of viral meningitis. This is because there is no specific therapy for any of them except for herpes simplex. Herpes simplex can cause viral meningitis; however, because there is often prompt resolution without additional therapy, testing is rarely done.

> NSAIDs at high doses can cause aseptic meningitis.

Etiology of CSF Lymphocytosis			
When this is in the history or physical...	**Then this is the "most likely diagnosis"**	**Best initial and most accurate test**	**Treatment**
AIDS, <50 CD4 cells	Cryptococcal meningitis	India ink, cryptococcal antigen	Amphotericin, then fluconazole
Immigrant, lung lesions, very high CSF protein	Tuberculous meningitis	Acid fast stain and mycobacterial culture	Add steroids to usual TB treatment, extend length of treatment
Camper/hiker with rash moving toward the trunk	Rocky Mountain spotted fever	Serology 95% sensitive over time; skin biopsy immediate with 70% sensitivity	Doxycycline
Tick bite, rash, joint pain, or carditis in the past	Lyme	Serology	IV ceftriaxone, cefotaxime
Eosinophils on CSF, travel in Southeast Asia	*Angiostrongylus cantonensis*	ELISA	Prednisone
None	Viral	None needed	None
NSAIDs, IVIG	Drug-induced	Exclude other causes	Stop drug

Encephalitis

Although there are many causes of encephalitis, the most common—and most treatable—cause is herpes simplex. Look for the acute onset of:

- **Fever**
- **Headache**
- **Confusion**, altered mental status, disorientation

Patients may also have nuchal rigidity and focal neurological abnormalities, but there is no way to confirm a diagnosis of encephalitis if all of these findings are present simultaneously.

> Encephalitis increases CSF lymphocyte count.

Best initial test: CT scan of the head may show abnormalities of the temporal lobe in 20% to 50% of patients. MRI is abnormal in 90%.

Most accurate test: PCR of the CSF for herpes simplex is 95% to 99% sensitive and specific. The PCR is more accurate than a brain biopsy.

Best initial therapy: Begin with acyclovir.

> In patients with encephalitis, 85% will have an increased number of CSF red blood cells.

▶ **TIP**

EEG will be one of the choices for "best diagnostic test." Although 80% of patients will show an abnormality, the EEG is neither sensitive nor specific enough to be useful.

Brain Abscess

ETIOLOGY

Brain abscess can arise from any cause of bacteremia in which seeding of the brain occurs. In addition, local infection in the sinuses or otitis media can spread contiguously into the brain. The microbiology is incredibly diverse:

- Anaerobes: 65%
- Streptococci: 35%
- Staphylococci: 35%
- Gram-negative bacilli: 35%

How can the causative organisms add up to 170%? Because brain abscess is polymicrobial in one-third to two-thirds of patients.

PRESENTATION/"WHAT IS THE MOST LIKELY DIAGNOSIS?"

Brain abscess presents with:

- Fever (50%)
- Headache (more than 80%)
- Focal neurological deficits (50%)
- Papilledema (25%)

Although **stiff neck (15%)** and **seizures (25%)** occur, their presence will not help you confirm a diagnosis before performing CT or MRI of the brain. If the question describes nuchal rigidity in addition to fever, headache, and focal findings, it is impossible to answer the "most likely diagnosis" question without imaging studies.

DIAGNOSTIC TESTS

The best initial test is either a CT or an MRI. The most accurate test is a brain biopsy. Neuroimaging cannot distinguish cancer from infection. Both can give contrast-enhancing mass lesions of the brain. Brain biopsy is indispensible in order to guide therapy. Brain biopsy is not essential if:

- Blood cultures are positive
- The patient has AIDS with fewer than 100 CD4 cells/μl

Local infection spread into brain is the most common route of brain abscess.

TREATMENT

It is impossible to construct empiric therapy for a clinical entity with such diverse microbiologic causes. In fact, there is no way to be sure from CT or MRI alone whether the lesion is cancer or infection. While awaiting biopsy results, empiric treatment is with:

> Empiric therapy is temporary only until culture results from a biopsy or blood culture are known.

- **Cefepime** (or ceftriaxone)

and

- **Metronidazole**

and

- **Vancomycin** (or linezolid)

Diagnosis of Contrast-enhancing Brain Lesions in AIDS

If the question describes a patient with a "ring" or **contrast-enhancing mass** lesion of the brain and **AIDS with fewer than 100 CD4** cells, then the "next best step in management" is:

1. Treat with pyrimethamine and sulfadiazine for 10 to 14 days.
2. Repeat the scan after treatment.
3. If smaller, continue treatment indefinitely.
4. If unchanged or larger, perform a brain biopsy.

In general, the response to a specific therapy is a very poor method of confirming a diagnosis; however, it is acceptable in the case of AIDS. Ring-enhancing mass lesions in patients with low CD4 cell counts are caused by either toxoplasmosis (60%) or lymphoma (30%). In addition, pyrimethamine and sulfadiazine is extremely narrow-range therapy. Nothing else except toxoplasmosis should respond to these medications.

Nocardiosis

ETIOLOGY

Nocardiosis is an infection of the lung, brain, and skin from the aerobic, Gram-positive actinomycete *Nocardia*. Nocardiosis is much **more common in immunocompromised people**. The primary portal of entry is **the lungs**. *Nocardia* then disseminates to the:

- **Brain (meningitis, abscess)**
- **Skin**

DIAGNOSTIC TESTS/TREATMENT

Nocardia is a unique organism. It is Gram-positive, but appears as:

- Branching and filamentous
- **Partially acid-fast positive**

Detection is best performed on a biopsy specimen rather than an expectorated sputum sample.

Treat with TMP-SMX. Alternative therapy is with:

- Third-generation cephalosporins (ceftriaxone, cefotaxime)
- Imipenem
- Amikacin

HEAD AND NECK INFECTIONS

Otitis Media

Since there is no radiologic test of otitis media, the diagnosis is based entirely on the physical examination. The most sensitive physical finding is **immobility of the tympanic membrane**.

Otitis media is associated with **redness, bulging, decreased light reflex**, pain, and sometimes fever. However, if the tympanic membrane is freely mobile on pneumatic insufflation (otoscopy), otitis media is not present.

ETIOLOGY

Otitis media is caused by:

- *Streptococcus pneumoniae*
- *Haemophilus influenzae*
- *Moraxella catarrhalis*

TREATMENT

The best initial therapy is amoxicillin.

Penicillin Allergic Patients

Rash only: cefdinir, ceftibuten, cefpodoxime, cefuroxime

Anaphylaxis: azithromycin, clarithromycin

If Amoxicillin Fails:
- Amoxicillin-clavulanate (Augmentin)
- Cefuroxime
- Cefdinir
- Ceftriaxone

Sinusitis

Sinusitis is most often an acute viral infection that resolves spontaneously either without treatment or with decongestants to open drainage.

Signs of a more serious infection that needs testing and antibiotics are:

1. • Discolored nasal discharge
2. • Fever
3. • Headache, face pain, tooth pain

When these symptoms are clear, there is no need for imaging studies and the answer to the "next best step in management" question is give antibiotics.

Which of the following is the most accurate diagnostic test of sinusitis?

a. X-ray
b. CT
c. MRI
d. Culture of the nasal discharge
e. Sinus aspirate/biopsy for culture

Answer: The correct answer is (e). A radiologic test is never the most accurate diagnostic test in infectious diseases. Culturing the discharge of the sinuses is useless since it will not tell what is inside the sinuses. Although not often necessary, the aspirate of the sinuses is the most accurate test.

TREATMENT

The majority of sinusitis cases are viral in etiology and do not require antibiotics. They will resolve spontaneously. Look for a case with:

• No fever
• No face tenderness
• Clear or whitish nasal discharge

The answer for these cases is:

1. Inhaled steroids
2. No antibiotics
3. Decongestants

There is no single distinct first therapy. Correct choices are:

• Amoxicillin with clavulanic acid
• TMP/SMZ
• Cefdinir, cefuroxime, or cefpodoxime

▶ **TIP**

The strongest educational interest of the boards is to make sure you know who **does not need antibiotics. Prevention of overtreatment is** the main educational objective.

Pharyngitis

Pharyngitis presents with:

- Sore throat/pain
- Adenopathy
- Exudate
- Possible fever
- The **absence** of hoarseness and cough

When all of these features are present, there is an extremely high likelihood of the presence of Group A beta-hemolytic streptococci (or *Streptococcus pyogenes*).

The best initial test is rapid antigen detection testing. This is a latex agglutination test that becomes positive with the specific strains of streptococci that are associated with rheumatic fever and glomerulonephritis.

The most accurate test is a throat culture and the best initial therapy is a penicillin (pen VK, ampicillin, amoxicillin).

> **Treat strep pharyngitis to prevent rheumatic fever.**

▶ **TIP**

Gram stain of the throat is never a correct answer; everyone has streptococci in the throat.

The key issue for pharyngitis is: Do we have to do a throat culture if the rapid antigen detection test is negative? The answer to this question in adults is is yes if most of the other features of pharyngitis are there.

In adults, we need to confirm each negative rapid strep test with a culture. This is if there is exudate, adenopathy, and fever. High pretest likelihood of strep means you need to confirm negative rapid strep test with a culture.

> **Positive rapid strep test = positive culture**

Influenza

Influenza presents with the abrupt onset of:

- Fever, myalgia, headache
- Malaise, cough, sore throat

Diagnostic Tests

When the diagnosis is unclear, the best initial tests are:

- Enzyme immunoassay (EIA) antigen detection
- Neuraminidase detection assay
- Real-time PCR (can be done in under 2 hours)
- Fluorescent antibody staining

> **Speed is essential in an influenza detection test.**

TREATMENT

Influenza A and B cannot be distinguished from clinical symptoms. Since amantadine is no longer indicated for routine use in influenza, there is no point in the speciation of the organism. The main issue for influenza is:

- Oseltamivir and zanamivir are indicated within the first 48 hours of the onset of symptoms.
- These agents have no benefit in the management of influenza pneumonia.

Influenza vaccine is recommended **yearly** for **everyone older than 6 months.** Use inactivated, injectable flu vaccine in everyone over age 50 or with underlying illness.

> Egg allergy is no longer a contraindication to flu vaccination injection.

> A test that returns a result in 2 days is useless if medications are to be given within 48 hours of the onset of symptoms.

LUNG INFECTIONS

"WHAT IS THE MOST LIKELY DIAGNOSIS?"

All lung infections present with fever and cough. What additional features are present to allow you to answer the "most likely diagnosis" questions?

Bronchitis:

- Modest amounts of sputum
- Minimal or absent fever
- Normal chest x-ray

Lung abscess:

- High fever
- Foul-smelling sputum
- Weight loss

> Pneumonia has a fever and cough with any degree of sputum.

> Yearly flu vaccine is universal in everyone older than 6 months.

▶ **TIP**

You cannot definitively answer the "most likely diagnosis" question for pneumonia by history and physical alone.

DIAGNOSTIC TESTS

The "best initial test" for all lung infections is a chest x-ray; however, this is not the same thing as assessing severity. You cannot assess the severity of pneumonia by chest x-ray. This is why chest x-ray findings are never part of the criteria to determine the need for admission.

The most accurate test for lung infections is first a sputum culture, but this test is enormously limited. Bronchoscopy and lung biopsy are both more accurate.

Limitations on the Sputum Testing

Sputum analysis is 50% sensitive at best.

Sputum testing is controversial. It is not necessary for routine cases of bronchitis. Even for cases of community-acquired pneumonia (CAP), it is **not clear** whether sputum Gram stain and culture should be done routinely. Many forms of pneumonia and bronchitis are not visible on Gram stain and do not grow on routine blood agar culture media. For abscess, sputum is not accurate because anaerobes are part of commensal oral flora. Even when you stain, culture, and evaluate sputum in every way, a diagnosis is obtained in only about 50% of patients.

▶ **TIP**

The most important question for respiratory infection is not the etiology, but determining the severity.

Critical Tests for Respiratory Infection

Blood pressure and respiratory rate are more important in assessing any respiratory infection.

In infectious diseases, you rarely have the determination of a specific organism at the time the decision is made for either admission or the choice of antibiotics. The most important tests are therefore the ones that determine a need for admission.

- ABG/oximeter
- Sodium
- BUN and creatinine

Summary of Lung Infections			
	Bronchitis	**Pneumonia**	**Abscess**
Past history	Can be healthy, but more frequent with COPD and underlying lung disease	Older smokers with chronic heart, lung, liver, or kidney disease or cancer	Alcoholics who aspirate and those with seizures, stroke, intoxication, or intubation
Fever	Absent to mild	Mild to severe	Severe and persistent
Sputum	Clear to purulent	Variable	High volume, foul smelling
Chest x-ray	Normal	Lobar infiltrates vs. bilateral interstitial infiltrates	Cavity that can have an air-fluid level and a thick wall

Bronchitis

DEFINITION

Bronchitis is defined as an acute, mild respiratory illness with a normal chest x-ray. It is important to distinguish:

- Acute bronchitis in healthy adults
- Exacerbation of COPD induced by acute bronchitis (or worsening of chronic bronchitis)

PRESENTATION

Acute bronchitis in a generally healthy adult is an extremely **benign, self-limited infection** often caused by viruses that does not need antibiotic treatment. These patients:

- Are **not hypoxic**
- Have normal pulse, blood pressure, and respiratory rate

Acute bronchitis as a cause of an exacerbation of COPD can induce:

- High-volume sputum
- Change in sputum character (becoming purulent)
- Abnormal auscultory findings on lung examination
- Hypoxia

DIAGNOSTIC TESTS

The answer for most causes of acute bronchitis is:

- No sputum stain
- No sputum culture
- No chest x-ray

You will answer "x-ray" if the case describes:

- Respiratory distress/hyperventilation
- Tachycardia or hypotension
- Consolidation on lung examination (e.g., rales and rhonchi)

TREATMENT

Acute, uncomplicated bronchitis in a generally healthy patient should not routinely be treated with antibiotics. There is no convincing evidence that azithromycin, doxycycline, or TMP-SMX is better than placebo or vitamin C.

> Acute bronchitis in a healthy person needs no antibiotics.

Bronchitis as a cause of COPD exacerbation is treated with antibiotics if the patient has:

- Increased dyspnea
- Increased sputum volume
- Increased sputum purulence

Pneumonia

Pneumonia is separated into:

- Community-acquired pneumonia
- Hospital-acquired pneumonia

• Ventilator-associated pneumonia

All forms of pneumonia present with fever, cough, and sputum, and are diagnosed with x-ray. The main difference between them is:

• Severity
• Microbiology

Community-Acquired Pneumonia

DEFINITION/ETIOLOGY

Community-acquired pneumonia (CAP) is defined as pneumonia developing before admission or within 48 hours of admission. The most common cause of CAP in adults is *Streptococcus pneumoniae*. Pneumococcus is the most common cause no matter what the group or the underlying illness. The other causes may alter based on underlying disease, but the most common cause is always pneumococcus.

> There is no utility in learning to match any particular sputum color with any specific organism.

Other Causes of CAP and Their Associations	
Predisposing condition/Unique presentation	**Organism**
Recent viral syndrome	*Staphylococcus aureus*
Young, healthy patients, hemolysis	*Mycoplasma pneumoniae*
Animal exposure	*Coxiella burnetii* (Q fever)
Dry environments, joint pain, erythema nodosum	Coccidioidomycoses
GI symptoms: nausea, vomiting, abdominal pain, diarrhea CNS symptoms: headache, lethargy Hyponatremia	*Legionella*
Alcoholism	*Klebsiella pneumoniae*

> Hyponatremia is most often associated with *Legionella*.

DIAGNOSTIC TESTS

The best initial test for any serious respiratory illness is an x-ray.

"Lobar" infiltrates are most likely associated with bacterial organisms such as:

• Pneumococcus
• *Staphylococcus*
• *Haemophilus*
• *Klebsiella*

"Bilateral interstitial" infiltrates are most likely associated with organisms such as:

- *Pneumocystis jirovecii* (pneumocystis pneumonia, or PCP)
- *Mycoplasma*
- *Chlamydophila* (formerly *Chlamydia*)
- Viral
- *Coxiella*

Specific Diagnostic Tests for Each Organism	
Organism	**Specific diagnostic test**
Mycoplasma	Cold agglutinins, serology
Legionella	Urine antigen
Coxiella	Serology
Pneumococcus	Urine antigen
Pneumocystis	Bronchoalveolar lavage

TREATMENT

Treatment of pneumonia is based on the severity of disease. It is extraordinarily unlikely to have a specific organism identified at the time that a treatment decision is made.

Criteria for Inpatient Treatment

Admission to the hospital is based on severity of disease. It is not based on the specific organism, since **you don't know the organism at the time of admission**, or on the chest x-ray findings although pleural effusion is a sign of greater severity. Severity is not based on the number of lobes of the lung involved.

Pneumonia is considered "severe" when there is:

- **Hypoxia** or respiratory distress
- **Hypotension**
- Tachycardia and fever
- **Altered mental status** or confusion
- Hyponatremia
- Elevated BUN and creatinine from dehydration

Additional criteria for severity are "risks" for a poor outcome such as:

- Advanced age
- Chronic heart, lung, liver, or kidney disease
- Malignancy
- Steroid use, AIDS, or diabetes
- Splenectomy

Initial treatment in infectious disease is almost always empiric except for:
- AIDS
- Tuberculosis
- Syphilis

It's not based on the etiology; it's based on the severity.

> Individual presentation is more important than risk factors in answering questions.

These criteria represent an increased likelihood of progression to severe pneumonia. They are not as important as the signs of severe infection described before them. For example, COPD is a risk for severe disease, while hypoxia actually means there is severe disease now. Diabetes, steroid use, or AIDS is a risk factor for bacteremia and severe disease. Hypotension, high fever, and confusion actually mean there is severe disease now.

CURB65 and Measures of Severity

The CURB65 score is a handy way of quickly assessing the severity of a patient's pneumonia. It has fewer criteria to remember than the "pneumonia severity index," which is basically the complete list of criteria previously described. CURB65 is a way of assessing who should be admitted to the hospital for inpatient intravenous antibiotics.

C = Confusion

U = Urea (BUN above 20)

R = Respiratory rate above 30 per minute

B = Blood pressure (systolic below 90, diastolic below 60)

65 = age above 65

Those with none or only one of these criteria can be managed safely as an outpatient. It is equivocal about what to do with two of the criteria. Those with three or more criteria should definitely be admitted to the hospital and possibly to the intensive care unit. CURB65 criteria are also an accurate way to assess who can be safely switched from intravenous to oral therapy. If the patient's respiratory distress and hypotension resolve, it is safe to switch to oral therapy.

| CURB65 Criteria as a Guide to Treatment Location ||
Number of criteria present	Treatment location
0–1	Outpatient
2	Inpatient, general floor
3–5	Intensive care unit

Pneumococcal Vaccine

The risk factors for severe disease just described happen to also be the criteria for the use of pneumococcal vaccine. Pneumococcal vaccine should be given to everyone above the **age of 65** and those with:

- Chronic heart (CHF), lung (COPD), liver (cirrhosis), or kidney disease (dialysis)
- Malignancy
- Steroid use, AIDS, or diabetes
- Splenectomy

The people in these risk groups should be revaccinated once after 5 years. In the general population without underlying illness, a single dose of pneumococcal vaccine is given at the age of 65 without the need for revaccination.

Treatment by Location

Outpatient treatment: The best initial therapy for outpatient treatment of CAP is with a macrolide such as:

- Azithromycin
- Clarithromycin

If the case describes previous antibiotic treatment within the last few weeks or chronic heart or lung disease, the best initial therapy is with:

- Levofloxacin
- Moxifloxacin
- Doxycycline

Inpatient treatment: The best initial inpatient therapy for pneumonia is:

- Respiratory fluoroquinolone (levofloxacin, moxifloxacin, gemifloxacin) or
- Ceftriaxone **and** azithromycin (or doxycycline)

Diagnosis of Hospital-Acquired and Ventilator-Associated Pneumonia

By definition:

Hospital-acquired pneumonia (HAP): pneumonia developing at least 48 hours after hospitalization

Ventilator-associated pneumonia (VAP): pneumonia developing at least 48 hours after placement of an endotracheal tube

Hospitals, and especially the intensive care unit, are dangerous places. Endotracheal intubation can be associated with a rate of pneumonia as high as 35% a week. This is about 5% a day for the first few days. This is the reason that **it is always preferable to use noninvasive positive pressure ventilation** such as CPAP or BiPAP when possible.

The best initial test is a chest x-ray. Sputum stain and culture are of even less value for HAP and VAP than for CAP because of the difficulty distinguishing colonization of the endotracheal (ET) tube from a genuine infection of the lungs.

Diagnostic Procedures for VAP

- **Tracheal aspirate:** Placing a suction catheter into the ET tube and aspirating the contents below the trachea, when the catheter is past the end of the ET tube
- **Bronchoalveolar lavage (BAL):** A bronchoscope placed deeper into the lungs, where there are not supposed to be any organisms. Can be contaminated when passed through the nasopharynx.

Of people with CAP, 80% can be treated as outpatients.

Respiratory fluoroquinolones are not needed for the majority of CAP patients.

239

- **Protected brush specimen:** The tip of the bronchoscope is covered when passed through the nasopharynx, then uncovered only inside the lungs. Much more specific because of decreased contamination.
- **Video-assisted thoracoscopy (VAT):** A scope is placed through the chest wall, and a sample of the lung is biopsied. This allows a large piece of lung to be taken without the need for cutting the chest open (thoracotomy). It is like sigmoidoscopy of the chest.
- **Open lung biopsy:** The most accurate diagnostic test of VAP, but with much greater morbidity and potential complication of the procedure because of the need for thoracotomy.

Treatment of VAP

1. Anti-pseudomonal beta-lactam
   - Cephalosporin (ceftazidime or cefepime)

or

   - Penicillin (piperacillin/tazobactam)

or

   - Carbapenem (imipenem or meropenem or doripenem)

Plus:

2. Second anti-pseudomonal agent
   - Aminoglycoside (gentamicin or tobramycin or amikacin)

or

   - Fluoroquinolone (ciprofloxacin or levofloxacin)

Plus:

3. Methicillin-resistant anti-staphylococcal agent
   - Vancomycin

or

   - Linezolid

> Although they cover MRSA, daptomycin and tigecyline are not appropriate choices for treatment of VAP.

Pneumocystis Pneumonia

The organism name has been changed to *Pneumocystis jiroveci* (instead of *P carinii*), but the name of the lung infection is still pneumocystis pneumonia or PCP.

PCP occurs almost exclusively in those with AIDS with fewer than 200 CD4 cells/μl. Patients present with:

- Dyspnea on exertion increasing over several days to weeks
- Dry cough
- Fever

Diagnostic Tests

The best initial test is the chest x-ray, which shows bilateral interstitial infiltrates. The chest x-ray in PCP is identical to that found in:

- *Mycoplasma*
- *Chlamydophila*
- Viruses
- *Coxiella*

The most accurate test is bronchoscopy for bronchoalveolar lavage.

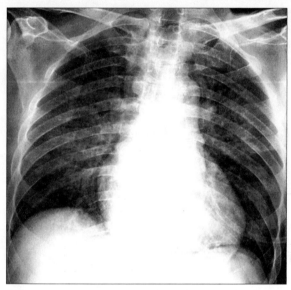

Figure 9.2: Chest x-ray: Bilateral interstitial infiltrates. You cannot distinguish PCP from mycoplasma or viral pneumonia by x-ray.

Source: Mohammad Babury, MD, and Mahendra C. Patel, MD

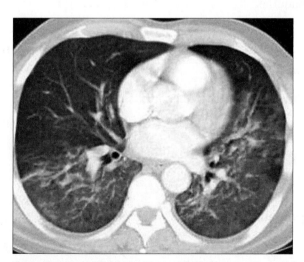

Figure 9.3: Chest CT: Bilateral interstitial infiltrates. The radiologic test is never the most accurate test in infectious diseases.

Source: Moe Sann, MD

PCP is almost always associated with an elevated LDH level. Although LDH is a rather nonspecific test when it is abnormal, a normal LDH has enormous negative predictive value. Because the chest x-ray can be normal in 25% of those with PCP on initial presentation, **a normal LDH is very useful to help exclude PCP.**

Sputum induction is a method of inhaling hypertonic saline to create sputum to expectorate. The specificity of sputum induction is essentially 100%. The problem with this method is a false negative rate of 20% to 50%.

Sputum "induction" is a way to produce sputum in a person with a dry or nonproductive cough.

TREATMENT

The best initial therapy is TMP-SMX.

Steroids decrease mortality by 50% in severe PCP.

Steroids are the answer when there is:

1. pO$_2$ below 70

or

2. A-a gradient above 35

Treatment of PCP in Sulfa Allergic Patients

Sulfa allergy is defined as:

- Rash
- Neutropenia

Alternate therapy for acute, active PCP is:

- Intravenous pentamidine

or

- Oral atovaquone (for mild PCP)

or

- Clindamycin and primaquine

PCP Prophylaxis

Prophylaxis is started when the CD4 drops below 200 CD4/μl. The best PCP prophylaxis is unquestionably TMP-SMX.

When a patient is sulfa allergic, you can use either:

- Atovaquone

or

Exclude G6PD deficiency before starting dapsone.

- Dapsone

The efficacy of these two medications is nearly equal. **They are both superior in efficacy to aerosolized pentamidine.**

▶ **TIP**

Aerosolized pentamidine should never be the right answer to anything.

Discontinuation of Prophylaxis

Prophylaxis for PCP can be discontinued when antiretroviral medication has maintained the CD4 above 200/μl for 3 to 6 months.

Tuberculosis

Epidemiology

Tuberculosis is extremely rare in the United States outside of specified risk groups. TB rarely occurs in the general population, and that is why PPD skin testing for latent TB is not indicated for the general population.

TB is found in:

- Recent immigrants (in the past 5 years)
- Homeless alcoholics
- Healthcare workers
- Prisoners
- People with HIV/AIDS
- Transplant recipients, those undergoing dialysis, and patients with silicosis
- Close contacts of those with TB

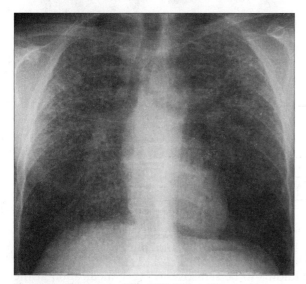

Figure 9.4: Chest x-ray: Miliary TB. Miliary TB cannot be definitively diagnosed from an x-ray.

Source: Mohammad Babury, MD, and Mahendra C. Patel, MD

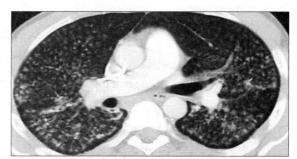

Figure 9.5: Chest CT: Miliary TB. Miliary TB is one of the few types of TB that need more than 6 months of therapy.

Source: Mohammad Babury, MD, and Mahendra C. Patel, MD

> Beware of reactivation of TB in anti-TNF users.

These are also the people who should undergo testing for latent TB.

PRESENTATION

TB presents as any other chronic lung disease/infection with:

- Fever, cough, and sputum
- Weight loss
- Signs of lung consolidation on examination

> Pleural biopsy is the single most accurate test of tuberculosis if there is effusion.

DIAGNOSTIC TESTS

- Chest x-ray with apical infiltrates and cavity formation
- Acid-fast stain and culture of sputum

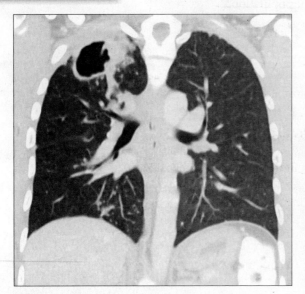

Figure 9.6: Chest CT: Cavitary TB. Cavitary TB may need longer than 6 months of therapy.

Source: Eduardo Andre, MD, and Giselle Debs, MD

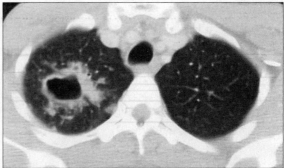

Figure 9.7: Chest CT: Cavitary TB. Only sputum testing or biopsy can distinguish active TB from an inactive cavity.

Source: Eduardo Andre, MD, and Giselle Debs, MD

TREATMENT

The best initial therapy for TB is a **four-drug regimen for the first 2 months**. After 2 months, the sensitivity of the organism should be known and two of the medications (ethambutol and pyrazinamide) can be stopped. Isoniazid and rifampin are continued for 4 more months for **a total of 6 months** of therapy.

> All the TB medications are hepatotoxic.

Even if the organism were known to be sensitive to every medication at the beginning of therapy, pyrazinamide is still used to allow the total length of therapy to be reduced from 9 months to 6 months. If the organism is pansensitive, ethambutal can be stopped.

Drug Therapy of Tuberculosis		
Initial drug treatment	**Adverse effects**	**After 2 months**
Rifampin	Red/orange body fluids (benign)	Continue
Isoniazid	Neurological toxicity	Continue
Pyrazinamide	Hyperuricemia	Stop
Ethambutol	Optic neuritis	Stop

Who Is Treated for More than 6 Months?

- Osteomyelitis
- Meningitis
- Miliary disease
- Pregnant patients cannot take pyrizinamide. Pyrizinamide is what takes us from 9 months of therapy down to 6 months.
- Cavitary disease

▶ **TIP**

Steroids are the answer for TB meningitis and TB pericarditis.

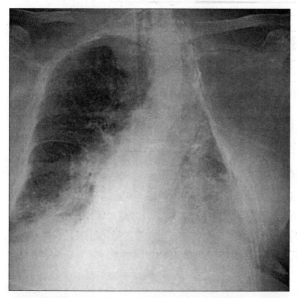

Figure 9.8: TB after throracoplasty in the distant past. Prior to the 1950s, TB was routinely treated with surgery. You will still find this x-ray in older patients. Notice the thoracoplasty with a large part of the left chest missing.

Source: Mohammad Babury, MD, and Mahendra C. Patel, MD

The PPD does not become negative after treatment.

Latent Tuberculosis

In the United States, targeted testing in high-risk populations for latent tuberculosis has been successful in helping to reduce the incidence of TB to the lowest level since reporting began.

Bacillus Calmette-Guérin (BCG) is not to be used for TB in the United States.

PPD skin testing or interferon gamma release assays (IGRAs) can be used interchangeably to detect prior exposure to TB. The only difference between their clinical utility is that prior BCG vaccination can make PPD testing falsely positive. The IGRA does not cross-react with BCG.

Booster Effect

If the person has never had a PPD test and the first test is negative, a second test should be done within 1 to 2 weeks to make sure the first test was truly negative. If the second test is positive, this indicates a "booster effect." The booster effect means that the first test was falsely negative. IGRAs do not need a second test.

Defining a Positive PPD

Larger than 5 mm:

- HIV-positive patients
- Close contacts of those with TB
- Steroid users (>15 mg/day)
- Organ transplant recipients

Larger than 10 mm: All the other risk groups such as those with silicosis, alcoholics, healthcare workers, homeless people, and prisoners.

Larger than 15 mm: People with no risks for TB, who should never have been tested in the first place. With low pretest likelihood, we increase the cutoff for a positive test.

TREATMENT

Treatment for latent tuberculosis is with isoniazid for 9 months. Afterward, there is no point in repeating a PPD test since it will always be positive.

- "Latent TB" testing is either a PPD or IGRA.
- Testing is done only in groups with an increased risk of TB.
- A positive PPD confers only a **10%** lifetime risk of developing TB.
- Treatment eliminates 90% of the risk of developing TB associated with either a positive PPD or IGRA.

SEXUALLY TRANSMITTED DISEASES

Urethritis

Urethritis presents with:

- Dysuria (frequency, urgency, burning)
- Discharge

Only test for latent TB in high-risk groups, not the general population.

BCG will only cause PPD reactivity for 5 years after the vaccination.

If the PPD is done yearly, a second test is not needed.

Prior to treatment, all patients should have a chest x-ray to exclude active TB infection.

Once a PPD is positive, it should never be repeated.

Urethritis and cervicitis can be treated with a single dose of antibiotics.

The most accurate test is a swab of the urethra for stain, culture, or nucleic acid amplification. Voided urine nucleic acid amplification test (NAAT) is best in men. Self-administered vaginal swab NAAT for cervicitis in women.

Treatment is for:

- **Gonorrhea:** ceftriaxone. Cefixime should be used only when it is not possible to inject ceftriaxone.
- **Chlamydia:** azithromycin or doxycycline. Quinolones are always wrong.

Ulcerative Genital Lesions

Gonorrhea does not produce ulcerative genital lesions. All of the causes of ulcerative genital lesions also produce inguinal adenopathy. The presence of lymph nodes does not help answer the "most likely diagnosis" question.

Ulcerative Genital Lesions with Adenopathy			
Presentation	**Most likely diagnosis**	**Diagnostic test**	**Treatment**
Vesicles	Herpes	Tzanck prep, viral culture	Acyclovir, famciclovir, valacyclovir
Tender nodes	Lymphogranuloma venereum	Serology, aspiration of a lymph node	Doxycycline
Soft, tender ulcer	Chancroid	Stain and culture on specialized media	Single dose azithromycin or ceftriaxone
Firm, painless ulcer and painless nodes	Syphilis	Dark-field, RPR/VDRL with 75%–80% sensitivity	Single dose IM penicillin or doxycycline

URINARY TRACT INFECTIONS

DEFINITION/ETIOLOGY

Anatomic lesions in the genitourinary system predispose to all of the urinary tract infections. Cystitis, pyelonephritis, and perinephric abscesses are all most commonly caused by *E coli*. The organism is more likely to lead to an infection if there is some foreign body or obstruction to the flow of urine.

> Routine testing of cure is not needed if ceftriaxone and azithromycin are used for urethritis.

Predisposing factors for urinary tract infections are:

- Stones
- Strictures
- Tumor (prostate, cervix, bladder)
- Obstruction (neurogenic bladder, pregnancy)
- Foreign body (catheters)
- Diabetes

PRESENTATION

All of the urinary infections can present with dysuria and symptoms of burning, urinary frequency, and an intense urge to urinate immediately.

Localizing Symptoms of Urinary Tract Infections			
	Cystitis	**Pyelonephritis**	**Perinephric abscess**
Localizing symptom	Suprapubic pain and tenderness, mild or absent fever	Flank (costovertebroangle) tenderness and pain, high fever	Signs of pyelonephritis persisting for several days to weeks despite appropriate therapy
Testing	None beyond the urinalysis	Renal sonogram or CT	Imaging with sonogram or CT followed by biopsy

DIAGNOSTIC TESTS

The best initial test for all urinary tract infections is:

1. Urinalysis
2. Urine culture

On the **urinalysis**, the most important clue is **white blood cells**. Protein is nonspecific, as are red cells. The presence of bacteria in the urine (asymptomatic bacteriuria) is important only for pregnant women and in those about to undergo urinary tract instrumentation such as urologic procedures.

Biopsy or aspirate is indispensible for perinephric abscess because the infection developed while the person was on antibiotics. Therefore, the only way to guide therapy is to have a clearly documented organism with its sensitivities.

> Bacteria on UA is important only in pregnant women and those about to get a urinary tract surgical procedure.

TREATMENT

Cystitis:

- Give **TMP-SMX**, fosfomycin, or **nitrofurantoin**.
- Extend the length of therapy to 7 days if it is "complicated" by anatomic abnormalities such as stones, strictures, or foreign bodies.
- Empiric treatment is routine (ie, not waiting for culture results).
- Fluoroquinolones are not the first-line therapy for cystitis.

Pyelonephritis:

- Give **TMP-SMX**, fluoroquinolones, cephalosporins, or aminoglycosides for 7 to 14 days of therapy. The range of antibiotics for pyelonephritis is extensive because any cephalosporin could cover *E coli*.
- **Oral** ciprofloxacin has the **same efficacy as intravenous medications** even if bacteremia occurs.

> Bacteremia can cause perinephric abscess.

Abscess:

- Unlike cystitis or pyelonephritis, specific microbiological evaluation to guide therapy is indispensible. Because perinephric abscess often develops while on therapy for pyelonephritis, there is a "selection pressure" for an increased amount of staphylococci to grow from a perinephric abscess. Antibiotics effective against Gram-negative bacteria will suppress or eradicate only these organisms, but leave Gram-positive organisms untouched. This will select out for a Gram-positive organism that grows around therapy. These untreated Gram-positive organisms often cause the abscess.

OSTEOMYELITIS

DEFINITION/ETIOLOGY

Osteomyelitis is an infection of the bone. The most common organism is *Staphylococcus aureus*, but numerous other organisms can cause osteomyelitis, including Gram-negative bacilli, fungi, and mycobacteria. Acute osteomyelitis is caused by trauma and the hematogenous spread of bacteria into the bone. In adults, the most common predisposing conditions are:

> Many other organisms besides *Staph aureus* cause osteomyelitis.

- **Peripheral arterial disease**
- **Diabetes**
- Skin **ulcer** and **local infection**

In adults, the most common cause of osteomyelitis is a spread of contiguous infection into the bone.

PRESENTATION

The infected bone presents with:

- Pain and tenderness at the site of involvement
- Local **redness**, **warmth**, and **tenderness**

Severe osteomyelitis may lead to the development of a **draining sinus tract**. It will drain through the surface of the ulcer.

Systemic signs of infection such as fever are rare (about 10% of cases).

DIAGNOSTIC TESTS

The best initial test is an x-ray. The x-ray can show:

- Destroyed bone
- Periosteal elevation
- Periosteal new bone formation

Although the x-ray can take 2 to 3 weeks to become abnormal, it is still the "best initial test." This is because:

- An abnormal bone x-ray eliminates the need for further radiologic testing. In other words, **you don't need an MRI or nuclear bone scan if the x-ray clearly shows the infection.**

- The majority of cases of adult osteomyelitis are chronic infections that have often been there long enough to make the bone x-ray abnormal.

If the x-ray is normal, the "next best step" is an MRI of the bone. Bone MRI is both 90% to 95% sensitive and specific.

The most accurate test is a bone biopsy. The only way to guide appropriate therapy is to have either:

- Bone biopsy that grows an organism
- Positive blood cultures (about 10% of cases)

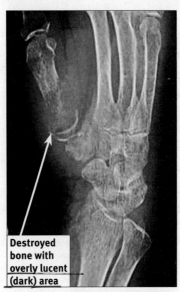

Destroyed bone with overly lucent (dark) area

Figure 9.9: Osteomyelitis. If the x-ray shows osteomyelitis, an MRI is not needed. Do the biopsy.

Source: Derek DeSa and Anuraag Sahai, MD

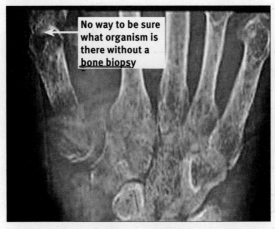

No way to be sure what organism is there without a bone biopsy

Figure 9.10: Osteomyelitis. You cannot adequately treat osteomyelitis without knowing the specific organism.

Source: Derek DeSa and Anuraag Sahai, MD

Adjunctive Diagnostic Tests

When is nuclear bone scan the answer?

- When an MRI is not possible (e.g., pacemaker in place)

When is an ESR or C-reactive protein (CRP) the answer?

- To follow the response to therapy
- To determine the duration of therapy, such as when to stop
- To determine the need for surgical therapy for debridement

> Probing to the bone indicates the presence of osteomyelitis, but you still have to biopsy to get the organism.

TREATMENT

Therapy is guided by the bone biopsy. Empiric therapy should be avoided because you cannot construct an empiric regimen that will cover all the possibilities. Although ciprofloxacin and vancomycin are acceptable as empiric therapy, you still cannot determine who needs different treatment.

If the organism is:

- **Sensitive staphylococcus:** The best initial therapy is oxacillin, nafcillin, or a first-generation cephalosporin such as cefazolin.
- **Resistant staphylococcus:** Use vancomycin, linezolid, or daptomycin. You just cannot be sure without either an open or a percutaneous biopsy.
- **Sensitive Gram-negative bacilli:** Give oral ciprofloxacin.

> Gram-negative bacilli can be treated with oral quinolones.

ENDOCARDITIS

DEFINITION/ETIOLOGY

Endocarditis is an infection of the heart valves that is most commonly caused by viridans group streptococci in native valves and by staphylococci in those with prosthetic valves. Injection drug use is also associated with staphylococci as the most common cause.

The majority of endocarditis arises without a clear etiology. Although valve disease and cardiac anatomic disease predispose one to endocarditis, the risk of individual valvular lesions is not as great as it once seemed. For example, although aortic stenosis and bicuspid aortic valve are associated with a greater risk of endocarditis than a normal heart valve, this risk is so small that routine endocarditis prophylaxis is no longer indicated for these anatomic defects when a patient is undergoing a bacteremia-causing procedure.

> Most cardiac lesions do not constitute a significant increase in risk of endocarditis.

The procedures and events that are associated with developing endocarditis have also been reconsidered recently. Although almost any cause of bacteremia is associated with an increased risk of endocarditis, only a few specific procedures need endocarditis prophylaxis anymore. The only procedures that are an indication for endocarditis prophylaxis are those that involve cutting the upper respiratory tract or dental procedures that elicit blood.

> Brushing your teeth with a hard toothbrush regularly is more dangerous than occasional dental extraction.

PRESENTATION

Endocarditis presents with:

Fever and a new or changed murmur

In addition, on rare occasion, endocarditis is associated with embolic phenomena such as:

- Janeway lesions: **flat and painless** in hands and feet
- Osler nodes: **raised and painful** in hands and feet
- Roth spots: retina
- Splinter hemorrhages: in the nail beds
- Hematuria: from emboli to the kidneys and glomerulonephritis
- Mycotic aneurysm: weakening of blood vessels of the brain

DIAGNOSTIC TESTS

The best initial test is a blood culture. If the blood cultures grow bacteria, the next best step is an echocardiogram. Transthoracic echocardiography (TTE) is done first. If the TTE is normal, then a transesophageal echocardiogram (TEE) should be performed.

Positive blood cultures + positive echocardiogram = endocarditis

▶ **TIP**

Blood cultures are the answer to "best initial test" because they are 95% to 99% sensitive (ie, a false negative rate of 1% to 5%).

Echocardiography

The TEE and TTE are equally specific. Positive blood cultures combined with a vegetation on either study is diagnostic of endocarditis.

However, the TTE is far less sensitive. There is a 40% false negative rate on the TTE. If a patient has blood cultures positive for an organism typical of endocarditis (e.g., viridans group streptococci, *Staphylococcus*, or *Streptococcus bovis*) and the TTE is normal, the answer is "perform TEE."

Accuracy of Echocardiography		
	TTE	**TEE**
Sensitivity	60%	90%–95%
Specificity	95%	95%

Endocarditis gives postinfectious glomerulonephritis from immune complexes depositing in the glomeruli.

Fever + murmur = endocarditis

Vegetation on either TEE or TTE is a "major criterion" for endocarditis. Positive blood cultures is a "major criterion" for endocarditis.

Two major criteria = endocarditis

Additional Diagnostic Testing in Endocarditis

- Normocytic **anemia** found in 90% of patients
- **Elevated ESR**
- Urinalysis with proteinuria, hematuria, and occasional red cell casts

Culture-Negative Endocarditis

How do we establish the diagnosis of endocarditis in the 1% to 5% who have negative blood cultures? A vegetation on an echocardiogram alone is not endocarditis. If blood cultures do not grow an organism, endocarditis is established with vegetation on echo (one "major" criterion), **plus any** three minor criteria:

- **Fever**
- **Risk** such as a prosthetic valve or injection drug use
- **Vascular phenomena:** major arterial emboli, septic pulmonary infarcts, mycotic aneurysm, intracranial hemorrhage, conjunctival hemorrhages, or Janeway lesions
- **Immunologic phenomena:** glomerulonephritis, Osler nodes, Roth spots, rheumatoid factor
- **Atypical organisms grown**

> The only real reason to know about embolic events in endocarditis is to diagnose culture-negative endocarditis.

TREATMENT

The best initial **empiric therapy is vancomycin and gentamicin**. This therapy is immediately changed once the organism and its sensitivity pattern are identified from blood cultures.

Treatment by Specific Culture Results

Viridans Group Strep

- Sensitive organisms get penicillin, ampicillin, or ceftriaxone as a single agent for 4 weeks.
- Partial resistance: Give penicillin or ampicillin for 4 weeks with gentamicin for the first 2 weeks.

Enterococci

- Ampicillin **and** gentamicin **both** for 6 weeks

Staphylococci (Sensitive Organisms)

- Oxacillin or nafcillin for 6 weeks (possibly with gentamicin for 3 to 5 days)

Staphylococci (Resistant Organisms)

- Vancomycin for 6 weeks

HACEK Group

HACEK: *Haemophilus, Actinobacillus, Cardiobacterium, Eikenella, Kingella*

- Ceftriaxone for 4 weeks

or

- Ampicillin/sulbactam for 4 weeks

Surgery for Endocarditis

The strongest indication for surgery in endocarditis is acute rupture of the valve or chordae tendineae and acute congestive failure. Other indications for surgery are:

- Abscess
- Fungal endocarditis
- AV block
- Recurrent of major embolic events while on antibiotics

Streptococcus bovis and Colonoscopy

All patients with *Streptococcus bovis* or *Clostridium septicum* endocarditis should undergo colonoscopy. There is a strong association of colon cancer with *S bovis* or *C septicum* for unknown reasons.

The medical management of *S bovis* is identical to the management of any other sensitive streptococcus in terms of antibiotic choice and duration: The organism is rarely resistant, so the patient should receive penicillin, ampicillin, or ceftriaxone for 4 weeks.

> *Streptococcus bovis* or *Clostridium septicum* = colonoscopy to exclude colon cancer

Endocarditis Prophylaxis

The indication for antibiotic prophylaxis for endocarditis is to have:

1. An anatomic defect with **significant** increased risk of endocarditis

plus

2. A bacteremia-causing procedure

The only anatomic defects thought to cause "significant risk" of endocarditis are:

- Prosthetic valves
- Unrepaired cyanotic heart disease (or first 6 months after repair)
- Cardiac transplant recipients with valvulopathy
- Previous endocarditis

> Mitral valve prolapse is not an indication for endocarditis prophylaxis, even if there is a murmur.

Prophylactic antibiotics are indicated only if there is both one of these risks **and** a bacteremia-causing procedure such as:

- Dental work that produces blood (such as an extraction)
- Respiratory tract surgery (such as tonsillectomy or adenoid removal)
- Procedures through infected urinary, skin, or GI areas

> Dental fillings are not an indication for endocarditis prophylaxis.

Choice of Antibiotics for Prophylaxis

- Amoxicillin 1 hour before the procedure
- Penicillin-allergic patients: clindamycin, azithromycin, or cephalexin

> Urinary, GI, and skin procedures need endocarditis prophylaxis only when infection present.

▶ **TIP**

Endocarditis prophylaxis has become considerably simplified compared with the past. If you can't remember what to do, just answer "no prophylaxis required."

LYME

PRESENTATION

The most common manifestation of Lyme disease is a rash. The rash of Lyme (erythema migrans) is:

- Round
- Red
- Pale center
- Large (wider than 5 cm)

If the question describes a rash such as this, the answer is amoxicillin or doxycycline.

You do **not** need to do serologic tests to confirm the presence of Lyme when there is a clear target-shaped (bull's-eye) erythema migrans rash.

Late Complications/Presentation of Lyme

The most common late complication of Lyme is joint pain. Other manifestations are:

- **Neurological:** Anything is possible, but seventh cranial nerve palsy is the most common.
- **Cardiac:** Anything is possible, but AV block is the most common.

DIAGNOSTIC TESTS

The Lyme rash does not need a confirmatory serologic test. All the other manifestations of Lyme must be confirmed with serologic tests prior to treatment. There are many causes of seventh cranial nerve palsy, joint pain, and AV block; confirm the diagnosis as Lyme.

> Erythema migrans rash has greater specificity than the Lyme serology.

There is nothing else that gives a 5-centimeter round, red rash with a pale center besides Lyme.

Best initial test is ELISA. Confirm with Western blot. Use of PCR is occasional.

Treatment of Lyme	
Manifestation	**Treatment**
Asymptomatic tick bite	None
Rash	Doxycycline or amoxicillin
Joint	Doxycycline or amoxicillin
Seventh cranial nerve palsy	Doxycycline or amoxicillin
Cardiac	Ceftriaxone
CNS	Ceftriaxone

Cefuroxime is an alternate therapy for Lyme.

Asymptomatic Tick Bite

The vast majority of asymptomatic tick bites should not receive antibiotic therapy. It is indicated in only a small number of cases:

- The tick is **attached for more than 24 to 36 hours**.
- You know it is an *Ixodes* tick.
- More than 20% of the ticks in the local environment are infected with Lyme.

HIV/AIDS

Opportunistic Infections

The most important point concerning AIDS-related opportunistic infections (OIs) is the need for prophylaxis. There are only two routine prophylactic medications for OIs in AIDS:

Primary prophylaxis means using a medication to prevent a disease from ever happening.

- At or **below 200** CD4/µl: **PCP** prophylaxis with TMP-SMX
- At or **below 50** CD4 /µl: **MAI/MAC** (atypical mycobacterial prophylaxis) with azithromycin

▶ **TIP**

The wrong answers for OI prophylaxis will be for cytomegalovirus, cryptococcosis, or herpes simplex. There is no indication for routine primary prophylaxis with ganciclovir, fluconazole, or acyclovir.

Cytomegalovirus Retinitis

CMV IgG levels and viral culture are wrong answers.

Cytomegalovirus (CMV) retinitis presents with blurry vision in a person with AIDS and fewer than 50 CD4 cells/µl. The best initial test is a dilated ophthalmologic exam to directly visualize the retinal lesion.

The best initial therapy is with oral valganciclovir. If the question specifically describes "sight-threatening" lesions near the fovea or optic nerve head, then intravenous ganciclovir with an intraocular ganciclovir implant are used first to control the disease. Oral valganciclovir would then be used afterward to maintain suppression of the lesion.

Discontinuing Treatment

If antiretroviral therapy brings the CD4 count above 100 for at least 3 to 6 months, oral ganciclovir can be discontinued.

> When the CD4 is corrected with antiretroviral medications, OI treatment can eventually be stopped.

Mycobacterium Avium Complex

Mycobacterium avium complex (MAC) presents as:

- Wasting syndrome (weight loss, fever, malaise)
- Lymphadenopathy
- Anemia
- Elevated alkaline phosphatase and GGTP with normal bilirubin

MAC occurs exclusively in those with far advanced AIDS and fewer than 50 CD4 cells/µl. The diagnostic tests are:

- Blood cultures for mycobacteria
- Lymph node biopsy
- Bone marrow biopsy
- Liver biopsy

> Azithromycin can be stopped if antiretroviral medication brings the CD4 count up above 100/µl for several months.

Treatment is with clarithromycin and ethambutol. Primary prophylaxis with azithromycin is begun when the CD4 level drops below 50/µl.

Progressive Multifocal Leukoencephalopathy

Progressive multifocal leukoencephalopathy (**PML**) presents with severe neurological damage exclusively to the brain in those with **fewer than 50 CD4** cells/µl. PML is occasionally seen in other immune disorders, such as with the use of **natalizumab** in multiple sclerosis.

> PML is from reactivation of the JC virus, which is a polyomavirus.

The best initial test is an MRI of the brain that shows lesions with:

- **No mass effect**
- **No contrast enhancement**

The most accurate test of PML is a brain biopsy; however, **CSF for PCR** for the JC virus can directly detect the DNA of the virus, without needing to biopsy the brain.

There is **no specific antiviral treatment** for PML. The only treatment is to raise the CD4 count with antiretroviral medications.

Immune Reconstitution Inflammatory Syndrome

Immune reconstitution inflammatory syndrome (**IRIS**) is a **paradoxical worsening** of AIDS as an idiosyncratic effect of initiating antiretroviral therapy. As the CD4 count improves and the immune system "reconstitutes," dormant opportunistic infections sometimes become "expressed." This is unpredictable and unavoidable. IRIS is the reason the antiretroviral medication is often deferred during the treatment of an acute OI.

IRIS can cause almost any of the AIDS-related OIs to become manifest, including MAI, cryptococcosis, CMV, PCP, herpes zoster, or hepatitis. IRIS may respond to steroids.

Vaccinations

Routine vaccinations in HIV/AIDS are:

- **Pneumococcus** (one booster at 5 years)
- **Influenza** (yearly)
- **Hepatitis B**
- **Hepatitis A**

Vaccines that are contraindicated in AIDS are:

- Varicella vaccine at fewer than 200 CD4 cells/µl
- Zoster vaccine at fewer than 200 CD4 cells/µl

> The zoster vaccine is the same as the varicella vaccine except that the dose is higher.

Antiretroviral Medication

Antiretroviral medication should be initiated when the CD4 count begins to decrease. OIs begin as CD4 counts drop below 200/µl; however, there is concern that the immune system will not recover normally if antiretroviral therapy (ART) is delayed until the CD4 becomes profoundly low.

There is universal agreement that antiretroviral therapy should begin below 350 CD4 cells/µl. Between 350 and 500 CD4 cells/µl, ART is probably beneficial as well. Therefore, a CD4 <500 is when ART is started.

> ART is to be started at <500 CD4 cells

Pregnancy

ART should be used in all pregnant HIV-positive women, regardless of the CD4 count. ART is used in pregnancy both to preserve the health of the mother and to prevent perinatal transmission. If the mother has a low CD4 count (below 500), then the ART should be continued lifelong even after the child is born. If the CD4 count is high (above 500), then ART is used only during pregnancy in order to prevent transmission to the baby. Start 3 antiretrovirals as soon as you know pregnancy is there.

> Do *not* wait for second trimester to start antiretrovirals in pregnancy. Start immediately.

Genotype Resistance Testing

Resistance to individual antiretroviral medications can be predicted from specific genetic mutations in the virus. Genotyping is routinely performed:

- Prior to initiating ART to be sure that the patient's virus is sensitive to the medications to be used
- When medications seem to be failing in order to assess the appropriate medications to switch to

What to Start?

The best initial antiretroviral therapy is:

- Efavirenz/tenofovir/emtricitabine

or

- Ritonavir-boosted atazanavir + tenofovir/emtricitabine

or

- Ritonavir-boosted darunavir + tenofovir/emtricitabine

or

- Raltegravir + tenofovir/emtricitabine

HLA-B*5701 is done before starting patients on an abacavir-containing regimen to reduce the risk of hypersensitivity reaction.

Adverse Effects

The most important question for Internal Medicine is the adverse effects of ART.

Protease inhibitors: hyperglycemia, hyperlipidemia

Nucleoside reverse transcriptase inhibitors (RTI): lactic acidosis, hepatic steatosis

Zidovudine: macrocytic anemia

Stavudine and didanosine: pancreatitis and peripheral neuropathy

Abacavir: skin hypersensitivity, Stevens-Johnson syndrome

Indinavir: nephrolithiasis

Tenofovir: renal toxicity

Non-nucleoside RTIs (Nevirapine): Stevens-Johnson syndrome

PCR RNA Viral Load Testing

Viral load testing should be performed at baseline and several times a year to assess effectiveness of therapy.

The first sign of drug failure is an increase in viral load.

Post-exposure Prophylaxis

All persons with serious exposures to HIV need to receive post-exposure prophylaxis in order to decrease the likelihood of transmission. The choice of medications is not as important as rapidly assessing the person exposed and initiating treatment. Any of the regimens previously described for 1 month post-exposure is acceptable, as is:

- Two nucleoside ARTs and efavirenz
- Two nucleoside ARTs and ritonavir/lopinavir

Risk of Transmission of HIV Based on Type of Exposure	
Exposure	**Risk of transmission**
Vaginal: Female to male	1 in 3,000
Vaginal: Male to female	1 in 1,000
Needle stick injury	1 in 300
Anal receptive	1 in 100
Mother to child	1 in 3 (no medication)

Perinatal Transmission

With no medications during pregnancy, the risk of perinatal transmission is about 25% to 30%. With medications, perinatal transmission is under 1%. Cesarean birth is indicated if the HIV is not well controlled on the day of delivery. If the CD4 is high (above 500/μl) and the viral load is low (less than 1,000 copies), there is no need to perform cesarean delivery. Other indications for cesarean delivery include absence of prenatal care or lack of ART administration through pregancy if the viral load is uncontrolled.

Only efavirenz is potentially teratogenic. Monotherapy in pregnancy is always incorrect for the mother. Use 3 medications through the entire pregnancy. Do not wait for the second trimester to start.

Cesarean delivery to prevent perinatal transmission is done if the viral load is above 1,000 copies.

NEPHROLOGY

10

ACUTE KIDNEY INJURY

DEFINITION

Acute kidney injury (AKI) replaces the term *acute renal failure*. AKI is a rise in the blood urea nitrogen (BUN) and creatinine over a short period of time such as 2 or 3 days. There is no precise definition in terms of exactly how much the creatinine must rise to qualify as AKI. AKI can be used interchangeably with terms such as azotemia or acute renal insufficiency. The term uremia implies a more severe form of AKI in which the buildup of nitrogenous waste products, fluid, acid, and potassium causes severe illness. Uremia is a term that generally implies the need for dialysis.

> Boards questions have to be clear. They will describe a rise in creatinine of at least 0.3 to 0.5 mg/dL over 2 to 3 days.

ETIOLOGY

AKI is best divided up into causes inside the kidney ("intrinsic" renal disease) and problems with perfusion or drainage of the kidney. Decreased perfusion of the kidney or prerenal azotemia means that the kidney itself is normal and would function normally if perfusion were restored. Problems with drainage of the kidney or postrenal disease is also a kidney that would be normal again if the obstruction were reversed. In both of these cases, the diagnostic tests are nearly identical. The answers to the "best initial" and "most accurate test" questions are the same.

With intrinsic renal failure, the etiologies are different; so the answers to the "best initial test" and "best initial therapy" questions are different.

Physical Findings

There are few physical findings unique to the different causes of AKI. Signs of fluid overload such as edema or rales can be found in any of them. In addition, signs of volume depletion such as tachycardia or hypotension are not present in half the cases of prerenal disease. Any specific physical findings would be those of the underlying systemic disease such as rales for CHF or edema with low albumin states. None of these is specific enough to be very helpful in answering the "most likely diagnosis" question.

▶ **TIP**

Nephrology is a laboratory-based specialty. You will not be able to answer questions without lab data.

DIAGNOSTIC TESTS

The "best initial test" for all questions is the BUN and creatinine. If the BUN and creatinine are given in the question, the "best initial test" is always a urinalysis (UA). The best initial imaging test is an ultrasound. The "most accurate test" depends on the disease.

| BUN-to-creatinine ratios |
| are not numerically precise. |
| These are approximations. |

How to Answer the "Best Initial Test" Question

Lab Results for Different Types of AKI		
	Prerenal azotemia	**Intrinsic renal disease**
BUN-to-creatinine ratio	>20:1	10:1
Urine osmolality	>500 mOsm/kg	<350 mOsm/kg
Specific gravity	High	Low
Urine sodium	<20 mEq/L	>40 mEq/L
FeNa (fractional excretion of sodium)	<1%	>1%

Urine osmolality and urine specific gravity are most often identical in terms of whether they are high or low.

High urine osmolality = concentrated urine = high specific gravity

Urine sodium and fractional excretion of sodium are most often identical in terms of whether they are high or low.

High **urine sodium = FeNa above 1%**

Low **urine sodium = FeNa below 1%**

▶ **TIP**

Choose the one that is closest to the correct answer. For example, 8:1 is closest to intrinsic disease. A ratio of 18:1 is closest to prerenal disease.

How to Answer the "Most Accurate Test" Question

Biopsy: The biopsy is always the **"most accurate test"** in **glomerulonephritis, nephrotic syndrome, and vasculitis.** This does not mean that the biopsy is always done in these cases. For instance, biopsy is the most accurate test of post-streptococcal glomerulonephritis and Henoch-Schönlein purpura, but it is rarely done.

> Biopsy is almost never correct for tubular diseases.

▶ **TIP**

"What is the most accurate" and **"what would you do"** are not always the same.

Urine eosinophils: acute (allergic) interstitial nephritis

Spiral CT scan: nephrolithiasis, renal obstruction

Angiography (arteriography): renal artery stenosis

Protein-to-creatinine ratio: presence of nephrotic range proteinuria

24-hour urine: creatinine clearance. Although the 24-hour urine may be very accurate for nephrotic range proteinuria, the technical difficulties of obtaining a precise collection decrease its accuracy. A single missed urination will underestimate the true level of proteinuria.

> The protein-to-creatinine ratio is equal to 24-hour urine for assessing proteinuria.

> The 24-hour urine is not needed to diagnose nephrotic syndrome, but it is still the "most accurate" way to determine creatinine clearance.

Casts

When they are in the stem, the presence of casts is extremely useful in answering the "most likely diagnosis" question. **Casts are often not present even when the person has the disease.** Testing for casts lacks sensitivity and negative predictive value. For instance, WBC casts are very specific for pyelonephritis; however, many patients with pyelonephritis do not have WBC casts. The same is true of granular casts and acute tubular necrosis (ATN). It helps if they are there, but granular casts are missing in 25% of those with ATN.

> Casts are specific, but not sensitive.

Casts and the "Most Likely Diagnosis"	
When this type of cast is present:	**This is the "most likely diagnosis":**
Red blood cell	Acute glomerulonephritis
White blood cell	Pyelonephritis
Eosinophil	Interstitial nephritis
Hyaline	Dehydration, prerenal azotemia
Granular or muddy brown	Acute tubular necrosis
Waxy	Nephrotic syndrome

▶ **TIP**

Intravenous pyelogram (IVP) is always the wrong answer.

The Urinalysis

Red blood cells (RBCs): RBCs are associated with all forms of **glomerulonephritis** as well as:

1. • Stones
4. • Hematologic disorders (thrombocytopenia, coagulopathy)
3. • Infections
2. • Tumors, Trauma, Treatments (e.g., cyclophosphamide)

Dysmorphic RBCs: glomerulonephritis. Although RBCs are found in many conditions, "dysmorphic" or misshapen RBCs are specific to glomerulonephritis.

Causes of inaccurate findings of hematuria	
False negative	**False positive**
• Large dose vitamin C (ascorbic acid)	• Foods: e.g., beets • Medications: rifampin or chloroquine • Pigments: hemoglobin or myoglobin

Nitrites: Gram-negative bacteria such as *E coli* produce nitrites on urinalysis.

Ketones: Diabetic ketoacidosis (DKA) and sometimes starvation. Ketones in the urine are not nearly as pathologically significant as ketones in the blood. Skipping two meals can put ketones in the urine. Ketones in blood indicate severe pathology such as DKA.

Bacteria: Bacteriuria has very little pathologic significance and often means the specimen is contaminated. **Bacteriuria is significant only for pregnant women**, who develop pyelonephritis 30% of the time, **and in those about to undergo surgery to the urinary system**.

▶ **TIP**

The most frequently asked bacteriuria question is about who **not** to treat. Do not treat bacteria in the urine unless the patient is pregnant or getting an invasive urologic procedure.

pH: Alkaline urine is significant for the risk of stone formation, particularly with infections with *Proteus*. Urine pH is also helpful in diagnosing the specific type of renal tubular acidosis (RTA). Distal RTA gives a high urine pH, while proximal RTA is variable but most often gives a low urine pH. Meat in the diet makes urine more acidic.

> Most stones (calcium oxalate) form in an alkaline urine.

WBCs: Besides infection, urine WBCs indicates acute interstitial nephritis. **Hansel stain or Wright stain is needed to detect eosinophils**.

> Do **not** get a urine culture unless there are **white cells** in the urine.

▶ **TIP**

The ordinary UA cannot distinguish if the WBCs are neutrophils or eosinophils.

An elderly, severely demented woman is transferred from a skilled nursing facility for respiratory distress. A urinary catheter has been in place for an indeterminate period of time. It was placed for the convenience of the nurses, who wished to avoid frequent diaper changes for the patient. Her urine culture grows Candida tropicalis. The UA shows 3 WBCs. Her temperature is 102 and the respiratory rate is 26 per minute.

What is the best management?

a. Change the urinary catheter plus fluconazole
b. Amphotericin bladder wash
c. Remove the catheter
d. No treatment necessary

Answer: The correct answer is (c). It is very common for a urinary catheter to become colonized with yeast. Only about a third of Candida infections will be with C albicans. It does not alter the management, which is to remove a urinary catheter that should never have been placed. If there were WBCs in the urine and signs of infection, fluconazole or amphotericin bladder washes would successfully treat the infection. The urinalysis in someone with a catheter in place can be difficult to interpret. Bacteria will colonize the catheter within 24 hours. In addition, just the presence of the catheter can be irritating to the bladder wall, resulting in the production of WBCs. In order to be certain that the organism that grows from a urinary catheter represents a genuine infection, you will need to see bacteria, WBCs, and another sign of infection. You must be careful to confirm that any sign of infection, such as a fever, is not explainable by the presence of another infection such as the respiratory infection described in this question.

Overnight on a Saturday, the junior resident admits a patient from a nursing home for "sepsis" and places the patient on levofloxacin. The patient is 72 with a history of prostate cancer producing obstructive uropathy, which necessitated the placement of a nephrostomy tube several months ago. The patient has no fever and a normal WBC count in the blood. UA shows 25 WBCs per high power field. A month prior to this admission, the UA had the same number of WBCs.

What would you do?

a. Switch levofloxacin to ciprofloxacin now
b. Stop the antibiotics
c. Continue levofloxacin and switch based on the results of the urine culture
d. Obtain renal ultrasound
e. Consult infectious diseases

Answer: The correct answer is (b). The patient does not have an infection. A nephrostomy tube by itself can lead to WBCs in urine. The key is that the patient is otherwise asymptomatic with no signs of infection. In addition, the UA has shown WBCs in the past.

> Chronic urinary catheters are always colonized with bacteria, fungi, or both. Do not treat without clear signs of infection.

Prerenal Azotemia

DEFINITION

Prerenal azotemia is a form of AKI caused by a decrease in the effective perfusion of the kidney. It does not matter what the total body water is. It only matters how much is in the intravascular space and is participating in filtration and reabsorption.

An edematous person, such as someone with heart failure, can have low renal perfusion.

ETIOLOGY

All forms of prerenal azotemia decrease effective renal perfusion. Hypovolemia is the same to the kidney as hypotension, congestive heart failure, or renal artery stenosis. Renal artery stenosis is an example of when the blood pressure can be elevated, but the glomerular capillary perfusion is decreased.

Causes of prerenal azotemia are:

- Hypotension, including any form of shock
- Hypovolemia
- Low oncotic pressure
- Congestive heart failure (CHF) and constrictive pericarditis

Hepatorenal Syndrome

Hepatorenal syndrome is elevated BUN and creatinine caused entirely by liver failure. The kidney itself is normal. The BUN-to-creatinine ratio is greater than 20:1 and the urine sodium is low (below 20 mEq/L). If you transplanted the kidney from a person with hepatorenal syndrome into another person, the kidney would function normally.

Treatment is with midodrine and octreotide. Volume expansion with albumin infusion is effective as well.

DIAGNOSTIC TESTS/TREATMENT

There are no unique physical findings in prerenal azotemia to allow you to answer the "most likely diagnosis" question. Treatment is based on correcting the underlying cause.

Prerenal azotemia can be associated with edema, signs of dehydration, or normal volume status.

▶ TIP

All the questions on prerenal azotemia will focus on specific diagnostic tests.

The best initial test is the BUN-to-creatinine ratio, which is elevated at more than 20:1. This is because there is increased urea absorption in the proximal tubule when the kidney is volume depleted. The urine sodium is low and

Increased aldosterone levels in volume depletion and other prerenal states remove sodium from the urine.

therefore the FeNa is low. Because the body is trying to retain fluid, the urine osmolality will be increased secondary to increased ADH secretion.

Postrenal Disease

DEFINITION/ETIOLOGY

Postrenal causes of AKI are, by definition, in a **normal kidney** in which there is **impairment of urine flow**. This back-pressure increases the hydrostatic pressure in the glomerular space of the Bowman capsule. Since all filtration is based on the hydrostatic pressure in the glomerular capillary being greater than the hydrostatic pressure in the Bowman capsule, an increase in the pressure in the Bowman capsule is the same as a decrease in glomerular filtration pressure.

Renal insufficiency with an increased creatinine will occur only if **both kidneys are obstructed**. Common causes are:

- Bladder **stones**
- Ureteral **strictures**
- **Tumor** (e.g., prostate, bladder, or cervical cancer)
- Retroperitoneal fibrosis
- Neurogenic or atonic bladder

DIAGNOSTIC TESTS

- Palpable bladder on examination
- Hydronephrosis on ultrasound or CT scan
- Large volume of urine elicited after placement of a urinary catheter

The laboratory values are similar to prerenal azotemia in that the BUN-to-creatinine ratio is greater than 20:1 and the urine sodium is low.

TREATMENT

Correct the underlying cause, which often results in chronic use of a urinary (Foley) catheter.

> Postrenal disease rapidly reverses if the obstruction is short term (a few days).

Intrinsic Renal Disease

These are all the causes of AKI that are either from exposing the renal tubules to toxins or from ischemia of the kidney. Because the toxins, tests, and treatments differ, they have to be addressed separately.

▶ **TIP**

We always address each disease based on extracting questions:

- What is the most likely diagnosis?
- What is the best initial test?
- What is the most accurate test?
- Which of the following physical findings is most likely to be found in this patient?
- What is the best initial therapy?

Acute Tubular Necrosis

Acute tubular necrosis (ATN) is AKI due to renal ischemia, often combined with a toxin. Toxins that cause ATN are:

- **Cumulative** (more toxicity with more use over time)
- **Not** associated with rash, fever, or eosinophilia
- **Not** treatable (no medication exists to reverse the effect)
- More likely to occur with dehydration and underlying renal disease

> The sicker the kidney, the easier it is to get ATN from a toxin.

Medications that Can Cause ATN

- Acyclovir
- Aminoglycosides (associated with **low magnesium** levels)
- Amphotericin
- Cisplatin, carboplatin
- Contrast agents
- Foscarnet
- Lithium
- Methotrexate
- NSAIDs
- Pentamidine

PRESENTATION/DIAGNOSTIC TESTS

There are **no unique physical findings with ATN**.

The best initial diagnostic tests are:

- BUN-to-creatinine ratio near 10:1
- Urine sodium above 40 and FeNa above 1%
- Urine osmolality below 350
- Granular (muddy) casts on UA

The reason the urine sodium is high is that a live and working proximal tubule is necessary to absorb sodium. Two-thirds of sodium is absorbed in the proximal tubule. If ischemia and toxins have "killed" the tubular cell, then:

1. The sloughed tubular cells go into the urine as granular or "muddy brown" casts.
2. The tubule cannot absorb sodium and it leaks into the urine as a high FeNa or high urine sodium.

▶ **TIP**

Biopsy is never the right answer for ATN.

TREATMENT

There is no specific therapy to reverse ATN. Patients are managed supportively. Supportive management means:

- If hypotensive, give normal saline.
- Make sure the potassium level is normal.
- Stop any other nephrotoxic substances or medications.
- Use dialysis if severe renal failure develops (acidosis, hyperkalemia, fluid overload, pericarditis, encephalopathy).
- If the drug causing the toxicity is critical, lower the dose, hydrate, and continue using it.

A patient with fever and confusion was admitted to your service 4 days ago. She was started on acyclovir as empiric treatment for herpes encephalitis. The PCR for herpes comes back today as positive. Her creatinine has started to rise from 1.0 mg/dL to 2.1 mg/dL over the last 3 days.

What would you do?

a. Continue acyclovir at a lower dose and hydrate
b. Stop acyclovir until the creatinine returns to normal
c. Continue at the same dose and hydrate
d. Switch the acyclovir to foscarnet
e. Use N-acetylcysteine

Answer: The correct answer is (a). When you have an absolute need to treat a disease such as herpes encephalitis, you cannot stop therapy. Foscarnet is even more nephrotoxic than acyclovir. You cannot wait for the creatinine to return to normal. N-acetylcysteine is worthless for acyclovir-related toxicity. Herpes encephalitis can cause permanent brain damage and death. You must treat even if the creatinine rises.

Cyclosporine and tacrolimus cause renal failure in 10% of users.

▶ **TIP**

Kidneys can be dialyzed; brain damage and death, on the other hand, cannot be reversed.

Wrong Answers in ATN Management

The questions on an exam must be clear. The clearest questions are about what is **not effective** since we have **no specific medication or treatment to reverse ATN.**

Furosemide can worsen AKI.

- Mannitol
- Furosemide
- Low-dose dopamine

Prevention of Contrast-induced AKI

Contrast agents are directly toxic to the kidney tubule as well as provoking a vasoconstriction of the afferent arteriole of the glomerulus. This is why contrast causes ATN, yet the urine sodium is low and the BUN-to-creatinine ratio is 20:1.

A young healthy person with no underlying renal disease has less than a 1 in 10,000 chance of acute renal failure from contrast.

After the age of 40, people lose 1% of their nephrons per year. Therefore, a person who is 70 or 80 years old is missing 30% to 40% of functioning nephrons just because of age. If you add in diabetes or hypertension, the patient is missing even more. **Dehydration** is the **worst risk** for contrast-induced AKI.

> Creatinine clearance is multiplied by 0.85 for women.

Creatinine Clearance Using Cockcroft-Gault Equation:

$$\text{Creatinine Clearance} = \frac{140 - \text{age} \times \text{Weight (kg)}}{72 \times \text{Creatinine (mg/dl)}}$$

What Do I Answer When Bicarbonate and N-acetylcysteine Are Controversial?

The answer is:

- Hydrate with normal saline.
- Use nonionic contrast agents.

The boards are not going to engage with controversies such as the use of N-acetylcysteine or bicarbonate. The evidence for the benefit of bicarbonate is better than for N-acetylcysteine, but neither is conclusive. Both are considered "with little harm and **possible** benefit."

Hydration with **normal saline is conclusive** in preventing contrast-induced AKI. That will be the answer.

Allergic (Acute) Interstitial Nephritis

DEFINITION/ETIOLOGY

Allergic (acute) interstitial nephritis (AIN) is a type of AKI that is from toxins to the kidney, but on a different basis. Drugs cause 70% of AIN cases. Common associations are penicillins, **NSAIDS**, sulfa drugs, allopurinol, rifampin, lamotrigine, quinolones, and **proton pump inhibitors**.

Toxins need time to damage the kidney tubule via ATN. **It takes 5 to 10 days for gentamicin or amphotericin to raise the creatinine.** Penicillin, on the other hand, can cause AIN with a single dose since it is an "allergic" phenomenon. The medications that cause AIN are the same that cause:

- Drug-induced rash
- Stevens-Johnson syndrome
- Toxic epidermal necrolysis
- Hemolysis

In the same way that beta blockers or calcium blockers are unlikely to cause a rash, they are also unlikely to cause AIN or hemolysis. Some drugs, like penicillins and sulfa drugs, are allergenic and some, like SSRIs, are not.

In addition to medications, other causes of AIN are:

- Autoimmune disorders (lupus, Sjögren, sarcoidosis)
- Infections
- Metals (lead, mercury)

> Allergenic substances cause rash, renal effects, and blood effects.

> Lead causes ATN, AIN, and proximal renal tubular acidosis.

Infection as a Cause of AIN

Infections can cause AIN. Infections do not just cause postinfectious glomerulonephritis. Examples include:

- Streptococcal infections
- Leptospirosis
- Cytomegalovirus
- Rocky Mountain spotted fever

PRESENTATION/DIAGNOSTIC TESTS

AIN can present with:

- Fever
- Rash
- Eosino**philia** and eosino**philuria**

Although most patients do not have this complete triad, if the question wants you to know the answer, they will have to put it in. Otherwise, no one could answer the question.

The most accurate test is the Hansel or Wright stain of the urine showing eosinophils. The UA cannot tell that the WBC is an eosinophil.

TREATMENT

The majority will resolve with stopping the offending drug or toxin, in the same way that most drug-induced rashes will resolve with stopping the drug. If the question describes a person whose condition is continuing to worsen despite stopping the offending medication, then the answer is prednisone (or other glucocorticoids).

Pigment (Hemoglobin/Myoglobin) in the Urine

PRESENTATION/"WHAT IS THE MOST LIKELY DIAGNOSIS?"

Hemoglobinuria: Only an ABO blood incompatibility or severe intravascular hemolysis is likely to cause sufficient hemoglobin release to cause AKI. Extravascular hemolysis does not release enough hemoglobin at a rapid enough rate to damage the kidney.

Myoglobin: Rhabdomyolysis from seizures, burns, trauma, statin medications, and crush injury should be clear from the history. The causes that are most often missed are:

- **Immobility** (pressure over several hours leads to muscle necrosis)
- **Heat disorders** ("malignant" hyperthermia, heat stroke, fever caused by neuroleptic malignant syndrome)
- **Hypokalemia**
- **Thyroid disorders** (both high and low)

> Pressure on a hard surface such as with syncope or stroke is very damaging to muscle. The patient doesn't have to seize to necrose.

DIAGNOSTIC TESTS

The main issue is for you to distinguish is whether the question is asking "What is the first test to establish a diagnosis?" or "What is the most urgent test?"

The first test to establish a diagnosis is a UA with the **dipstick positive for blood, but no cells are seen.** For rhabdomyolysis, the most accurate test is a urine myoglobin and elevated CPK level. The urine dipstick cannot distinguish between hemoglobin, myoglobin, and red blood cells. That is why the dipstick is positive with all of them. The CPK level can be up, but that does not mean it is spilling into the urine to damage the kidneys.

> For rhabdomyolysis, CPK level is not as specific as myoglobin in urine.

The "most urgent test" is either a potassium level or an EKG. This question tests whether you know how patients die from rhabdomyolysis. Rhabdomyolysis causes hypocalcemia. Damaged muscle "absorbs" calcium. Muscles have a sarcoplasmic endoplasmic reticulum with a powerful sodium-calcium pump that "sucks" calcium out of the cytosol into storage. When the wall of muscle cells is damaged, it sucks calcium right out of plasma and into storage, causing hypocalcemia.

TREATMENT

If the EKG shows the peaked T waves of hyperkalemia, the best initial therapy is calcium chloride or calcium gluconate.

The best initial therapy to prevent AKI is:

- Hydration with normal saline
- Mannitol
- Bicarbonate

Bicarbonate prevents the precipitation of myoglobin at the kidney tubules and prevents the oxidative stress to the tubule cells.

Tumor Lysis Syndrome

Prevention of AKI from Tumor Lysis

Chemotherapy for hematologic malignancies such as leukemia and lymphoma can be very damaging to kidneys because of the **sudden release of uric acid** and potassium. This is from rapid-growing, large-volume disease, such as acute leukemia with very high WBC counts or bulky lymphomas.

Prevention of AKI is with:

- **Hydration**
- **Allopurinol** or **rasburicase** to prevent uric acid toxicity. Allopurinol decreases uric acid formation. Rasburicase increases its breakdown.

▶ **TIP**

In tumor lysis syndrome, isotonic saline is the right answer, and alkalinization is the most common wrong answer.

Myeloma

The most common cause of death in multiple myeloma is infection and renal failure. Myeloma has many ways to kill the kidney such as:

- **Hyperuricemia** precipitating in the kidney tubule
- **Bence-Jones proteinuria** (light chain disease)
- **Hypercalcemia** causing ATN and nephrogenic diabetes insipidus
- **Amyloidosis**
- Excess immunoglobulins clogging up the glomeruli

▶ **TIP**

Bence-Jones protein will not show up on a dipstick. You must do urine immunoelectrophoresis.

Hypercalcemia

Hypercalcemia from any cause will cause AKI. Calcium will cause:

- ATN from direct toxicity to the tubules
- Nephrogenic diabetes insipidus

Pigments are like putting a hand on a hot stove. Decrease the duration of contact and run it under water.

Rasburicase is a recombinant urate-oxidase stimulator. It prevents AKI from tumor lysis syndrome.

Urate-oxidase increases metabolism and degradation of uric acid.

The only protein a dipstick will detect is albumin.

- Renal tubular acidosis
- Nephrocalcinosis

The best initial therapy for hypercalcemia is always hydration with large volumes of normal saline. Only if volume deficit is replaced and urine output is adequate should you answer a loop diuretic such as furosemide.

Crystals

Uric acid and oxalate are the two most common crystals to cause ATN. Uric acid is from gout or tumor lysis syndrome. Oxalate is the answer when you see an overdose of ethylene glycol from antifreeze in the history. The best initial test for both of them is the UA. Unlike joint fluid, you do not need a polarizing microscope to detect uric acid crystals in urine. Oxalate crystals have a distinct shape like an envelope.

The "best initial therapy" for ethylene glycol overdose is with fomepizole, which blocks the production of oxalic acid. It is the oxalic acid or oxalate that is damaging to the kidney. Dialysis is then used to remove the ethylene glycol. Rasburicase is proven to prevent only the development of AKI from tumor lysis syndrome. If severe hyperuricemia and renal failure develop, dialysis must be performed.

Atheroembolic Disease

Look for a patient with atherosclerotic disease who develops AKI just after a vascular catheter procedure. When the catheter goes into the aorta or the coronary ostia, cholesterol plaques get knocked off the vessel and embolize to the kidney and the skin. Look for:

- **Livedo reticularis**
- **Blue spots** in the toes
- AKI
- **Eosinophilia, eosinophiluria,** low serum complement levels

There is no specific therapy that is clear beyond managing lipids with statins.

> Atheroembolic disease is like reaching up on a shelf and knocking off a plate that breaks on the floor: The pieces embolize.

> Warfarin does not help atheroemboli.

Analgesic Nephropathy

Analgesics are toxic to the kidney through multiple mechanisms such as:

- Direct toxicity (ATN)
- Allergic interstitial nephritis
- Papillary necrosis
- Membranous glomerulonephropathy
- Vasoconstriction of the afferent arteriole

Prostaglandins normally function to dilate the afferent arteriole. NSAIDs will inhibit this, leading to vasoconstriction of the afferent arteriole. In young, healthy people, this has little relevance. In an elderly person with underlying renal insufficiency, this can be quite damaging and provoke a sudden bump up in creatinine.

There is no specific therapy for any form of analgesic nephropathy.

Nephrogenic Systemic Fibrosis

Gadolinium is the contrast agent used with **MRI**. Gadolinium was long thought to be extremely benign. As the number of MRI procedures has soared, a very rare hypersensitivity reaction called nephrogenic systemic fibrosis has been described. This syndrome:

- Occurs **in those with renal insufficiency** (90%)
- Produces epidermal fibrotic plaques resembling scleroderma as well as systemic fibrosis
- Has no clear treatment

Do not give gadolinium to patients with severe renal dysfunction unless you are willing to dialyze them immediately after the procedure.

Papillary Necrosis

Papillary necrosis is a rare disorder occurring in those with chronic renal disease such as sickle cell, chronic pyelonephritis, or tubulointerstitial disease. It is an acute event often precipitated by the use of NSAIDs, which constrict the afferent arteriole leading to ischemia of the papillae. The papillae then slough off and are found in the urine. The most accurate test is a CT scan showing an abnormal "bumpy" contour of the inside of the kidney. There is no treatment.

Papillary necrosis presents like pyelonephritis. Look for:

- Chronic renal disease (diabetes, sickle cell, obstructive uropathy)
- Sudden onset of flank pain and fever **without tenderness**
- **Necrotic material** in the urine
- Occurrence immediately **after the use of NSAIDs**

GLOMERULONEPHRITIS

Common Principles

Glomerulonephritis (GN) is an inflammatory disorder of the glomeruli. It is associated with a number of vasculitic diseases (Wegener, systemic lupus erythematosus, Henoch-Schönlein, Churg-Strauss, polyarteris nodosa) as well as streptococcal and other infections. All forms of glomerulonephritis have the following in common:

> GN has a low urine sodium and FeNa initially below 1%.

- **Dysmorphic RBCs** on UA
- RBC casts

- Proteinuria
- The potential to progress to nephrotic syndrome
- Most accurately diagnosed with a renal biopsy
- Often treated with steroids or cytotoxic medications such as cyclophosphamide

Pulmonary-Renal Syndromes

Several disorders predominantly affect the lung and kidney. These are:

- Goodpasture syndrome
- Wegener granulomatosis
- Microscopic polyangiitis
- Churg-Strauss syndrome

All of them present with cough, hemoptysis, fever, weight loss, hematuria, and red cell casts. They all have blood tests to help establish a diagnosis, but they are most accurately diagnosed with a kidney biopsy. **Steroids and cyclophosphamide** are the treatment for all of them.

What Is Different?/How Do I Answer the "Most Likely Diagnosis" Question?

Goodpasture

- **Limited only to lung and kidney** with no other organs involved
- May involve only the lung or only the kidney
- "Best initial test" is blood for **anti-basement membrane antibodies**
- Severe disease (pulmonary hemorrhage) is treated with **plasmapheresis** in addition to steroids and cyclophosphamide
- **Linear deposits** on kidney biopsy

Wegener Granulomatosis

- Systemic vasculitis than **can involve almost any organ**
- Prominent **upper respiratory tract involvement** (otitis, sinusitis)
- **Granulomas** on biopsy
- **Anti-proteinase-3 positive** (c-ANCA)

Microscopic Polyangiitis

- **Less upper respiratory tract involvement** than Wegener although it is a systemic vasculitis as well
- **No granulomas**
- **Anti-myeloperoxidase positive** (p-ANCA)

Churg-Strauss Syndrome

- **Asthma**
- **Eosinophilia**

Polyarteritis Nodosa

Polyarteritis nodosa (PAN) is a disorder of medium-sized vessels. The main difference between PAN and the disorders previously mentioned is:

- **PAN has no lung involvement**.
- **Abdominal pain** is a strong clue, particularly **worsened by eating**.
- There is no accurate blood test.
- PAN is strongly associated with **chronic hepatitis B or C**.
- **Angiography** of the **mesenteric**, renal, or hepatic artery is characteristic enough to establish a diagnosis without the need for renal biopsy.

▶ **TIP**

The presence of ANCA should prompt you to look for one of the other diagnoses previously described, not PAN.

Common Features of Vasculitis

All forms of vasculitis discussed here (Wegener, microscopic polyangiitis, Churg-Strauss, and PAN) have the following features in common:

1. Fever, weight loss, joint pain, and myalgia
2. Stroke in a young person
3. Mononeuritis multiplex
4. Gastrointestinal bleeding
5. Skin lesions (petechiae, purpura, livedo reticularis)
6. Eye involvement (iritis, uveitis)
7. Anemia and leukocytosis

> Goodpasture is not a vasculitis. There is only lung and kidney involvement.

They all respond to steroids and cyclophosphamide. They can all cause nephrotic syndrome.

Henoch-Schönlein Purpura

Henoch-Schönlein purpura (HSP) is related to the deposition of IgA in multiple tissues, but the most common are:

- Gastrointestinal (abdominal pain, diarrhea, bleeding)
- Joint pain/arthralgia
- Skin (purpura, petechiae), more on the lower extremities
- Renal (glomerulonephritis)

The **most accurate test is a biopsy**. IgA levels are not useful. **No treatment** is usually necessary since resolution is spontaneous. If proteinuria is present, the answer is ACE inhibitors (or ARBs). If "progressive renal failure" is described, the answer is trial of steroids.

> IgA levels don't help in HSP. Steroid use is of unproven benefit.

(Berger's Disease)

IgA Nephropathy

This is the most common cause of acute glomerulonephritis in the United States. Look for "recent upper respiratory tract infection" in the stem of the question. "Recent" for IgA nephropathy means in the last 1 to 2 **days**. Post-streptococcal glomerulonephritis is 1 to 2 **weeks** after the infection.

- **Hematuria** is the most prominent feature.
- There are **no unique physical findings**.
- There is **no blood test**.
- Biopsy is the most accurate test.

TREATMENT

Treatment questions for IgA nephropathy are extremely dependent on the precise wording. There is a difference between what is used and what will benefit the patient. **There is no proven therapy to reverse or stop the progression of IgA nephropathy.**

Hematuria Alone with Normal Glomerular Filtration Rate

- No treatment is necessary.

Mild Proteinuria

- Use **ACE inhibitors** or ARBs as you would for almost any patient with proteinuria.
- **Fish oil** can be used with any person in whom ACE inhibitors is indicated.

| Fish oil is unproven. |

Progressive Disease/Severe Proteinuria

- ACE inhibitors and corticosteroids
- Cyclophosphamide, azathioprine, or mycophenolate to get the patient off of steroids

| No treatment is proven in IgA nephropathy. ACE inhibitors, fish oil, and a trial of steroids are used. |

Post-streptococcal Glomerulonephritis

Post-streptococcal glomerulonephritis (PSGN) occurs 1 to 2 weeks after streptococcal infection of either the pharynx or the skin. The time between the infection and the renal disease is longer after a skin infection than after a pharyngeal infection.

| Skin infections can cause renal disease, but not rheumatic fever. |

Characteristic features are:

- **Periorbital** and scrotal **edema**
- "Cola" or "tea" **colored urine** (from the proteinuria and hematuria)
- **Hypertension in** 50% to 90%

The best initial tests are:

(1) • Anti-streptolysin O

(2) • Anti-DNAse antibodies

(3) • Anti-hyaluronidase

(3) • Low complement level

The "best initial therapy" is:

• Diuretics

• Antibiotics, if there is evidence of persistent streptococcal infection

Biopsy is not necessary.

Lupus Nephritis

Systemic lupus erythematosus (SLE) can be diagnosed from blood tests with an ANA and double-stranded DNA antibody. **Renal biopsy is essential in lupus nephritis to determine the severity of the disease**, not to establish a diagnosis. If the urine shows protein, red cells, or red cell casts, the "next best step in management" is a renal biopsy. Glomerulo**sclerosis** is scarring of the kidney and will not respond to medical treatment with prednisone. Severe disease with membranous (class V) lupus nephritis can be detected only by renal biopsy. Membranous disease is treated with both prednisone and either cyclophosphamide or mycophenolate. Mycophenolate has less adverse effects and is more effective in establishing remission, but there are more recurrences of disease after stopping treatment than with cyclophosphamide.

Cryoglobulinemia

Cryoglobulinemia is associated with chronic hepatitis C and sometimes hepatitis B. In addition to renal involvement, there is:

Rheumatoid factor is a marker for cryoglobulins. Both are IgM.

• Joint pain → Palpable Purpura (Raynaud Phenomen

• Skin lesions → Kidney (MPGM), nervous System motor sensory Axono Pathy

• Hepatosplenomegaly

Diagnosis by confirmed by Serology (crioglobuling (↓ complement levels)

The **best initial tests are a cryoglobulin level** and a rheumatoid factor and low serum complement levels. The best initial therapy is to **control the hepatitis with interferon and ribavirin**. For cryoglobulins not caused by hepatitis C, use plasmapheresis, steroids, and rituximab.

Severe cryoglobulinemia not caused by hepatitis C gets steroids, cyclophosphamide, and acute plasmapheresis.

Cold agglutinins = hemolysis

Cryoglobulins = glomerulonephritis

or skin biopsy

Alport Syndrome *X-linked*

This is **glomerulonephritis with eye and ear problems**. Patients have a genetic defect in collagen production. They experience visual problems because of displacement of the lens of the eye. Sensorineural hearing loss occurs. This is an **X-linked** disorder that has **no specific treatment.**

Thin Basement Membrane Disease

This is a defect in type IV collagen like Alport syndrome, but it is not severe enough to cause renal failure. There are recurrent episodes of hematuria. Biopsy is the only way to confirm the diagnosis. No treatment is needed. The main point of knowing about this disorder is to be able to **reassure patients they do not have a dangerous disease.**

Fabry Disease

Fabry disease is an X-linked recessive disorder in which the patient is **deficient in the alpha-galactosidase enzyme**. There is an abnormal buildup of **lipids** (globotriaosylceramide) in blood vessels.

The main organs affected are:

- **Kidney:** Mild proteinuria progresses to end stage renal disease (ESRD) by age 20 to 40.
- **Heart:** Premature coronary disease and hypertension may result.
- **Skin:** Angiokeratomas are tiny painless papules. They occur anywhere.

▶ **TIP**

"Foamy urine" is your tip to the diagnosis.

The most accurate test is the **alpha-galactosidase enzyme**. Treatment is with infusion of a recombinant version of the alpha-galactosidase enzyme.

Rapidly Progressive Glomerulonephritis

Rapidly progressive glomerulonephritis (RPGN) is not a separate disease. RPGN refers to the most severe and rapidly progressive form of the diseases described in this section. The terms RPGN and "crescentic glomerulonephritis" are essentially interchangeable.

Some diseases like Goodpasture (anti-GBM disease) frequently become rapidly progressive. Some, like PSGN, rarely become progressive.

>50% crescents + >50% decline in GFR in 3 months = RPGN

> X-linked disorders predominantly affect men. It is much more unusual to be homozygous and express an X-linked disorder in a woman.

> Proteinuria = Foamy-uria

Diagnostic Tests/Treatment

Test as you would for each individual disease. Biopsy is the most accurate diagnostic test

The best initial therapy is high-dose **corticosteroids**, often with **cyclophosphamide** and **plasmapheresis**.

Complement Levels

Complement levels can help somewhat in establishing a diagnosis. In terms of SLE, they can be used to assess the presence of an acute exacerbation or worsening of disease.

Interpretation of Complement Levels	
Low complement levels	**Normal complement levels**
• Postinfectious glomerulonephritis	• IgA
• Lupus nephritis	• Anti-GBM disease
• Membranoproliferative glomerulonephritis	• PAN
• Cryoglobulinemia	• Wegener
	• Henoch-Schönlein

EVALUATION OF PROTEINURIA

Mild proteinuria is very common and may occur in 2% to 10% of the general population at any given time. Your question is: "Who has mild, transient proteinuria? And who needs a kidney biopsy to detect serious, treatable disease?"

▶ **TIP**

These questions apply exclusively to the asymptomatic patient with no edema or signs of nephrotic syndrome.

For mild proteinuria in the asymptomatic patient:

1. Repeat the UA.
2. Assess for CHF, fever, or vigorous exercise. These all cause transient proteinuria without pathologic significance.
3. If the repeat UA shows no proteinuria, then disregard this initial specimen. No further evaluation is needed.

For persistent proteinuria:

1. Assess for orthostatic proteinuria.
2. Split the sample. Measure a protein-to-creatinine ratio on a 16-hour sample from 7 A.M. to 11 P.M., then a separate sample in the morning.

3. If there is proteinuria only on the daytime sample, no further evaluation is needed.

4. If the proteinuria is persistent (not related to body position), renal biopsy may be indicated.

Summary of Mild Proteinuria Evaluation

1. Repeat the sample—it may go away.
2. Assess for fever, exercise, and CHF, which all cause benign proteinuria.
3. Consider splitting the sample for orthostatic proteinuria.
4. Biopsy the kidney if the proteinuria is persistent and is not related to a known cause or orthostasis.

NEPHROTIC SYNDROME

DEFINITION

Nephrotic syndrome is not a single specific disease, but rather a term describing such severe damage to the glomeruli that massive proteinuria has developed that exceeds the ability of the liver to replace it. When a person urinates under 3.5 grams of protein per day, the liver increases the output of protein to compensate. When a person urinates more than 3.5 grams of protein per day, the liver cannot compensate and the blood level of albumin falls.

Hyperlipidemia occurs because it is lipoprotein signals that control the blood level of triglycerides and cholesterol. If the lipoprotein signals have been urinated out with all the other protein, the body loses the ability to control cholesterol levels and they elevate.

Nephrotic syndrome is defined as:

- **Proteinuria** in excess of 3.5 g/1.73 m^2 of body surface area per 24 hours
- **Hypoalbuminemia**
- **Edema**
- **Hyperlipidemia**

ETIOLOGY

Any of the glomerular disorders described in the previous section can cause nephrotic syndrome. The **most common cause in adults is membranous nephropathy**. In addition, nephrotic syndrome is caused by other systemic diseases such as:

- Diabetes
- Amyloidosis
- Myeloma

RPGN = time course
Nephrotic = severity of proteinuria

PRESENTATION

Besides edema, nephrotic syndrome also presents with:

- **Thromboembolic disease:** This is from the urinary loss of protein C, protein S, and antithrombin.
- **Infection:** Immunoglobulins are lost, increasing infection particularly with pneumococcus.

DIAGNOSTIC TESTS

The best initial test is UA that shows 4+ protein or, **if the UA with proteinuria is already given**, the answer is:

- Test protein-to-creatinine ratio on a spot urine.
- 24-hour urine collection for protein is not necessary. The protein-to-creatinine ratio on a single urine specimen is sufficient. If the ratio of protein to creatinine is 2, then the patient is excreting 2 g per 24 hours. If the ratio is 5, then he or she is excreting 5 g per 24 hours.

The most accurate test is renal biopsy.

> The "Maltese cross" is an oval fat body seen under polarized light in the urine with nephrotic syndrome.

Laboratory Abnormalities in Nephrotic Syndrome

- Elevated triglyceride and cholesterol level
- Low vitamin D levels
- Low thyroid hormone levels from urinary loss
- Low copper, iron, and zinc levels from urinary loss of carrier proteins

When Do I Answer "Renal Biopsy"?

If the cause of nephrotic syndrome is clear from systemic manifestations such as a long history of hypertension and diabetes, renal biopsy is **not** needed.

Renal biopsy is the answer if:

- The diagnosis is not clear.
- There is a primary renal disorder such as IgA nephropathy, membranous nephropathy, focal-segmental, or minimal change disease in which there is **no blood test** and **no specific physical findings** to suggest the disorder.

TREATMENT

Nephrotic syndrome is managed by treating the underlying cause and using:

- Diuretics
- Statins to control hyperlipidemia
- ACEIs or ARBs to reduce proteinuria and decrease the rate of decline in GFR

CAUSES OF NEPHROTIC SYNDROME

Besides the systemic diseases previously described, there are several primary renal disorders causing nephrotic syndrome. These include:

- Membranous nephropathy
- Focal segmental glomerulosclerosis
- Minimal change disease
- Mesangial proliferative glomerulonephritis
- Membranoproliferative glomerulonephritis

You **cannot distinguish between these disorders by physical examination, urinalysis, or symptoms**. The only way to distinguish them is by renal biopsy. They are all **treated with steroids** and immunosuppressive medication such as cyclophosphamide or cyclosporine.

Membranous Nephropathy

This is the most common in adults. Membranous nephropathy is also associated with:

- Cancer
- Hepatitis B and C
- ACE inhibitors, NSAIDs, penicillamine, and gold
- SLE

Testing and treatment is as previously described for nephrotic syndrome. The **best initial test is a UA and protein-to-creatinine ratio**. There is no way to confirm a diagnosis without renal biopsy.

TREATMENT

The **best initial therapy is with prednisone**. If there is severe proteinuria after prednisone, the next best step in management is **cyclophosphamide**. When there is no response to steroids and cyclophosphamide, the answer is less clear; cyclosporine, tacrolimus, and mycophenolate can all be correct.

All patients with nephrotic range proteinuria should be managed with:

- ACE inhibitors or ARBs
- Statins for hyperlipidemia
- Blood pressure target of 130/80 or below

Focal Segmental Glomerulosclerosis

Focal segmental glomerulosclerosis (FSGS) occurs in association with **injection drug use, heroin use, or HIV**. Testing and treatment is the same as for membranous nephropathy, but the response is usually worse.

③ Minimal Change Disease and Mesangial Nephropathy

Mesangial nephropathy is likely just a variant of minimal change disease (MCD). Although they are more common in children, they still occur in adults, especially in those with **lymphoma, leukemia,** or **NSAID use.** Hypertension and ESRD are uncommon in MCD. Unlike FSGS, which is extremely treatment resistant, **less than 10% of those with MCD are treatment resistant.**

④ Membranoproliferative Glomerulonephritis

This disorder is really a final common pathway toward ESRD for chronic hepatitis, SLE, **Sjögren syndrome,** post-streptococcal infection, or **endocarditis.** Complement levels are low. Treat the underlying disease, especially infections such as hepatitis C. Otherwise, trials of prednisone, cyclophosphamide, and cyclosporine will work in about half of cases.

> In the pre-antibiotic era, glomerulonephritis was the most common cause of death from endocarditis.

⑤ Diabetic Nephropathy

Screening for proteinuria in diabetes mellitus should occur annually. If the UA is negative, the "next best step" is testing the urine for microalbumin.

ACE inhibitors and ARBs are used in all those with any degree of proteinuria in diabetes mellitus. The goal of BP in diabetes is below 130/80.

> ACE inhibitors are **not** recommended for diabetics with normal blood pressure and no microalbuminuria.

HIV Nephropathy

HIV causes hyponatremia, thrombotic thrombocytopenic purpura, and nephrotic syndrome. If HIV-associated nephrotic syndrome is described, **the right answer is antiretroviral therapy. The wrong answer is prednisone.** When CD4 cells rise with the use of antiretrovirals, there should be prompt improvement in both the nephrotic syndrome and renal function as long at the disease has not progressed to ESRD. ACE inhibitors or ARBs are beneficial.

> Indinavir causes kidney stones, not nephrotic syndrome.

Amyloidosis

DEFINITION

Amyloidosis is the deposition of abnormal proteins throughout the body. When amyloidosis originates from myeloma, Waldenström, or lymphoma, it is called "AL" for **a**myloid **l**ight chain. When amyloidosis originates from amyloid A protein, an acute phase reactant from chronic inflammatory conditions such as rheumatoid arthritis, inflammatory bowel, or chronic infections, it is called "AA" for **a**myloid **A.**

AL Disease (Light Chains)

Causes are:

- Myeloma and monoclonal gammopathy of unknown significance (MGUS)
- Waldenström macroglobulinemia

AA Disease (Amyloid A)

Causes are:

- Rheumatoid arthritis or ankylosing spondylitis
- SLE
- **Familial Mediterranean fever**
- **Chronic infection** of any kind
- Hereditary

PRESENTATION

Amyloidosis presents with involvement of the following organs:

- **Renal:** Nephrotic syndrome develops.
- **Heart:** Restrictive cardiomyopathy occurs.
- **Neurological:** Peripheral neuropathy develops because the nerves become enlarged and then they become compressed.
- **Joint and muscle:** Weakness, pain, and enlargement of the tongue occur.
- **Bleeding:** Factors lost (causing prolonged bleeding times).

DIAGNOSTIC TESTS

There is **no blood test** for amyloidosis. The test is a biopsy obtained from:

- Abdominal fat pad (greatest sensitivity)
- Rectum
- Marrow
- The involved organ

The most accurate test on the biopsy is a Congo red stain.

TREATMENT

There is no specific therapy for amyloidosis. Treatment is based on correcting the underlying cause. AL disease is treated with the alkylating agents that you would use for myeloma, such as melphalan and prednisone. All the other treatments mimic those for myeloma (thalidomide, lenalidomide, bortezomib, bone marrow transplantation). AA disease that is not responsive after correcting the underlying cause is managed with colchicine and cyclophosphamide.

END STAGE RENAL DISEASE/DIALYSIS

DEFINITION

Any form of renal failure without reversible cause that is severe enough to need dialysis is referred to as ESRD. ESRD is most commonly caused by diabetes and hypertension; however, glomerulonephritis, cystic disease, or virtually any of the disorders described in this section can lead to ESRD.

PRESENTATION

Hypertension/accelerated atherosclerosis: The most common cause of death in ESRD is cardiac. Patients develop coronary artery disease and myocardial infarction prematurely. BP is hard to control without an intact kidney. Lymphocytes normally function to monitor lipid accumulation and endothelial cell damage in the coronary arteries. Lymphocytes do not work normally in ESRD and there is accelerated atherosclerosis. **The goal of BP with kidney damage is below 130/80.**

Metabolic acidosis: The body makes 1 mEq of organic acid per kilogram per day. If the kidney fails, this accumulates and metabolic acidosis with an increased anion gap develops. Although there is no medical therapy for this, some data suggest that bicarbonate therapy is beneficial.

Anemia: Loss of erythropoietin leads to normochromic, normocytic anemia. It is the only form of anemia of chronic disease in which erythropoietin is useful. Maintain the hemoglobin between 10 and 12 g/dL. Higher levels do not help.

Hyperkalemia: Potassium is normally excreted by the kidney. Dead kidneys lead to the accumulation of potassium.

Hypocalcemia/bone disease: The kidney activates vitamin D to its most active form, which is 1,25 dihydroxy-vitamin D. ESRD is associated with low vitamin D levels that cause an increase in parathyroid hormone (PTH) levels. This secondary hyperparathyroidism will leach calcium and phosphate out of the bones, making them soft. This condition, known as renal osteodystrophy, manifests as osteomalacia (vitamin D deficiency) and osteitis fibrosis cystica (high PTH).

Hyperphosphatemia develops because PTH takes phosphate out of the bone, but the kidneys can't excrete it. All of these disorders are controlled with phosphate binders, vitamin D, and calcium replacement.

Hyperphosphatemia: This is treated with oral phosphate binders such as calcium carbonate or calcium acetate. Sevelamer and lanthanum are two oral phosphate binders that do not contain calcium. Cinacalcet is a mimic of calcium that inhibits the parathyroid gland, decreases levels of PTH, and helps control hyperphosphatemia and osteitis fibrosa cystica.

Pericarditis: Uremia is irritating to the pericardium. The only treatment for the pericarditis of uremia is dialysis.

Encephalopathy: Renal failure results in the accumulation of waste products that interfere with normal cognitive function and result in delirium. This can be treated only with dialysis.

Bleeding: Platelets work abnormally in a uremic environment: They do not degranulate. Platelets must release the contents of their alpha and dense granules in order to work. Uremia-induced bleeding presents like von Willebrand disease. This is treated with desmopressin, which will stimulate increased platelet function. It is used only in acute bleeding associated with uremia. Platelet function is also improved by dialysis and erythropoietin.

Infections: WBCs do not work normally in a uremic environment. In addition, the most important risk for infection is vascular access. In order to do dialysis, the patient must have a shunt, a fistula, or a catheter in place through which to perform dialysis. These patients are at high risk for infection with *Staphylococcus aureus* and *Staphylococcus epidermidis*.

A patient is admitted for fever. The patient has been on dialysis through a temporary central venous catheter for the last few weeks. There is no murmur. The patient is started on vancomycin and gentamicin and the catheter is removed. Blood cultures grow S. aureus that is sensitive to oxacillin. The vancomycin is changed to oxacillin. Two days later, the patient is still febrile and the blood cultures are still positive.

What is the most appropriate management in this case?

a. Switch the oxacillin back to vancomycin
b. Echocardiography
c. Add rifampin
d. Cardiothoracic surgery evaluation

Answer: The correct answer is (b). The most common infection in those on dialysis is related to vascular access. Central venous catheters in particular have a high risk of infectious complications and endocarditis. Endocarditis presents as a sustained bacteremia even though this case does not describe a murmur. There is no point in switching back to vancomycin; if the organism is sensitive to oxacillin, then vancomycin has twice the failure rate of a beta-lactam antibiotic such as oxacillin. It is not very distressing to still have bacteremia despite the use of antibiotics in a person with endocarditis. It is important to confirm with the echocardiogram, however, that it really is endocarditis. You must increase the length of therapy in those with endocarditis or they will recur after stopping the antibiotics.

If the organism is sensitive, vancomycin has a greater failure rate than penicillins or cephalosporins.

Vascular Access

The more permanent and "natural" the access, the less the chance of infection. Dialysis through a catheter has the highest risk of infection and bacteremia. Catheters should be used only for short durations while awaiting more permanent access such as an arteriovenous (AV) graft or AV fistula. The AV graft can be ready to use in a much shorter period of time (1 to 2 weeks). An AV fistula takes several months to mature enough to be usable.

> It is dangerous to use a catheter for dialysis in the long term.

Dialysis

Absolute Indications

- Pericarditis
- Altered mental status
- Uncontrollable hypervolemia or hyperkalemia
- Metabolic acidosis
- Bleeding from uremia-induced platelet dysfunction

Complications

Dialysis accelerates atherosclerotic disease. Coronary artery disease and infection are the most common causes of death on dialysis. Dialysis also leads to renal cyst formation for unclear reasons.

Transplantation

Transplantation is amazingly superior to being maintained on dialysis in the long term. There are about 80,000 to 100,000 people on the transplant list. Mortality on the list is 6% to 10% per year.

Five-year Survival Rates	
Live related donor	90%
Cadaver donor	82%
Dialysis alone	40%
Diabetic on dialysis	20%

Immunosuppressive Medications

The average waiting time for a matched organ for transplantation is 2 to 4 years. When the transplantation occurs, it is indispensible to use immunosuppressive agents in the recipient to prevent organ rejection. Here is what is used, in order from most used to least used:

- Tacrolimus
- Mycophenolate
- Corticosteroids

- Cyclosporine
- Sirolimus
- Azathioprine

Which of the following is most likely to recur after kidney transplantation?

a. Focal segmental glomerulosclerosis
b. IgA nephropathy
c. Diabetic nephropathy
d. Lupus nephritis
e. Membranous nephropathy

Answer: The correct answer is (a). Focal segmental glomerulosclerosis often recurs after transplantation. The next most likely is diabetic nephropathy. The others all can recur; they just do so less often than FSGS.

Adverse Effects of Immunosuppressive Therapy

The death rate on dialysis is very high, about 10% per year. Therefore, preventing organ transplant rejection with immunosuppressive medication is so important that you would stop medication only with the most severe adverse effect. In other words, the adverse effect of a medication is better than the adverse effect of death from dialysis.

> Renal transplantation increases the risk of skin cancer and lymphoma. Skin is more common than lymphoma.

| Adverse Effects of Immunosuppressive Drugs ||
Medication	Adverse effects
Tacrolimus	Nephrotoxicity, hyperkalemia
Mycophenolate	Diarrhea
Cyclosporine	Nephrotoxicity
Sirolimus	Leukopenia, hyperlipidemia
Azathioprine	Leukopenia

ELECTROLYTE DISORDERS

Hyponatremia

ETIOLOGY

Hyponatremia is extremely common. Treatment is based on the etiology.

Hypervolemic Causes

> Perfusion pressure is more important than a normal sodium level.

These patients have edema and ascites and may have rales as a sign of pulmonary congestion. They are all from increased ADH as a part of the underlying disease. For instance, in CHF, if the volume receptors in the atria sense a diminished intravascular volume, it is appropriate to increase ADH to restore volume. The body will always choose to retain water to maintain perfusion—even if it causes sodium levels to drop. Common causes of hyper-volemic hyponatremia are:

Normal Serum Osmolality = 285-295 mOsm/kg H2O

- Cirrhosis
- Nephrotic syndrome
- Congestive heart failure
- Renal failure

Hypovolemic Causes

These patients first lose water and sodium through the skin, GI tract, or urine. ADH increases, causing thirst, so the patient drinks water. Renal water reabsorption is increased by the ADH. Over time, hyponatremia develops. Addison disease (hypoadrenalism) causes hyponatremia from hypovolemia due to inadequate aldosterone production, which in turn increases ADH release, thirst, and renal water retention. Causes are:

> Skin, urine, and GI fluid losses cause hyponatremia only if combined with free water replacement.

- **Skin losses:** sweating, burns, severe exercise
- **Urine losses:** thiazide diuretics, renal insufficiency
- **Gastrointestinal losses:** diarrhea, vomiting, nasogastric suction
- **Hypoadrenalism:** Addison disease

Extrarenal losses are characterized by a urine sodium [ ] less than 10meq/L

Renal tubular Necrosis may result in adverse renal failure which can result hypervolemia hypotonic hyponatremia urine Na ↑ the 20mg/L

Euvolemic Causes

These patients have no physical examination findings of volume overload or dehydration.

- **SIADH**
- **Hypothyroidism:** low thyroid hormone levels leading to decreased free water clearance
- **Psychogenic polydipsia** or beer potomania
- **Pseudohyponatremia:** hyperlipidemia or myeloma with increased paraprotein

Hyperglycemia

High glucose levels will pull water out of cells into the vascular space. Since the cell membrane is relatively impermeable to sodium, the increased free water coming out of the cells will lower the serum sodium level. Treat this by correcting the glucose level.

> High glucose levels decrease sodium levels.

> **For every 100 mg/dL increase in glucose, there is a 1.6 mEq/L decrease in sodium.**

If you miss the hyperglycemia as the cause of hyponatremia, you will harm the patient and give the wrong answer on your test.

Syndrome of Inappropriate Secretion of Antidiuretic Hormone

Abbreviated SIADH, this syndrome is caused by any disease of the CNS or lung. It is not clear why lung pathology causes SIADH. Cancer of the pancreas, lung, or thymus can also cause SIADH. Medications causing SIADH include:

- SSRIs
- Sulfonylureas
- Carbamazepine
- Tricyclic antidepressants
- Chemotherapy: cyclophosphamide, cisplatin, vincristine, vinblastine

Other causes of SIADH, all of them idiopathic, are:

- AIDS
- Surgery
- Pain

PRESENTATION

All sodium disorders cause **CNS symptoms**. They range from mild **confusion** or nausea to lethargy, **disorientation**, stupor, seizures, and **coma**. This is from either hypernatremia or hyponatremia.

> Symptoms are based on severity, not etiology, of hyponatremia.

▶ **TIP**

You cannot determine the etiology of hyponatremia by the symptoms.

DIAGNOSTIC TESTS

If the etiology of hyponatremia is not clear from the history, the "best initial test" is a urine sodium level, not a serum osmolality. Low serum sodium is nearly synonymous with low serum osmolality. Therefore, a serum osmolality measurement is unlikely to help establish a diagnosis.

| Using Urine Sodium to Establish the Etiology of Hyponatremia ||
Low urine sodium (<10 mEq/L)	High urine sodium (>10 mEq/L)
Dehydration	Diuretics
Vomiting	ACE inhibitors
Diarrhea	Renal salt wasting
Sweating and other skin losses	Addison disease

Diagnosing SIADH

SIADH is associated with an inappropriately **high urine sodium** and **high urine osmolality**. A healthy person with hyponatremia should excrete urine with a low sodium and low osmolality. The diagnosis of SIADH depends on the presence of **euvolemia** and an inappropriately high urine sodium and osmolarity.

Lab findings in SIADH include:

- High urine sodium (often above 40 mEq/L)
- High urine osmolality (anything above 100 mOsm/kg is abnormal)
- **Low uric acid** level and **low BUN**

TREATMENT

Besides correcting the underlying cause, hyponatremia is managed with:

Mild disease (no symptoms): Restrict fluids. Correct at a rate less than 10 mEq per 24 hours.

Moderate disease (nausea, headache, minimal confusion): Saline infusion with a loop diuretic is indicated.

Severe disease (severe confusion, seizures, coma): Correct at a rate of 1 to 2 mEq per hour for the first several hours using:

- Hypertonic saline

or

- Vasopressin V2 receptor antagonists such as conivaptan or tolvaptan

Look at the type of symptoms to answer the treatment questions for hyponatremia. Don't use just the sodium level to determine the answer to the treatment question. A slow drop in sodium can produce no symptoms with a level of 110 mEq/L. Raise the sodium at 10 mEq per 24 hours. A rapid drop in sodium from 140 to 120 mEq/L can produce a seizure. With seizures and coma, raise the sodium much faster.

Osmotic Demyelination Syndrome (Central Pontine Myelinolysis)

When sodium levels are brought up too quickly, osmotic demyelination syndrome occurs. This disorder is idiopathic and presents with:

- Dysarthria
- Dysphagia
- Paraparesis or quadriparesis
- Behavioral disturbances

Lethargy, coma, and seizures may also be seen but are less common.

Desmopressin and water by mouth or IV is used to re-lower the sodium level should this syndrome occur.

Treating Chronic Hyponatremia

When SIADH cannot be cured because of unresectable malignancy, ectopic focus, or chronic lung disease, treatment is with tolvaptan, an oral ADH receptor antagonist. Since the advent of the ADH (V2) receptor antagonists, lithium has become obsolete for this indication if tolvaptan can be obtained.

Lithium has no greater efficacy and more adverse effects such as tremor, leukocytosis, hyperparathyroidism, and permanent diabetes insipidus.

Hypernatremia

Hypernatremia is a much simpler disorder to learn. There are fewer causes, and the symptoms are exactly the same as for hyponatremia. Acute treatment is based on hydrating the patient and, in the case of diabetes insipidus, administering desmopressin (ADH) as well.

ETIOLOGY

Hypernatremia is caused by many of the disorders that result in hypovolemic hyponatremia. If the patient loses high volumes of fluid through the skin, urine, or bowel, and does not replace water, he or she will develop hypernatremia. Diabetes insipidus (DI) is either a deficiency in the amount or the effect of ADH. Central DI is caused by any damage to the brain that will destroy the cells in the hypothalamus that produce ADH for storage in the posterior pituitary.

Nephrogenic DI is caused by:

- Hypercalcemia
- Hypokalemia
- Chronic tubulointerstitial disease (lithium toxicity, lead, Sjögren)

DIAGNOSTIC TESTS

Only DI requires specific diagnostic tests. Every form of hypernatremia is associated with hyperosmolality because the majority of serum osmolality is sodium.

$$\text{Serum osmolality} = (2 \times \text{Na}) + \text{BUN}/2.8 + \text{glucose}/18$$

To confirm the type of DI, the patient is observed for a response to the injection of ADH. If the urine volume goes down and the urine osmolality goes up, the patient has central DI. If there is no response, the diagnosis is nephrogenic DI.

TREATMENT

1. Replace volume losses.
2. Correct the underlying cause, particularly the cause of nephrogenic DI.

3. Chronic central DI is managed with intranasal ADH replacement as desmopressin.

4. Chronic nephrogenic DI is managed with thiazide diuretics.

Hyperkalemia

ETIOLOGY

Hyperkalemia is caused by anything that decreases urine output, destroys large numbers of cells, inhibits aldosterone, or creates acidosis. In addition, medications that inhibit the sodium/potassium ATPase pump will increase potassium levels.

Cell Breakdown

- Tumor lysis syndrome
- Rhabdomyolysis
- Hemolysis
- Pseudohyperkalemia: specimens left out too long, causing WBCs or platelets to release potassium in the sample. **A tourniquet left on too long will falsely elevate potassium**. An under-anticoagulated specimen will cause hemolysis in the specimen, falsely elevating the potassium level.
- Succinylcholine and neuromuscular blockade

> Hemolyzed blood specimens have high potassium levels. Repeat it, don't treat it.

Aldosterone Inhibition or Deficiency

- ACE inhibitors or ARBs
- Addison disease
- Spironolactone or eplerenone, amiloride
- Heparin (inhibits the production of aldosterone)
- Type IV RTA
- Oliguric renal failure

Inhibition of the Sodium/Potassium ATPase

- Digoxin
- Beta blockers

Transcellular Shift

- Diabetes or insulin deficiency allows potassium to accumulate outside the cell.
- Acidosis. Normally hydrogen ions are taken up into the cells in exchange for the release of potassium. For every decrease of 0.1 point in the pH, the potassium level should increase by 0.7 mEq/L.

PRESENTATION

Hyperkalemia is often asymptomatic until the moment it interferes with the cardiac conduction system, resulting in a fatal arrhythmia. Alterations in potassium levels (either up or down) interfere with the ability for muscles to perform normally.

> Potassium problems do not cause seizures.

DIAGNOSTIC TESTS

The most urgent diagnostic test when there is a high potassium level is an EKG. The earliest finding of hyperkalemia on an EKG is "peaked T waves." Widening of the QRS can occur as the conduction system is further impaired.

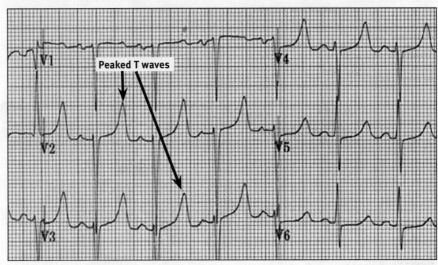

Figure 10.1: EKG with peaked T waves. Peaked T waves are critical in determining therapy with calcium chloride.

Source: Eduardo Andre, MD, and Giselle Debs, MD

TREATMENT

1. **Calcium chloride** or **calcium gluconate** is the best initial therapy when hyperkalemia and **EKG abnormalities** are present.
2. When there is severe hyperkalemia, but the EKG is normal, the best initial therapy is with **insulin and glucose** to drive potassium into cells. It needs 20 to 30 minutes to work. Or, use **sodium bicarbonate**, which drives potassium into cells in the same way that acidosis shifts potassium out of cells. Bicarbonate is not used as much in the urgent management of hyperkalemia because metabolic alkalosis can be dangerous to the conduction system and sodium bicarbonate can cause volume overload.
3. Beta agonists such as **albuterol** drive potassium into cells. They are **slower** than—and not as potent as—giving insulin and glucose, and can cause tachyarrhythmias.
4. Sodium polystyrene sulfonate (Kayexalate®) is a sodium/potassium cation exchange resin. It is used orally or as a retention enema in those who

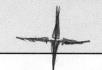

cannot take oral medication. **Sodium polystyrene sulfonate removes potassium from the body via the bowels**. It is slower than the other therapies and requires several hours to work, but it removes potassium from the body. Even though this agent is slow, it is certainly preferable to waiting for dialysis.

Hypokalemia

ETIOLOGY

The causes of hypokalemia are divided into the same categories as the causes of hyperkalemia, just in the opposite direction, so to speak. If acidosis causes hyperkalemia, then alkalosis causes hypokalemia.

The single biggest difference in etiology between high and low potassium disorders is the effect on the gastrointestinal (GI) system. There is only loss of potassium from the GI system.

Gastrointestinal Losses

- Diarrhea: The colon secretes potassium. More colon activity means more potassium loss.
- Vomiting: Gastric fluid is low in potassium, but the volume loss and concomitant alkalosis lead to potassium loss from the kidney. Hypovolemia stimulates aldosterone, which stimulates potassium secretion in response to sodium reabsorption.

Skin Loss

Sweat is low in potassium, so hypokalemia can occur only with very **high-volume sweating** combined with decreased dietary ingestion. Again, losses are primarily from the kidney if hypovolemia stimulates aldosterone.

Hypomagnesemia

When magnesium levels are low, potassium channels open in the kidney tubule, leading to increased potassium loss in the urine.

> Look for a patient whose potassium level does not rise after vigorous replacement to suggest hypomagnesemia.

Aldosterone Excess

- Primary hyperaldosteronism (Conn syndrome)
- Licorice
- Bartter syndrome
- Cushing syndrome (hypercortisolism)
- Secondary hyperaldosteronism with decreased renal perfusion

Stimulation of the Sodium/Potassium ATPase

- Beta agonists (albuterol)

Transcellular Shift

- Excess insulin allows potassium to accumulate inside the cell.
- Alkalosis occurs.

Comparison of Etiology of Potassium Disorders	
Hyperkalemia	**Hypokalemia**
Cell lysis: hemolysis, rhabdomyolysis	Formation of blood with B12 or folate replacement
Decreased aldosterone	Increased aldosterone
Decreased Na/K ATPase	Increased Na/K ATPase
Decreased insulin	Increased insulin
Acidosis	Alkalosis
Potassium-sparing diuretics	Loop diuretics
Oliguric renal failure: accumulation RTA type IV	Renal: RTA, proximal and distal
Succinylcholine	GI and skin losses
	Low magnesium

PRESENTATION

All potassium disorders present with muscular and cardiac conduction abnormalities. Hypokalemia presents with weakness that can be so profound that rhabdomyolysis develops. Other manifestations are:

- Cardiac conduction defects: U waves, T wave flattening
- Ileus
- Nephrogenic diabetes insipidus

> **Periodic paralysis can be with either high or low potassium.**

▶ TIP

Look for sudden weakness after administering fluids containing dextrose. Sugar increases insulin release, which drives potassium into cells and causes hypokalemia-induced muscle weakness.

TREATMENT

Oral: There is no maximum rate of replacement. The GI tract will regulate absorption. When the kidneys are intact, the GI tract cannot absorb potassium faster than the kidney can excrete it. If the level does not rise after replacement, look for hypomagnesemia.

> **Avoid glucose-containing solutions with hypokalemia.**

IV: Rates of IV potassium replacement must be kept low to give time for the potassium to enter the cell. Rapid potassium replacement above 20 mEq/hour can cause depolarization of the cardiac conduction system, resulting in death.

Phosphate Disorders

ETIOLOGY

Hypophosphatemia is caused by nutritional deficiencies, increased urinary loss, decreased GI absorption, and transcellular shift.

Urinary loss:

- Hyperparathyroidism: PTH increases excretion of phosphate.
- Fanconi syndrome: Everything is malabsorbed at the proximal tubule.

Decreased GI absorption:

- Vitamin D deficiency: Vitamin D controls absorption of both calcium and phosphate.
- Fat malabsorption leads to decreased vitamin D.

Transcellular shift:

- Alkalosis
- Insulin and administering glucose

These all function to rapidly activate enzymes in the biochemical pathways that put glucose into storage as glycogen and other pathways that bind phosphate to glucose. Alkalosis, insulin, and glucose essentially "use up" all the available phosphate.

Low phosphate decreases 2,3-DPG. Low 2,3-DPG shifts the oxygen dissociation curve to the left increasing hemoglobin's affinity for oxygen and making it harder for oxygen to be delivered to the tissues. Therefore,

Low phosphate = tissue hypoxia

PRESENTATION/TREATMENT

Hypophosphatemia presents as rhabdomyolysis, muscle weakness, cardiac weakness, hemolysis, and CNS abnormalities. The CNS manifestations all mimic **global ischemia.** If the body doesn't have phosphate, it can't make ATP and it can't deliver energy to tissue. Hence, muscle breaks down, and the brain becomes confused. Seizures, lethargy, and coma can occur.

Replace phosphate slowly so that it does not precipitate out with calcium.

ACID-BASE DISORDERS

Metabolic Acidosis

Every time there is a large decrease in the serum bicarbonate, it implies a metabolic acidosis. You cannot tell just from that one lab value whether metabolic acidosis is the primary disorder or whether it is compensation for chronic

> Alcoholics are the most likely group to be nutritionally deficient.

respiratory alkalosis, although the latter is a rare condition. The pH will allow you to determine what is the primary disorder and what is compensation, as the pH is always closer to what is expected with the primary disorder. If the pH is acidotic (below 7.35) and the serum bicarbonate is low, then the primary disorder is metabolic acidosis.

ETIOLOGY

All forms of metabolic acidosis are characterized by a decrease in the serum bicarbonate. Because it is almost impossible to have a metabolic disorder without some respiratory compensation, you should expect to see a low pCO_2 (below 40 mmHg) with metabolic acidosis.

Anion Gap

The first step in determining the etiology of the metabolic acidosis is the anion gap.

The anion gap is:

$$Na^+ \text{ minus } (HCO_3^- \text{ plus } Cl^-).$$

The difference between the measured cations (sodium) and the measured anions (bicarbonate and chloride) is usually albumin, which is an "unmeasured anion." If a toxic, acidic substance such as lactate, formic acid, acetone, oxalic acid, or beta-hydroxybutyric acid is added to the body, then the total anions (bicarbonate/chloride) are decreased. Since electrical neutrality is mandatory, if sodium stays constant but you add **extra cations**, then the bicarbonate plus chloride must go down. One acid molecule uses up (is buffered by) one bicarbonate molecule, decreasing the value of bicarbonate plus chloride.

Causes of Metabolic Acidosis with an Increased Anion Gap

- Lactic acidosis
- Aspirin toxicity
- Methanol poisoning
- Uremia
- DKA
- Isoniazid toxicity
- Ethylene glycol poisoning
- Starvation

> An increased anion gap means something new and bad is in there.

In each of these, there is an extra acid or toxic substance introduced, accumulated, or produced in the body. This substance reacts with bicarbonate (one of the measured anions), hence the "gap" or difference between sodium (the cation) and the anions increases.

Causes of Metabolic Acidosis with a Normal Anion Gap

- Renal tubular acidosis
- Diarrhea
- Ureterosigmoidostomy

Metabolic acidosis with a normal anion gap has a decreased serum bicarbonate, as do all types of metabolic acidosis. The difference is that in these conditions, **the chloride level is increased**, so the gap between the cations (sodium) and anions (bicarbonate and chloride) is **normal**. These conditions are based on the loss of bicarbonate from the urine or bowel. When the anion gap is increased, it is based on the addition of a substance into the body that is abnormal.

Normal anion gap acidosis = hyperchloremic acidosis

Lactic Acid

Any cause of **hypotension, hypovolemia**, or **hypoperfusion** can lead to lactic acidosis. When salicylates cause metabolic acidosis, it is actually through the production of lactic acidosis as well. All causes of lactic acidosis should be accompanied by a respiratory alkalosis which is compensatory. **If a person has a low serum bicarbonate, it would be abnormal not to have a low pCO$_2$.** The management of lactic acidosis is based on correcting the underlying cause.

Severity of lactic acidosis is directly correlated to how low the serum bicarbonate is.

Aspirin or Salicylate Toxicity

Look for a patient with hyperventilation and tinnitus. The question will often give a clear reason for aspirin toxicity such as rheumatoid arthritis or osteoarthritis. Metabolic acidosis in aspirin toxicity is caused by the loss of oxidative phosphorylation in the mitochondria of all cells in the body. Without oxidative phosphorylation and Krebs cycle, the body is dependent on glycolysis for producing ATP. The metabolic waste of glycolysis is lactate. This is why the metabolic acidosis of salicylates is a lactic acidosis.

Acute overdose: respiratory alkalosis first
Chronic overdose: metabolic acidosis, with some respiratory alkalosis

Other manifestations are:

- Confusion/encephalopathy
- Acute kidney injury
- Decreased hearing
- Respiratory injury, from direct stimulation of the brainstem or from lung injury (ARDS)
- Seizures and coma in severe cases

The respiratory alkalosis of salicylates is not compensation. It is a second primary problem. **Salicylates directly stimulate the brainstem**, causing hyperventilation.

The treatment of salicylate overdose is with alkalinization of the urine to increase excretion of aspirin and dialysis.

Toxic Alcohols: Methanol, Ethanol, Ethylene Glycol

All of these produce:

- Inebriation
- Metabolic acidosis with an increased anion gap
- Respiratory alkalosis to compensate

Differences Between Toxic Alcohols		
	Methanol	**Ethylene glycol**
Etiology	Windshield wiper fluid, photocopier fluid, wood alcohol	Suicide attempt with antifreeze
Physical findings	**Visual disturbance**, blurry vision	Inebriation, seizures, coma
Specific test	Retinal exam with hyperemia	Hypocalcemia, oxalate crystals on UA, renal

TREATMENT

There is no specific therapy to reverse ethanol. Those who are seizing from severe toxicity can have the alcohol removed by dialysis. For methanol and ethylene glycol, the management is based on blocking the production of the toxic metabolite. It is not the methanol itself that produces retinal damage; it is the formic acid or formaldehyde to which it is metabolized. It is not the ethylene glycol that produces the kidney failure and ATN; it is the oxalic acid or oxalate.

The best initial therapy is with **fomepizole**. Fomepizole interacts with alcohol dehydrogenase to block the production of the toxic metabolite. **Dialysis** is then used to remove the substance from the body.

Starvation and Diabetic Ketoacidosis

Both starvation and DKA lead to metabolic acidosis because cells do not have glucose to consume as an energy source. The cells use free fatty acids, and the ketone bodies or ketoacids that come with them, instead. In DKA, this is because there is no insulin to get the glucose into the cell. In starvation, there is just a shortage of glucose, particularly after hepatic stores of glycogen are depleted.

The best initial therapy for DKA is insulin and fluids, while simply giving glucose for starvation solves the problem. This is why **alcoholic and starvation ketoacidosis is best treated with glucose or dextrose-containing fluids**. Once you give the cells the glucose they need, they will stop producing ketoacids as a by-product of pathological fatty acid consumption.

Normal Anion Gap Acidosis

Since diarrhea and renal tubular acidosis (RTA) both give a normal anion gap and an elevated chloride level, the question will be: "How do I distinguish them from the labs?"

This, of course, precludes the idea of simply asking patients if they have diarrhea. It may also be, perhaps, that the diagnosis is not clear from the history or they may have both conditions.

Urinary Anion Gap

If a patient has diarrhea, his or her kidney will still retain the ability to excrete acid. A patient who has a metabolic acidosis on the basis of a GI problem should have a low urine pH. In some forms of RTA (proximal), the urine pH will also be low.

> Urine pH alone is not sufficient to distinguish between diarrhea and RTA.

In RTA, the patient has lost the ability to excrete acid (H^+) through the kidney tubule. With proximal RTA, the kidney cannot reabsorb all of the filtered bicarbonate but can excrete acid normally. This is true of both proximal RTA, in which bicarbonate is lost, and distal RTA, in which acid cannot be excreted. **The urinary anion gap (UAG) is a way of telling whether the kidney can excrete acid.**

In diarrhea, the kidney can still properly acidify urine; in RTA, the kidney cannot. The UAG tells if there is a normal amount of acid in the urine. When the kidney excretes acid, it is bound to NH_3, or ammonia. When bound to acid, the NH_3 becomes ammon**ium**, or NH_4^+. Acid (H^+) is buffered in the urine with ammonia (NH_3).

> NH_4^+ = acid excreted into urine

$$\text{Urine anion gap} = \text{sodium } (Na^+) - \text{chloride } (Cl^-)$$

If the **UAG is positive**, the kidney **is not properly excreting acid**. This is **RTA distal type**. If the **UAG is negative**, the kidney is **properly excreting acid**. This is **diarrhea**.

Distinguishing Types of RTA

Proximal RTA (type II): These patients have lost the ability to reabsorb bicarbonate that has just been filtered at the glomerulus. Bicarbonate is freely filtered, and 80% to 90% of it should be reabsorbed at the proximal tubule. When the body loses the ability to reabsorb bicarbonate:

1. There is a massive bicarbonaturia and high urine pH.
2. When the body becomes depleted of bicarbonate, the distal tubule is able to excrete acid.
3. The urine pH becomes negative.
4. Any bicarbonate given to the patient will be filtered at the glomerulus and then **lost in the urine** because the defect is the inability to reabsorb bicarbonate proximally.

5. Treatment is difficult, because you can't just give bicarbonate and solve the problem (it will keep being lost).

6. Treatment is based on giving a diuretic such as thiazide to provoke a volume contraction. If the proximal tubule reabsorbs more bicarbonate with volume contraction, then the concentration of bicarbonate in the body goes up. Volume contraction also increases aldosterone, which excretes acid from the distal tubule. **Anyone with a contraction of bodily volume in general has an increase in bicarbonate concentration** due to increased proximal bicarbonate absorption.

> Treatment of proximal RTA is based on creating a "contraction alkalosis" by increasing proximal bicarbonate reabsorption.

Because the urine pH is negative (below 5.5), stones and nephrocalcinosis do not form. However, because the blood is acidotic, calcium is leached out of the bones and they become soft. Other proximal tubular defects may be present, resulting in Fanconi syndrome, and include glycosuria without hyperglycemia, hypophosphatemia, hypouricemia, and amioaciduria.

Distal RTA (type I): These patients have lost the ability to excrete acid or hydrogen ions at the distal tubule. When the distal tubule excretes acid, it generates a new bicarbonate. The inability to excrete acid in the distal tubule results in the following:

1. Urine pH becomes alkaline (ie, no acid).
2. **Kidney stones form in an alkaline urine.**
3. If acid is infused into the body as ammonium chloride, the kidney cannot excrete it. Hence, the urine will stay basic despite an increasingly acidic body. This is why the urine anion gap (UAG) is positive in RTA. **There is no acid excretion, so urine ammonium chloride is low.**
4. Distal RTA is relatively easy to treat because the proximal tubule is intact. Because the proximal tubule is intact, you can give bicarbonate and it will be absorbed.

Hyporeninemic hypoaldosteronism (type IV): These patients almost always have diabetes mellitus and have a decrease in the effect on the distal tubule to aldosterone. Because of this, you find:

1. Hyperkalemia and acidosis
2. Persistent sodium loss into the urine, even if the diet is restricted in salt

Treatment is with replacing aldosterone, which is done by giving fludrocortisone.

Summary of Types of RTA			
	Proximal (Type II)	**Distal (Type I)**	**Hyperkalemic (Type IV)**
Clue in history	Fanconi syndrome Urinary loss of glucose and amino acids	Amphotericin use	Diabetes mellitus
Key feature	No stone	Yes, stones	Hyperkalemia
Urine pH	First high, then low	High >5.5	High >5.5
Diagnostic test	Give bicarbonate and find a high urine pH	Give ammonium chloride (acid) and find a basic (high) urine pH	High urine sodium on sodium-restricted diet
Treatment	Very high dose bicarbonate Diuretics	Bicarbonate	Fludrocortisone

Causes of Proximal and Distal RTA	
Proximal RTA	**Distal RTA**
• Myeloma • Amyloidosis • Carbonic anhydrase inhibitors • Heavy metals (copper, lead) • Vitamin D deficiency • Renal transplantation	• Sjögren syndrome • Amphotericin • SLE • Sickle cell • Hypercalciuria

Metabolic Alkalosis

Any time the serum bicarbonate is greatly elevated, it implies metabolic alkalosis. You cannot tell just from an elevated serum bicarbonate whether the metabolic alkalosis is the primary disorder or whether it is compensation for a chronic respiratory acidosis. In order to determine if the metabolic alkalosis is the primary disorder or if it is compensation, you look at the pH.

ETIOLOGY

Gastrointestinal Causes

Vomiting causes metabolic alkalosis because of:

- Direct loss of acid from the stomach
- Volume contraction leading to increased aldosterone and hypokalemia
- Increased aldosterone, which excretes hydrogen and potassium ions from the distal tubule

> **Alkalosis causes hypokalemia. Hypokalemia causes alkalosis.**

Milk-alkali syndrome from massive antacid ingestion is less common, but still occurs.

Urine Loss

Both thiazide and loop diuretics will cause metabolic alkalosis because:

- Any cause of volume contraction increases the renin-angiotensin-aldosterone system and proximal tubular bicarbonate reabsorption.
- Hypokalemia leads to alkalosis. Potassium will leave the cells to correct the serum hypokalemia. Hydrogen ions will go into the cells to maintain electrical neutrality. Hypokalemia increases proximal tubular bicarbonate reabsorption.

Hyperaldosteronism

> **Mineralocorticoid = aldosterone**

Aldosterone increases the reabsorption of sodium at the distal tubule. In exchange for the sodium reabsorbed, either a hydrogen ion or potassium will be excreted. Any cause of primary or secondary hyperaldosteronism will lead to both metabolic alkalosis and hypokalemia.

Causes of Primary Hyperaldosteronism:

- Conn syndrome
- Hypercortisolism has mineralocorticoid effect as well as glucocorticoid effect. Hypercortisolism can increase blood pressure.
- Renin-secreting tumor increases aldosterone.

Causes of Secondary Hyperaldosteronism:

- Any cause of intravascular volume contraction
- Diuretics, CHF
- Bartter syndrome

Bartter Syndrome

Bartter syndrome is an autosomal recessive disorder resulting in loss of salt and water from the loop of Henle. It is distinguished from primary hyperaldosteronism because the blood pressure is normal.

Bartter is associated with:

- Secondary hyperaldosteronism with high renin levels
- **Normal BP**
- Hypokalemia and metabolic alkalosis

High urine chloride distinguishes this from surreptitious vomiting.

> **Bartter syndrome is like being on furosemide all the time.**

It is **treated with NSAIDs** and a potassium-sparing diuretic (**spironolactone**, amiloride).

Gitelman Syndrome

Gitelman syndrome is similar to Bartter in that it is an autosomal recessive disease with secondary hyperaldosteronism, hypokalemia, and alkalosis. The main difference is the site of the defect: Gitelman is a defect at the **distal tubule**. Bartter and Gitelman present like diuretic abuse or someone surreptitiously vomiting.

> **Gitelman** is like being on a **thiazide** diuretic all the time.

Liddle Syndrome

Liddle syndrome is an overactivity of the sodium channel in the late distal/early collecting duct. There is:

> **Spironolactone** will not work in Liddle because it is a defect in the epithelial sodium channel, not the aldosterone receptor.

- Overabsorption of sodium, leading to hypertension
- Hypokalemia
- Metabolic alkalosis

Liddle is **treated with** a potassium-sparing diuretic such as **amiloride or triamterene**.

NEPHROLITHIASIS

Look for a patient with:

- Sudden onset of flank pain radiating to the groin, scrotum, or vulva
- Hematuria/dark urine

What Is the Question?
- What is the **next best step** in management? Answer: **analgesics**
- What is the **most accurate** test? Answer: **spiral (helical) CT**
- What is the **best initial** diagnostic test? Answer: spiral CT if it is a choice; ultrasound if the patient is pregnant or spiral CT is not in the choices
- What is the **best long-term therapy**? Answer: Wait for stones smaller than 5 mm to pass. Use thiazides to prevent recurrences in overexcretion of calcium
- When is a **stent** the answer? Answer: hydronephrosis from **ureteral obstruction**

Wrong Answers
- **Intravenous pyelogram (IVP) is always the wrong answer**.
- Plain x-ray (KUB) should be done only if you do not have the ability to do either a spiral CT or an ultrasound.
- Plain x-ray will not detect stones in the ureters.
- **Dietary calcium restriction is wrong**. Without calcium in the diet, more oxalate will be absorbed and more stones will form.

If the plain x-ray is normal, you have to do a spiral CT to detect the 20% of stones that might be missed on plain x-ray. If the plain x-ray is positive, you still have to do a spiral CT to see if there is an obstruction, such as hydronephrosis, that needs to be stented (you could do an ultrasound, which gives much less radiation, is less expensive, and is very sensitive for hydronephrosis). In addition, plain x-ray is completely inadequate to determine a precise stone size.

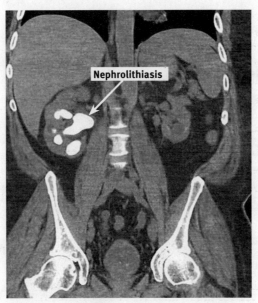

Figure 10.2: Abnormal CT scan with nephrolithiasis.
Stones appear white like a bone on a CT scan.
Source: Eduardo Andre, MD, and Giselle Debs, MD

A 46-year-old man comes to the emergency department with acute renal colic that resolves with ketorolac and morphine. A spiral CT shows a 1.5 cm stone in the renal pelvis. There is no sign of obstruction. This is his first episode of renal colic and all anatomy is normal.

What is the next best step in management?

a. Hydrate and strain the urine for 2 weeks
b. Lithotripsy
c. Thiazide use for 3 months
d. Measure 24-hour urine calcium
e. Surgical removal of the stone

Answer: The correct answer is (b). This stone is far too large to pass. It will not even get through the ureter. Stones above 20 to 30 mm should be removed surgically via percutaneous intervention. It is rare to do open surgery for stones. Even the largest staghorn calculi can be removed percutaneously. For very large stones, a lithotripter can be put directly into the kidney through the flank and then the stone is broken up and irrigated out of the kidney. Of stones smaller than 5 mm, 90% will pass spontaneously. If the case specifically describes a stone between 2 and 4 mm, then hydrate and strain the urine, waiting for it to pass spontaneously.

All long-term management is based on stone size and etiology.

Facilitating Stone Passage

For relatively small stones that have not passed spontaneously, calcium channel blockers and alpha-adrenergic blockers can aid the passage of stones.

Preventing Recurrences/Long-term Management

1. Exclude hypercalcemia, sarcoid, hyperparathyroidism, and all easily correctable causes of nephrolithiasis.
2. Increase hydration.
3. Increase calcium in the diet.
4. Give thiazides for calcium overexcreters.

Special Circumstances

- Struvite stones: Test and treat urinary infections.
- Uric acid stones: Diagnose with CT or ultrasound; they are not radiopaque. Use potassium citrate to alkalinize the urine. Some receive allopurinol.
- Cystine stone: Alkalinize with potassium citrate.

> Uric acid and cystine stones are treated by alkalinizing the urine.

CYSTIC KIDNEY DISEASE

Adult polycystic disease is more common than most people think. It accounts for about 5% of those on dialysis. Patients present with recurrent episodes of hematuria and pain. Over time there are more episodes of pyelonephritis and stones. Screening is with ultrasound so we can avoid contrast. There is no treatment to reverse the disease. The drug of choice for controlling hypertension is ACE inhibitors.

> The BP goal in cystic disease is below 130/80.

Frequently Asked Questions

- What is the most common **cause of death**? Answer: **ESRD** (not subarachnoid hemorrhage)
- What is the most common **extra-renal site** of cysts? Answer: **liver**
- What is the most common **cardiac abnormality**? Answer: **mitral valve prolapse**
- Should we **screen for cerebral aneurysm**? Answer: **not unless there is a family history**

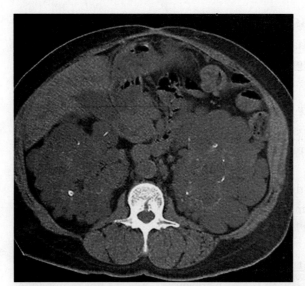

Figure 10.3: CT scan with polycystic kidney disease. Cysts occur through most of the body with polycystic kidney disease.

Source: Mohammad Babury, MD, and Mahendra C. Patel, MD

Extra-Renal Manifestations

Polycystic kidney disease is a systemic defect in collagen presenting with:

- Cysts of the liver, pancreas, and ovary
- Mitral valve prolapse
- Diverticuli
- Subarachnoid hemorrhage

Cerebral Aneurysm

The most common wrong answer is to answer "subarachnoid hemorrhage" as the most common cause of death in patients with polycystic kidney disease. It is not even clear if we should screen for aneurysm with a noninvasive modality such as magnetic resonance angiography (MRA). Remember that gadolinium is no longer to be considered benign in those with renal insufficiency because of nephrogenic systemic fibrosis.

A risk of unruptured cerebral aneurysm in polycystic kidney disease at 5% to 10% seems very high—until you realize that at least 2% of the general population has an unruptured aneurysm.

HYPERTENSION

Diagnosis

When the patient is asymptomatic, the best initial step is to establish a diagnosis. At least 20% to 30% of hypertension on a single reading will ultimately prove not to be chronic. **The higher the blood pressure, the more likely it is to be genuine hypertension.** Repeat the blood pressure measurements 3 to 6 times in an ambulatory office setting or use home blood pressure monitoring as an alternative.

> There is no rush in establishing a diagnosis of hypertension in an asymptomatic person.

Lifestyle Modifications

Once a diagnosis of hypertension is established, the next best step in management is to attempt to control blood pressure with non-pharmacologic methods. The definition of hypertension is:

BP greater than 140/90 in general population

BP greater than 130/80 in diabetics and those with renal disease

The most effective lifestyle modification is weight loss. The least effective modifications are sodium restriction and relaxation methods. Regular exercise and altering the diet to reduce meat and increase vegetables are effective (DASH diet), but not as effective as weight loss.

These modifications should be tried for 3 to 6 months before beginning drug therapy.

Drug Therapy

The best initial drug therapy is a thiazide diuretic. This can be either hydrochlorothiazide or chlorthalidone.

If a single medication is insufficient to control blood pressure, the next drug to add can be any of the following:

Beta blockers = calcium channel blockers = ACE inhibitors = angiotensin receptor blockers (ARBs)

In general, the specific medication used to control blood pressure is not nearly as important as achieving the goal of controlling the pressure. The therapeutic benefit of thiazides over the other classes for initial management is small. Here are the clearest facts:

- Thiazides are recommended first.
- If there is another compelling indication to use another class of medications, there is virtually no benefit lost by switching to the other class.

- At least **30% of patients will need two medications** to control blood pressure.
- If the BP at the outset is greater than 160/100, you should start with two medications.
- The goal of BP in a diabetic or patient with renal disease is below 130/80.

Compelling Indications	
Compelling indication	**Drug to use first**
Coronary disease	Beta blockers (BB)
CHF	ACE (ARB), BB
Osteoporosis	Thiazides
Peripheral arterial disease	Use BB if patient has coronary disease, CHF, or another disease with mortality benefit for BB
Depression, asthma	Avoid BB
Migraine	BB, calcium channel blockers

Hypertensive Crisis or Emergency or Accelerated or Urgency

Don't spend too much time on learning different definitions of these terms. The key issue is:

Hypertension + acute symptoms/end organ damage = immediate treatment with IV drugs

There is no significant difference between the following medications. The key issue is the route of administration:

- Labetalol
- Nitroprusside
- Enalaprilat
- Esmolol
- Nicardipine

Don't lower the blood pressure more than 25% per 24 hours.

Secondary Hypertension

Since 90% to 95% of those with hypertension have idiopathic or "essential" hypertension, when do we investigate for secondary hypertension?

- Those not controlled with two medications
- Age under 30 or over 60
- A clear feature of the history or physical suggesting secondary hypertension

The most common cause of secondary hypertension is renal artery (renovascular) stenosis.

Features in the History/Physical Suggesting Secondary Hypertension	
Historical/Physical feature	**Most likely diagnosis**
Diastolic bruit	Renal artery stenosis
Episodic hypertension	Pheochromocytoma
Hypokalemia	Hyperaldosteronism
Upper extremity BP > lower extremity BP	Coarctation of the aorta
Truncal obesity, hump, bruising	Hypercortisolism
Hirsutism, clitoromegaly	Congenital adrenal hyperplasia

Renal Artery Stenosis

Look for a young woman with fibromuscular dysplasia or an older person with atherosclerotic disease. When there is no clear feature to suggest another cause of secondary hypertension, this is the answer because it is more common than all the other causes put together.

The best initial test is an ultrasound of the kidneys to assess their size.

The single most accurate test is an angiogram. There are 3 less invasive tests:

1. MRA
2. Duplex ultrasound
3. Nuclear captopril renogram

When done properly, these tests are about equal in their accuracy. However, **duplex ultrasound lacks accuracy in obese patients**. Nuclear captopril renogram lacks accuracy in those with renal insufficiency.

TREATMENT

The answer to the "best initial therapy" question is not entirely clear at this time. Renal artery **angioplasty and stenting** is probably still the answer for young women with fibromuscular dysplasia. For older persons with atherosclerotic disease, the answer is less clear. Your questions must be clear so the questions may keep to simply asking the diagnostics. The other way to make the question clear is to include only wrong choices that are obviously incorrect, as in the following question:

What is the best initial therapy of renal artery stenosis?

a. Renal artery angioplasty and stenting
b. Minoxidil
c. Reserpine
d. Furosemide
e. Clonidine

Answer: The correct answer is (a).

This question is a good example of how the boards can make almost any answer correct, as long as the other choices are even more wrong. Relax. Boards don't ask unanswerable questions.

Neurology

11

CEREBROVASCULAR ACCIDENT (STROKE)

DEFINITION

Cerebrovascular accidents (CVAs) most often present as the sudden onset of neurological dysfunction related to an embolus or thrombus (more than 85%) or a hemorrhage. The deficit is entirely related to the anatomic location of the CVA. The most common location is the middle cerebral artery (MCA) because it has the largest circulation. There is no way to distinguish between hemorrhagic and nonhemorrhagic CVA without an imaging study of the brain.

Middle Cerebral Artery

CVA of the MCA results in contralateral weakness, sensory loss, and hyperreflexia. Reflexes may be reduced immediately after a stroke. Hyperreflexia may need time to develop. A homonymous hemianopsia is common. The patient looks away from the side of the hemiplegia and toward the side of the lesion. Aphasia will occur if the stroke occurs in the dominant hemisphere. Left cerebral dominance occurs in 90% of the population in the same way that 90% of the population is right-handed.

DIAGNOSTIC TESTS

The best initial test is a **CT scan without contrast**. This is because the most urgent step is to exclude a hemorrhage, which is essential prior to initiating any form of therapy. Hemorrhage will be visible instantaneously on a CT scan.

> History, physical examination, and a head CT should be performed and interpreted within 45 minutes of presentation to the emergency department.

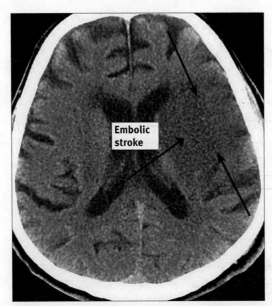

Figure 11.1: Head CT with non-hemorrhagic MCA stroke.
Embolic stroke or CVA needs 3–5 days to become visible on CT scan, but only 24 hours to be seen on MRI.
Source: Moe Sann, MD

The **most accurate test of a nonhemorrhagic stroke is an MRI**. Strokes will be detectable on an MRI within 24 hours in more than 95% of cases. Diffusion and perfusion studies of the brain by MRI, however, will detect a stroke within minutes of its occurrence.

The source of an embolic stroke should be evaluated by:

- Echocardiography
- Carotid dopplers
- EKG, Holter or telemetry monitoring

TREATMENT

CT shows blood instantly.

The best initial therapy of a CVA depends on the time course of the presentation. Thromobolytics are indicated up to 3 hours after the onset of the CVA. After 3 hours, the patient should be placed on aspirin. If the patient is already on aspirin, the answer is either:

Diffusion and perfusion MRI studies show ischemic stroke instantly.

- Switch the aspirin to clopidogrel, or
- Add dipyridamole

Statins are helpful in most thrombotic strokes.

Specific Treatments Based on Etiology

CHADS$_2$ score 0–1: Aspirin CHADS$_2$ score 2–5: Warfarin

Atrial fibrillation: Start warfarin to keep the INR between 2 and 3. The duration of therapy is permanent as long as the atrial fibrillation persists. Atrial flutter is managed in the same way. Anticoagulation should be delayed immediately after a large stroke because it may turn the patient's stroke hemorrhagic.

Carotid stenosis: Endarterectomy is the answer if carotid stenosis is greater than **70%**. It is not clear what to do with 50% to 70% stenosis. The management of asymptomatic carotid stenosis is similarly unclear. Carotid **angioplasty and stenting are inferior** to surgical endarterectomy.

Intracerebral thrombolytics: At the present time, IV thrombolytics are FDA approved only for strokes presenting to the emergency department within **3 hours** of onset. Intraarterial thrombolytics can be safely and effectively given for up to 6 hours after the stroke.

Ticlopidine: If the patient is allergic, or intolerant of both aspirin and clopidogrel, the answer is ticlopidine. The most common adverse effect of ticlopidine (besides bleeding) is neutropenia (0.4%) and thrombotic thrombocytopenic purpura (TTP).

> 70% stenosis + symptoms = surgery

Patent foramen ovale (PFO) closure: PFO closure is the answer if the patient has a deep vein thrombosis (DVT) and a PFO.

Heparin: Heparin is always wrong; it no longer has a role in the management of acute stroke. Heparin causes hemorrhagic stroke and thrombocytopenia (HIT), which is associated with the development of venous and arterial thrombi.

> Statins are helpful in most thrombotic strokes.

Catheter (endovascular) clot-reducing devices: Although several devices can be used after the 3-hour window, none is to be considered "standard of care" at this time. The use of these clot-removing catheters is available only in a very small number of centers.

Control of risk factors: Diabetes mellitus, hypertension, tobacco smoking, and hyperlipidemia should all be brought under control.

Treatments that Are Always Wrong

When you see the following as answer choices for the management of stroke, they are **never the right answer**:

> Oxygen is useful only if the patient is hypoxic.

- Heparin
- Hypothermia
- Glucocorticoids
- Barbiturate coma
- Antiepileptic medications
- Brain surgery (operative drainage of an intraparenchymal hemorrhage)

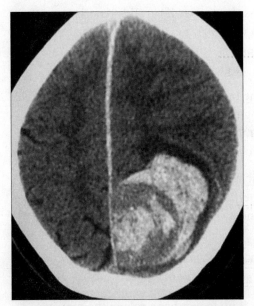

Figure 11.2: Head CT with hemorrhagic stroke. Recent blood appears white. This is why you do not need contrast to detect intracranial bleeding.

Source: Mayurkumar Gohel, MD

▶ **TIP**

Antiepileptic medications are used if a seizure occurs, not prophylactically.

Anterior Cerebral Artery

Stroke in the anterior cerebral artery leads to the triad of:

- Confusion and abulia (loss of initiative)
- Leg weakness on the contralateral side
- Urinary incontinence

Anterior cerebral artery stroke is diagnosed and treated in the same way as a middle cerebral artery stroke.

Posterior Circulation Syndromes

Unlike the middle and anterior cerebral arteries, disorders of the posterior circulation have bilateral abnormalities. **Isolated unilateral weakness is not a feature of posterior circulation** abnormalities.

Vertebrobasilar artery:

- Vertigo, diplopia, ataxia
- Bilateral sensory or motor symptoms

Wallenberg syndrome (posterior inferior cerebellar artery):

- Contralateral sensory (pain/temperature) loss of the trunk
- Ipsilateral sensory loss of the face

> Bilateral pinpoint pupils are most often found with basilar artery (pontine) stroke.

> Wallenberg syndrome is characterized by severe hiccups.

- Dysphagia, slurred speech, loss of gag reflex
- Ataxia
- Vertigo, diplopia, nystagmus, vomiting
- Horner syndrome

Weber syndrome:

- Ipsilateral third cranial nerve palsy
- Contralateral hemiplegia

Benedikt syndrome:

- Ipsilateral third cranial nerve palsy
- Contralateral ataxia

Basilar artery stroke: Severe disease produces the locked-in syndrome. These patients are quadriplegic and can communicate only with vertical eye movements.

> The only stroke that leads to loss of consciousness is the posterior circulation.

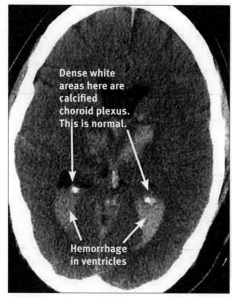

Figure 11.3: Hemorrhage. Acute blood is white, but so is the normal calcified choroid plexus. No treatment for intraventricular hemorrhage.
Source: Nirav Thakkar, MD, and Nihar Shah, MD

Diagnostic Testing of Posterior Circulation Syndromes

Besides the usual testing for all strokes such as head CT and MRI, specific testing issues for the posterior circulation syndromes are:

> Do not repair the carotids for posterior circulation issues.

- Carotid Doppler studies are misleading because carotid stenosis cannot occlude the vertebrobasilar system.
- **Transcranial Dopplers assess posterior circulation.**
- MRI is superior to CT scan in assessing the posterior circulation and cerebellum.

▶**TIP**

Beware answering "carotid endarterectomy" when significant (greater than 70%) carotid stenosis is found in association with posterior circulation syndromes.

Cerebral Vein Thrombosis

Occlusion of the sagittal venous sinus occurs in association with pregnancy and hypercoagulable states. Patients present with:

- Severe headache, papilledema, or seizures
- Normal CT of the brain in 30%; only nonspecific abnormalities found in most of the rest
- Negative lumbar puncture (normal cell count and protein)

The most accurate test is magnetic resonance venography. The most effective therapy is heparin.

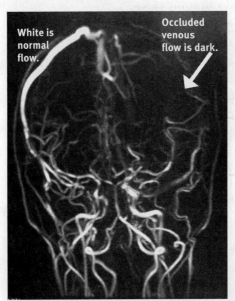

Figure 11.4: MRV showing occlusion of flow.
Normal blood flow appears white on MRV.

Source: Mayurkumar Gohel, MD

▶**TIP**

Cerebral vein thrombosis is the only type of CVA in which to use heparin.

Hemorrhagic CVA

There is generally no therapy for intraparenchymal hemorrhagic strokes. Surgical drainage is more harmful than helpful.

Stroke in a Young Person

CVA is rare in a person under the age of 60 who does not have clear risk factors such as:

- Hypertension
- Diabetes mellitus
- Tobacco smoking
- Hyperlipidemia

If you are presented a case of a young person (under 50 to 60) with a stroke without clear risk factors, you should look for vasculitis and thrombophilia. Testing should include:

- ANA, ESR, rheumatoid factor
- Protein C, protein S, antiphospholipid antibodies (lupus anticoagulant)
- Factor V Leiden mutation
- VDRL/RPR, Lyme serology, C-ANCA in some cases
- TEE

Subarachnoid Hemorrhage

Nontraumatic subarachnoid hemorrhage (SAH) is most often from the spontaneous rupture of aneurysm in the cerebral circulation. The most common site is the circle of Willis.

PRESENTATION/"WHAT IS THE MOST LIKELY DIAGNOSIS?"

Look for a patient with the sudden onset of:

- Severe, excruciating headache
- Fever, **photophobia**, neck stiffness
- Focal neurological findings in 30%
- **Loss of consciousness in 50%**

SAH presents like meningitis. In order to answer the "most likely diagnosis" question before obtaining the CT or lumbar puncture, the case will have to include **loss of consciousness** and say that the **onset was extremely rapid.**

> A "sentinel headache" precedes SAH in 10% to 40% of patients. This is a "thunderclap" headache that indicates the need for a head CT scan.

Cerebral T Waves

Myocardial injury can develop after an SAH for unclear reasons. Perhaps because of a massive outflow of sympathetic stimulation, patients can develop **inverted T waves on an EKG**, sometimes called cerebral T waves. This is because there are ischemic changes on the basis of head injury. There is **no specific therapy** for the cardiac problem.

DIAGNOSTIC TESTS

The best initial test for SAH is a **head CT without contrast**. On the first day, the CT is **95% sensitive**. Because the blood hemolyzes, the CT loses about 5% sensitivity each day. If the head CT is negative, the "most appropriate next step in management" is a lumbar puncture. The lumbar puncture is essentially 100% sensitive by 4 hours after rupture. If the question says the lumbar puncture is negative, there is no SAH.

> A 43-year-old man is brought to the emergency department with the sudden onset of an extremely severe headache. His temperature is 101°F. He has no history of headaches. He lies in bed staying very still, with his arm draped over his face. The head CT is normal. Lumbar puncture reveals 85 WBCs (normal level is less than 5).
>
> Which of the following should be done next to determine the etiology of his headache?
>
> a. MRI
> b. Cerebral angiogram
> c. Ratio of red blood cells to white cells greater than 500:1
> d. MR angiography
> e. CSF culture
>
> Answer: The correct answer is (c). The normal WBC count in blood is 5,000 to 10,000. The normal RBC count in blood is 5,000,000. Hence, the normal ratio is to have one WBC for every 500 to 1,000 red blood cells.

Localizing the Site of Bleeding

The most important initial therapy for SAH is to close off the site of the bleeding in order to **prevent rebleeding**. Of patients whose bleeding recurs, half will die. The first test for the location of the hemorrhage is CT or MR angiographies, which have a sensitivity of 95%. The single most accurate test, however, is traditional **angiography** with a catheter and injectable contrast material. The smaller the lesion, the less accurate the CT or MR angiography, and the greater the need for angiography with a catheter.

> Angiography is not used to detect SAH; it is used to localize the lesion in order to repair it.

TREATMENT

The best initial therapy is to close off the site of the bleeding. A catheter is placed into the cerebral vasculature, and a **platinum wire is coiled up inside the site of the bleeding**. This occludes the lesion so it cannot rebleed. Surgical clipping is not only far more invasive and complicated, but also has much greater operative morbidity. You must cut through the skull from the outside to perform clipping. Coiling with a platinum wire can be done easily in a few minutes with no more morbidity than any other catheter procedure of the brain such as an angiogram. Platinum is used because it never oxidizes or wears out.

> Occluding the site of bleeding by coiling a wire is superior to surgical clipping.

Nimodipine is a calcium channel blocker that is used just after the hemorrhage **to prevent ischemic stroke**. After bleeding, the natural response is that there is vasospasm of the vessel to decrease blood loss. This vasospasm can decrease perfusion sufficiently that an ischemic stroke may develop. Nimodipine is given routinely to all patients with SAH.

Some patients with SAH will develop hydrocephalus. This is from the blood in the subarachnoid granulations blocking off the drainage of CSF. If **hydrocephalus develops, a shunt is placed**.

> It is not necessary to screen family members for subarachnoid.

▶**TIP**

Standard SAH care is:

- Coiling
- Nimodipine
- Shunting hydrocephalus

> Steroids and antiepileptic therapy are incorrect answers in SAH.

Antifibrinolytic Therapy

Because SAH is a bleeding disorder, certain medications have been tried in an attempt to interrupt the fibrinolytic system. Epsilon aminocaproic acid and tranexamic acid have been used to interrupt the fibrinolytic system in the past and in orthopedic surgery. They have not proven to be beneficial in central nervous system (CNS) bleeding. When you see tranexamic acid and epsilon aminocaproic acid in the choices, they are **never right**.

Incidentally Found Cerebral Aneurysms

Aneurysms of the circle of Willis can be found in 1% to 2% of the general population. The larger they are, the more likely they are to rupture. Lesions smaller than 7 to 10 mm **do not** need intervention such as coiling or clipping.

> Incidentally found asymptomatic **small** aneurysms do **not need** to be repaired.

SPINE DISORDERS

Cord Compression

Cord compression presents with back pain associated with spine tenderness. Lumbosacral strain (low back pain) may be associated with discomfort of the paraspinal muscles, but there is no point tenderness of the spine. Cord compression is also associated with:

- Hyperreflexia/exaggerated deep tendon reflexes of the lower extremities
- Sensory low below the point of compression
- Extensor plantar reflex (upgoing toes)
- History of cancer

> When cord compression is clearly present, give steroids without waiting for an MRI.

The "most appropriate next step in management" is first to give glucocorticoids such as dexamethasone, not to do the MRI first. An MRI should be done, but relieving pressure on the spine is more urgent.

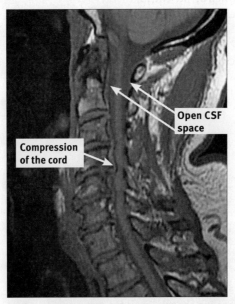

Figure 11.5: MRI of spinal cord compression. The spinal cord is slightly whiter than the surrounding CSF. Loss of the dark area around the cord means compression.

Source: Danny Guillen, MD

TREATMENT

Besides relieving swelling on the cord with steroids, treatment of cord compression is based on the cause of the compression (e.g., radiating lung cancer or giving chemotherapy for lymphoma).

▶ TIP

When is CT myelogram the answer? Only when an MRI is contraindicated.

Spinal Epidural Abscess

Epidural abscess is cord compression from a collection of pus pressing against the cord. It presents in the same way as cord compression, with the prominent addition of fever and the absence of a history of cancer. Testing and treatment are the same. This includes the "best initial step" of giving dexamethasone. **Relieving cord compression with steroids is more important than worrying about the risk of immunosuppression with dexamethasone.**

DIAGNOSTIC TESTS/TREATMENT

The most accurate test is a **biopsy or aspirate for culture**. The most common organism is *Staphylococcus*. Because of the severity of the disease and the risk of permanent paralysis, the best answer for initial therapy would be both **vancomycin and an antistaphylococcal beta-lactam antibiotic** such as oxacillin, nafcillin, cefazolin, or ceftriaxone. Empiric therapy with vancomycin and ceftriaxone (or cefotaxime) is also a good choice. Ceftriaxone and cefotaxime will have the same antistaphylococcal coverage as cefazolin, with the addition of greater Gram-negative coverage. Treatment is then modified based on culture results.

> Vancomycin fails more often for **sensitive** staphylococci compared with oxacillin or cefazolin.

Syringomyelia

Pain and temperature sensory fibers cross (decussate) at the level of the spinal cord that they enter. They then ascend to the brain on the opposite side of the spinal cord. A "syrinx" is a bubble or cavity, so syringomyelia simply means a cavity has developed in the center of the spinal cord at the level at which the pain and temperature fibers cross.

> The most common cause of spinal epidural abscess (65%) is *Staphylococcus aureus*.

PRESENTATION/"WHAT IS THE MOST LIKELY DIAGNOSIS?"

Syringomyelia presents with a unique **loss of pain and temperature sensation** that occurs in a **capelike distribution** across the back, neck, and both arms. Loss of reflexes also occurs. A **history of trauma** to the spine is a clue to the diagnosis.

DIAGNOSTIC TESTS/TREATMENT

MRI is both the "best initial" and the "most accurate" diagnostic test. Treatment is with **surgical decompression** and repair.

Subacute Combined Degeneration of the Spinal Cord

Subacute combined degeneration (SCD) of the spinal cord is damage of the posterior columns of the cord from vitamin B12 deficiency, **copper deficiency**, or syphilis. SCD presents with loss of proprioception (position) and vibratory sensation. Treat with B12 replacement when deficient.

> In B12 deficiency, SCD is not the most common neurological deficit; peripheral neuropathy is more common.

Anterior Spinal Artery Infarction

Anterior spinal artery infarction presents with **loss of everything except position and vibratory sensation**. Because the anterior spinal artery supplies everything except the posterior columns, the patient will lose pain, temperature, reflexes, motor strength, and touch. There is **no treatment.**

These patients have flaccid paralysis with preservation of position and vibratory sensation.

Tropical Spastic Paraparesis

Tropical spastic paraparesis (TSP) is a disorder of the central nervous system from **HTLV-I** infection that **mimics multiple sclerosis**. Patients present with weakness of the legs, hyperreflexia, and painful spasticity. White matter lesions develop in the spinal cord and are visible on MRI. The differences between TSP and multiple sclerosis are:

- Presence of antibodies against HTLV-I
- Almost exclusive involvement of the lower extremities only
- Residence or originating in the tropical regions, particularly the Caribbean
- Absence of optic neuritis

There is **no treatment for HTLV-I**. The antiretroviral medications used against HIV do **not** have an effect.

Brown-Séquard Syndrome

Hemisection of the spinal cord from trauma or a compressing tumor results in a loss of pain and temperature on the contralateral side from the injury and loss of position and vibratory sensation on the same side as the injury. Pain and temperature decussate; position and vibratory sensation do not. There is no specific therapy, except surgical decompression for the rare case of neoplastic compression.

Spasticity

Spasticity means **painful**, overly **contracted muscles** from injury to the spinal cord or upper motor neurons. There is an unopposed reflex arc that makes relaxation of the muscles difficult and impairs passive flexion of the muscles. Spasticity can occur from almost any damage of the spinal cord or brain that interrupts input from the upper motor neurons, such as stroke, trauma, or encephalitis, but it is especially common with multiple sclerosis.

Spasticity is not an incidental problem. For patients, it may be the most important manifestation of their disease.

DIAGNOSTIC TESTS/TREATMENT

Spasticity is diagnosed by physical examination. Spasticity presents as muscles with an **increased resistance to passive movement**. No laboratory test is necessary. The best initial treatment is physical therapy. When this is not effective, the "most appropriate next step in management" is one of the following:

- Baclofen (oral or intrathecal)
- Dantrolene
- Tizanidine (central-acting alpha agonist)
- Intramuscular phenol or botulinum toxin injections

Benzodiazepines are effective, but may cause relaxation to the point of sedation. When medical therapy previously described is not effective, the next step is to directly inject baclofen into the central nervous system (intrathecal).

"Tenotomy" is surgically cutting the tendons to release the muscles when all medical therapy fails.

SEIZURES

ETIOLOGY/DIAGNOSTIC TESTS

All of the things that cause altered mental status, confusion, or delirium may potentially cause seizures. When they are modest, they make the patient confused; when severe, they make the patient seize.

- Hypoxia, hypoglycemia, hypocalcemia, hypomagnesemia
- High or low sodium levels
- Cocaine toxicity
- Withdrawal from alcohol, benzodiazepines, or barbiturates
- Any anatomic abnormality of the brain
- Any brain infection (meningitis, encephalitis, abscess)

You should perform an electroencephalogram (EEG) only when the results of all of these tests are normal.

There is no point in doing an EEG for a seizure from a brain tumor.

TREATMENT

Despite the fact that the number of antiepileptic medications has expanded, there is still no clear answer for the "best initial therapy" of epilepsy. Only the management of status epilepticus is clear.

Who to Treat?

Do not treat those with only a **single seizure**. Antiepileptic drugs (AEDs) should be initiated only if:

- EEG results are abnormal.
- Abnormality is evident on brain imaging (MRI).
- Persistent abnormalities are present in the neurological examination.
- The patient is presenting in status epilepticus (the seizure did not resolve spontaneously).

Valproic acid increases insulin resistance.

What to Start?

There is no clear answer to this question, so it cannot be asked on the boards. **All** of the following are essentially **equal**: phenytoin, valproate, carbamazepine, phenobarbital, and levetiracetam.

Because the efficacy of these agents is close to equal, the lack of adverse effects has made levetiracetam popular. There is also no need to monitor drug levels with levetiracetam.

Specific Questions

1. **What is the best drug in pregnancy?** There is **no answer**. Guidelines essentially say, "We don't know what to tell you to use, but use the smallest amount of it."

2. **What is the most dangerous AED in pregnancy?** This answer is clear: Valproate acid has the most adverse effects in pregnancy in terms of potential malformations of the child.

3. What is the treatment of **absence seizures (petit mal)**? Ethosuxamide.

4. **When can I stop medications?** After 2 years of no seizures. If "**sleep deprivation EEG**" is in the choices, then that is the answer prior to stopping medications.

5. What is the rule on **seizures and driving**? The patient is not supposed to drive until 6 to 12 months have passed without a seizure. However, that does not mean you are able to restrict the patient's license or will be protected if you report him to the Department of Motor Vehicles. The rules or laws on seizures and driving vary by state. There is no single answer you can give on a national examination. Your answer is: "**Advise the patient not to drive**" and to "find an alternate means of transportation."

6. When do you answer "**surgery**"? Recurrent seizures despite the use of at least 2 different seizure medications.

> Valproic acid is most dangerous in pregnancy.

> Phenytoin causes osteoporosis and folate deficiency.

Status Epilepticus

The only truly clear therapy for seizures is the management of status epilepticus. In order of how they are used, therapy is:

1. Benzodiazepines (lorazepam, diazepam)
2. Fosphenytoin
3. Phenobarbital

If the seizure persists, then consider neuromuscular blockade, intubation, and treatment with:

4. General anesthesia: midazolam, propofol, pentobarbital, or thiopental

HEADACHES

PRESENTATION/"WHAT IS THE MOST LIKELY DIAGNOSIS?"

There is no specific test to prove the identity of the headache syndromes. Therefore, recognizing the symptom pattern is the "most accurate diagnostic test."

Tension headaches: Bilateral and described as "**squeezing**" or "**like a belt wrapped around my head.**" There are no physical finding abnormalities and no visual disturbances.

Migraine: Visual disturbance and aura (the sense that a headache is about to start) are the key to the diagnosis. **Visual disturbances** in migraine are photophobia, **flashing lights** (photopsia), "**black spots** in front of my eyes" (scotoma), and wavy, **hazy images** in front of the eyes (fortification spectra). Phonophobia, an intolerance of loud noises, is associated with migraines.

Nausea and vomiting are common in migraine. Look for the phrase "during menstruation" in the history, which is characteristic. **Chocolate**, **alcohol**, and **cheese** can trigger migraines.

Severe migraines may be associated with such severe vascular phenomena as to cause focal neurological deficits (complicated migraine).

Cluster headaches: The term "cluster" refers to the pattern of the timing of the headaches. There are **multiple, severe** headaches of **short duration** happening over a few days or weeks that ultimately stop happening. They can recur as a pattern of multiple short headaches the same time the following year. Cluster headaches occur almost exclusively in men (more than 90%) and are associated with a red, tearing eye; rhinorrhea; and nasal stuffiness.

> Only 20% with migraine get an aura.

TREATMENT

All forms of headaches can be treated with NSAIDs. **Abortive therapy** with a **triptan** (e.g., sumatriptan, almotriptan, rizatriptan, zolmitriptan) or ergotamine is useful in both cluster and migraine headaches. Abortive therapy with **100% oxygen will work only for cluster headaches**. Since cluster headaches will stop on their own after a while, there is often no point in starting prophylactic therapy with beta blockers. All forms of prophylactic therapy take several weeks to work. **Prophylactic propranolol is used in migraines** if they occur 4 or more times a month. Propranolol is the best of the prophylactic therapies in migraine. Almost every form of antiepileptic drug is effective in some people with neuropathic pain such as migraine or peripheral neuropathy. Agents with efficacy similar to propranolol are amitriptyline, valproic acid, topiramate, and other beta blockers such as metoprolol or timolol. It is unlikely that you will be asked to choose between them as a "best initial therapy" for prophylaxis of migraines.

> Triptans are contraindicated in:
> - Pregnancy
> - Coronary disease
> - Hypertensive crisis

Treatment for Cluster Headache

As with migraine, the best initial therapy to abort a cluster headache is a triptan (such as sumatriptan) or ergotamine. If this is ineffective, the "most appropriate next step in management" is the inhalation of **100% oxygen**, which is effective in about 80% of patients.

For cluster headache prophylaxis, use verapamil.

Other treatments for cluster headache that are useful but take some time to be effective are:

- Prednisone
- Lithium
- Valproic acid

These agents would be used for a cluster headache specifically only if a triptan, ergotamine, or 100% oxygen was not fully effective.

Migraine Prophylaxis Medications

The most effective migraine prophylaxis is with beta blockers. This is one of the last remaining indications for the nonspecific beta blocker propranolol.

Seizure medications: gabapentin, pregabalin, phenytoin, carbamazepine, topiramate

Calcium channel blocker: verapamil

Antidepressants: tricyclic antidepressants, SSRIs

Botulinum toxin: injected into the scalp

Summary of Headache Syndromes			
	Tension headache	**Migraine**	**Cluster**
Presentation	Bilateral, band-like pain	Aura in 20%, worsened by alcohol, chocolate, menstruation	Men 90% Sharp, always unilateral, like "an icepick stuck in my eye"
Visual findings	No visual disturbance	Photophobia, flashes, floaters	Red, injected, tearing eye leading to nasal stuffiness
Treatment	NSAIDs and analgesics	Abort with triptans or ergotamine, prophylaxis with propranolol	Abort with triptans or ergotamine. 100% oxygen as additional abortive therapy. Some respond to prednisone or lithium.

Pseudotumor Cerebri

ETIOLOGY

The cause of pseudotumor cerebri (idiopathic intracranial hypertension) is unknown. We know that it is associated with:

- Obesity
- Vitamin A toxicity
- Sagittal sinus thrombosis
- Oral contraceptives

PRESENTATION

Pseudotumor cerebri presents with severe headache and diplopia in association with:

- Papilledema
- Normal head CT
- Elevated CSF pressure on lumbar puncture with normal cell count, glucose, protein

An obese 27-year-old woman on contraceptives comes to the office with severe headaches. Ocular examination reveals papilledema. Head CT is normal and the LP shows markedly increased intracranial pressure.

Which of the following is most likely to be associated with this patient?

a. Seizures
b. Cerebral herniation
c. Inability to look outward
d. Dilated pupils
e. Respiratory distress

Answer: The correct answer is (c). Pseudotumor cerebri is associated with sixth cranial nerve (abducens) palsy. The reason for this is not clear. Seizures do not occur. Although intracranial pressure is elevated, cerebral herniation does not occur. This is because the pressure is elevated evenly throughout the brain. In order for herniation to occur, the pressure has to be elevated further in one side of the head than in the other. If it is diffusely increased, the brain cannot be "pushed" anywhere. Pseudotumor is not associated with evidence of brainstem compression such as respiratory distress or dilated pupils.

TREATMENT

The best initial therapy is a **carbonic anhydrase inhibitor** such as **acetazolamide**, which will block the production of CSF. In severe, acute circumstances, repeated lumbar puncture can be used to rapidly lower intracranial pressure. If acetazolamide does not lead to resolution, the "most appropriate next step in management" is **prednisone**. When all medical therapy fails, placing "fenestrations" or small holes in the optic nerve increases drainage of CSF. Ventriculoperitoneal shunts are also used.

> Always correct the underlying cause. Stop oral contraceptives, stop vitamin A, lose weight.

Trigeminal Neuralgia

The trigeminal nerve is an entirely sensory cranial nerve that can be pathologically compressed in its canal as it passes to the face. Look for **sudden**, **severe**, **overwhelming facial pain** that can be incapacitating. It can be triggered by relatively minor touch: chewing, stroking the face lightly, or the tongue hitting the back of the teeth. The presentation is so characteristic that no specific diagnostic test is generally indicated. The "best initial therapy" is **carbamazepine** or **oxcarbazepine**. If there is no response, switch the patient to one of the following until an effective medication is found:

> Multiple sclerosis is associated with trigeminal neuralgia.

- Pregabalin
- Gabapentin

- Valproic acid
- Baclofen
- Lamotrigine

If there is no improvement, surgery can decompress the nerve or the nerve can be cut (rhizotomy) to relieve the pain.

> Don't forget to exclude a posterior fossa tumor.

VERTIGO SYNDROMES

"WHAT IS THE MOST LIKELY DIAGNOSIS?"

Anything that causes vertigo will also cause nystagmus. The presence of nystagmus will not help you answer the "most likely diagnosis" question in patients with vertigo. If the patient perceives the world as spinning around her, it is understandable that her eyes will "bounce back and forth" to try to keep up with it. Vertigo also causes nausea, so the presence of nausea and vomiting will not help with the "most likely diagnosis" question either.

▶ **TIP**

The most common question on the boards is "What is the most likely diagnosis?"

The key to the "most likely diagnosis" question is:

> CNS causes of vertigo do not cause hearing loss or tinnitus.

- **Hearing loss and tinnitus (peripheral only)**
- Ataxia
- Does the vertigo change with a change in position?
- Are there focal neurological problems? (Central only)

Central Causes of Vertigo

"Central" means the central nervous system. Stroke, vertebrobasilar migraine, multiple sclerosis, and drug toxicity cause vertigo by damaging the central nervous system. When the defect is in the CNS, there is no hearing loss or tinnitus. A stroke causing a speech defect is common, but a stroke that causes the patient to lose hearing is very unusual. When there is hearing loss and tinnitus, it is a problem in the eighth cranial nerve or in the ear itself. Other clues to the presence of a CNS etiology are:

> Phenytoin toxicity is one of the few causes of both horizontal and vertical nystagmus. This happens at very high levels of phenytoin.

- Focal neurological deficits
- Vertical nystagmus

Focal neurological deficits, particularly dysarthria, hemifacial anesthesia, or ataxia, occur in association with nystagmus/vertigo in those who have a stroke of the brainstem or cerebellum. Phenytoin is associated with nystagmus.

Horizontal nystagmus is always a more benign finding than vertical nystagmus. Horizontal nystagmus can occur when the phenytoin level is at the high end of the normal therapeutic range. When the level is very high, the eyes will rapidly look up.

Peripheral Causes of Vertigo

Peripheral nerve defects of the eighth cranial nerve or the inner ear present with hearing loss and/or tinnitus.

Acoustic Neuroma

Tumors of the eighth cranial nerve are also known as acoustic neuroma, neuronoma, or schwannoma, and are associated with **ataxia** or **gait unsteadiness**. This is in addition to nystagmus, hearing loss, and tinnitus. The most accurate test is an **MRI** of the head with attention to the internal auditory canal. Treatment is with **mechanical decompression** with **surgery** or stereotactic **radiotherapy**. About 5% are bilateral, particularly in association with neurofibromatosis Type 2. MRI *of the head only* will miss it.

> Eighth cranial nerve tumor (acoustic neuroma) needs MRI of the auditory canal specifically, not just the head.

Labyrinthitis

Both labyrinthitis and Ménière disease present with vertigo and nystagmus in association with hearing loss and tinnitus. Labyrinthitis is more **acute** than Ménière. Labyrinthitis is usually a brief viral infection of the inner ear.

> Use steroids in acute hearing loss for labyrinthitis.

TREATMENT

Meclizine is useful for most causes of vertigo. Steroids are useful for labyrinth TTD with hearing loss.

Meclizine

Meclizine has anticholinergic and **antihistamine** effects and is useful for vertigo and as an antiemetic for nausea. It inhibits the chemoreceptor trigger zone at the base of the fourth ventricle. Its use may decrease endolymph production and relieve symptoms of pressure in the inner ear. Adverse effects are sedation and dry mouth.

Ménière Disease

Ménière disease is chronic and patients have a feeling of "fullness" in the ear. **Treat with sodium restriction and diuretics**. Treatment with hydrochlorothiazide or acetazolamide is used to decrease the production of endolymph. Refractory cases are treated with:

- Corticosteroid injections
- Gentamicin injections into the ear when medications fail
- **Surgical decompression** of the inner ear (endolymphatic sac decompression, sectioning of the vestibular nerve)

> Syphilis can cause endolymphatic hydrops of the inner ear like Ménière disease.

Perilymphatic Fistula

Perilymphatic fistula is a leak of endolymph from the inner ear that is secondary to **barotrauma** to the ear. There is **hearing loss**, **tinnitus**, **vertigo**, and **nystagmus**. The most common injury in an explosion is rupture of the tympanic membrane, with a number of people developing the fistula. Many patients will resolve spontaneously, but those who do not may need to have the site of leakage **repaired surgically.**

Benign Positional Vertigo

Benign positional vertigo (BPV) is exclusively vertigo and nystagmus without hearing loss or tinnitus. BPV is characterized by severe, acute attacks of vertigo brought on by a change in position of the head. Otoliths are calcium carbonate particles that normally function in the semicircular canals to move the endolymph so that the head's position in space can be determined as the body moves. In BPV, the otoliths become stuck, so the inner ear never "resets" after movement. Treatment is with the Epley maneuver, the rapid alternating movement of the head up and down and side to side, which reestablishes the stones in the canals. This is effective in 90% of patients.

Vestibulitis

Vestibulitis presents in almost the same way as BPV except that the **symptoms don't change dramatically with the position of the head**. There is nystagmus and vertigo without hearing loss or tinnitus. Treat with meclizine and wait for resolution, which should occur in a few days or weeks.

Labyrinthitis – hearing loss or tinnitus = vestibulitis

Summary of Peripheral Vertiginous Conditions						
	Acoustic neuroma	**Labyrinthitis**	**Ménière**	**Perilymph fistula**	**Benign positional vertigo**	**Vestibulitis**
Unique feature	Unsteady gait, ataxia	Acute hearing loss/tinnitus from a virus	Same as labyrinthitis, chronic, "fullness" in ear	Barotrauma	No hearing loss or tinnitus	Same as BPV without relationship to position
Treatment	Surgical decompression	Antibiotics if febrile, meclizine	Diuretics, salt restriction, ablating the inner ear with gentamicin, or surgery	Repair leaks that don't resolve	Meclizine, vigorous repositioning attempt (Epley maneuver)	Meclizine

PERIPHERAL NEUROPATHIES

Acute Inflammatory Polyneuropathy or Guillain-Barré Syndrome

DEFINITION/ETIOLOGY

Guillain-Barré syndrome (GBS) is an idiopathic disorder of multiple nerve roots that is associated with:

- *Campylobacter* infections
- Vaccinations

PRESENTATION/"WHAT IS THE MOST LIKELY DIAGNOSIS?"

Ascending weakness + areflexia = GBS

GBS starts as foot and leg weakness that "ascends" toward the trunk and upper extremities. It is sequential, with loss of ankle reflexes first, then loss of patellar reflexes. The weakness is flaccid, bilateral, and symmetrical. Sensory dysesthesia (abnormal sensation) can occur but it is much less prominent than the motor findings. Dysautonomia (sudden abnormal fluctuations in pulse and blood pressure) occurs in 20% of those with GBS.

> Dysautonomia causes blood pressure instability, arrhythmias, and constipation.

▶ **TIP**

Only polio and GBS give ascending weakness and loss of reflexes.

A patient comes to the emergency department with bilateral leg weakness that has been getting worse over the last few days. On physical examination there is loss of the ankle and patellar reflexes.

Which of the following is the most important to do first?

a. Lumbar puncture
b. Forced vital capacity on pulmonary function tests
c. Nerve conduction studies
d. Electromyography
e. Head CT
f. MRI of the spine

Answer: The correct answer is (b). GBS can affect the diaphragm as it ascends, and breathing can stop when the diaphragm is involved. The head CT and MRI of the spine will show nothing in GBS, which is exclusively a problem of the peripheral nervous system. Lumbar puncture is more useful to exclude infection than it is to confirm a diagnosis of GBS, since CSF can be normal in the first few days after GBS starts. GBS weakens the diaphragm, making it harder to inhale. Inhalation is active; exhalation is passive.

> Weakness from GBS is severe, but respiratory involvement is fatal.

▶ **TIP**

GBS decreases peak **inspiratory** pressure.

DIAGNOSTIC TESTS

The "most accurate test" of GBS is a **nerve conduction study/electromyography**. Since GBS is from loss of the myelin insulation surrounding peripheral nerves, the efficiency of nerve conduction is markedly impaired with GBS. You put two needles into a peripheral nerve and send a jolt of electricity down it, and see how fast (or slow) the impulse is conducted.

CSF shows a high protein with a normal cell count.

TREATMENT

The "best initial therapy" is **either intravenous immunoglobulin (IVIG) or plasmapheresis.** Combining them does not help. IVIG is more commonly done because plasmapheresis is harder to perform, since it is like dialysis.

▶ **TIP**

Steroids are the most common wrong answer for GBS.

Diabetic Peripheral Neuropathy

Patients present with **numbness, tingling**, and **burning** bilaterally. Although the most accurate diagnostic test is a nerve conduction study, this is rarely necessary with a clear history of diabetes. Treatment of all peripheral neuropathies is unsatisfying. The best of the therapies are **pregabalin**, duloxetine, and gabapentin. They usually produce about a 50% reduction in pain in about 50% of patients. Tricyclic antidepressants are no more efficacious and have more adverse effects.

Adverse effects of tricyclic antidepressants include:
• Sedation
• Dry mouth
• Orthostatic hypotension

Mononeuropathies

Most of the mononeuropathies are from trauma or compression of the nerve. There is little medical therapy to reverse them. The management, with the exception of facial palsy, is to remove the cause of pressure or compression.

Mononeuritis Multiplex

The term "mononeuritis multiplex" means the involvement of multiple peripheral nerves large enough to have names (e.g., an ulnar **and** a peroneal nerve, or a radial **and** a median nerve). This differs from the term "peripheral neuropathy," which describes diffuse, often bilateral involvement of tiny twigs of peripheral nerves. Examples of conditions resulting in peripheral neuropathy are diabetes, pyridoxine (B6) deficiency, or B12 deficiency.

"What Is the Most Likely Diagnosis?"

Multiple, asymmetrical neuropathies of large nerves = mononeuritis multiplex

Bilateral, symmetrical "glove and stocking," "numbness and tingling" = peripheral neuropathy

Mononeuritis multiplex should make you look for a systemic disease such as vasculitis. This is very important. The "best initial test" and "best initial therapy" questions will be of the underlying disease, not specifically a nerve conduction study.

> Mononeuritis multiplex cannot be fixed with decompression measures such as you would do for single nerve syndromes.

ETIOLOGY

Look for:

- Polyarteritis nodosa
- Wegener granulomatosis
- Churg-Strauss syndrome
- Vasculitis
- Liver and kidney failure
- Amyloidosis
- Paraneoplastic syndromes

TREATMENT

Besides correcting the underlying cause, the "best initial therapy" is with gabapentin, pregabalin, duloxetine, or tricyclics as you would treat peripheral neuropathy.

Radial Nerve Palsy

Look for injury to the axilla such as with crutches or the arm hanging over the back of a chair ("Saturday night palsy"). **"Wrist drop"** occurs because the radial nerve supplies the extensor muscles of the wrist and fingers.

> Radial nerve = wrist drop

Ulnar Neuropathy

Look for:

- Injury to the elbow
- Repetitive trauma to the palm (bike riders)
- Sensory loss of the fourth and fifth fingers
- Weakness of hand muscles near the fourth and fifth fingers
- Splints first, surgery last

> Pregnancy increases lumbar lordosis, which stretches L2/L3 nerve roots, causing pain.

Meralgia Paresthetica (Lateral Femoral Cutaneous Nerve)

This damage to the lateral femoral cutaneous nerve as it passes under the inguinal ligament occurs in obese or pregnant people who sit with their legs crossed. Look for pain and paresthesias along the outer aspect of the upper, outer part of the thigh.

Peroneal Neuropathy

The peroneal nerve passes behind the knee and supplies the muscles that dorsiflex the foot. High boots hit the back of the knee, causing **foot drop**. It also happens from sitting cross-legged for too long. The most common compression site is at the fibular head.

Tarsal Tunnel Syndrome

> Tarsal tunnel syndrome is like carpal tunnel syndrome, but it occurs in the foot.

The tibial nerve passes under the tarsal tunnel of the foot. Overuse or compression of the posterior tibial nerve leads to **pain**, **paresthesias**, **and numbness** on the **bottom of the foot**. The pain is worse at night. Tarsal tunnel syndrome spares the heel. Surgical release is curative.

Plantar Fasciitis

Plantar fasciitis can easily be confused with tarsal tunnel syndrome. Both cause **pain in the bottom of the foot**.

Clinical Pattern of Tarsal Tunnel Syndrome and Plantar Fasciitis	
Tarsal tunnel	**Plantar fasciitis**
Worse at night	Worse with first few steps in the morning
More use makes it worse	Stretching and use improve the pain
Spares the heel	Mainly affects the heel
May have muscle weakness	No muscle weakness

Bell (Seventh Cranial Nerve) Palsy

Besides paralysis of the entire half of the face, Bell palsy is associated with:

- Hyperacusis (loss of the "shock absorber" stapedius muscle in the middle ear)
- Face "feels stiff" or "pulled to one side"
- Impaired eye closure potentially causing corneal ulceration
- Loss of taste

TREATMENT

The best initial therapy is with **prednisone. Lubricating eye drops** are used because there is considerable difficulty in closing the eye: The orbicularis oculi muscle is innervated by the facial nerve.

▶**TIP**

Acyclovir is the most common wrong answer. It does not help.

MYASTHENIA GRAVIS

PRESENTATION

Look for a person with muscle weakness associated with:

- Worsening at the end of the day
- **Difficulty chewing** or finishing meals
- Difficulty swallowing leading to aspiration pneumonia
- **Diplopia** and **ptosis**

Myasthenia gravis has no effect on sensation. Reflexes also remain normal. The key is, sustained activity makes the weakness worse.

DIAGNOSTIC TESTS

The best initial test is **anti-acetylcholine receptor antibodies**. They are present in 90% of patients. For those with a negative test for acetylcholine receptor antibodies, the "most appropriate next step" is antibodies to muscle-specific tyrosine kinase. Anti-muscle specific kinase (anti-musk) is present in 50% of patients.

Edrophonium testing: If anti-acetylcholine receptor antibodies are not in the choice, the "best initial test" is to give edrophonium and observe for an improvement in muscle strength.

Single fiber electromyography: This is the **most accurate test** for myasthenia gravis. There will be decreased muscle response to stimulation.

Chest x-ray/CT/MRI: When the question asks, "What imaging study is most likely to benefit the patient?" the answer is "chest...something." This is to look for thymoma.

> Pupillary responses are normal in myasthenia.

> Myasthenia is first diagnosed with anti-acetylcholine receptor and anti-muscle specific kinase.

TREATMENT

The best initial therapy is with anti-acetylcholinesterase medications such as:

- Pyridostigmine
- Neostigmine

Although these medications will increase the level of acetylcholine and improve symptoms, they do nothing to alter the progression of the disease. Anti-acetylcholine receptor antibodies will continue to degrade the number of receptors at the neuromuscular junction. The disease will worsen and will be harder to control with pyridostigmine or neostigmine.

When anti-acetylcholinesterase medications do not control the disease, the "most appropriate next step in management" is thymectomy if the person is younger (less than 60). If the patient is older, thymectomy will not work and prednisone is started until other immunosuppressive medications, such as azathioprine, cyclosporine, cyclophosphamide, or mycophenolate, have time to take effect.

With **acute myasthenic crisis**, some patients present with sudden, extremely severe weakness. Severe acute disability is treated with **IVIG or plasmapheresis** in addition to pyridostigmine or neostigmine. Ventilatory support is given as needed.

AMYOTROPHIC LATERAL SCLEROSIS

Amyotrophic lateral sclerosis (ALS) is a disorder of upper and lower motor neurons producing the following problems:

Presentation of ALS	
Upper motor neuron finding	**Lower motor neuron finding**
Spasticity	Wasting
Hyperreflexia	Fasciculations
Upgoing toes (extensor plantar reflex)	

> Sensory, sexual, autonomic, and cognitive function are normal in ALS.

There is **no specific diagnostic test**. MRI of the head and spine will be normal. Treatment is with **riluzole**, which prevents glutamate accumulation at the motor neuron and decreases the rate of progression of disease.

Complications of Disease

- **Carbon dioxide accumulation:** Use CPAP or BiPAP as the best initial therapy. Some patients will become ventilator-dependent or need intubation.
- **Bulbar palsy:** This means damage to the nuclei of the cranial nerves. This gives difficulty swallowing, chewing, and coughing. This contributes to respiratory difficulty and aspiration pneumonia.

MULTIPLE SCLEROSIS

PRESENTATION/"WHAT IS THE MOST LIKELY DIAGNOSIS?"

> Internuclear ophthalmoplegia: inability to adduct one eye past the midline, with nystagmus of the other eye

Multiple sclerosis (MS) most commonly presents with **transient visual disturbance** in a young woman. The visual disturbance is due to **optic neuritis**. By definition, you cannot make a diagnosis of MS on only this single presentation. The **optic neuritis should largely resolve with steroids**. Subsequent defects will be:

- Motor weakness at any part of the body
- Sensory disturbance (weakness, numbness, tingling)
- Spastic paraparesis
- Urinary urgency
- Ataxia
- Worsened by increasing body heat

> Cognition stays intact in MS until the disease is very far advanced.

DIAGNOSTIC TESTS

The best initial and most accurate test is an MRI.

For MS, CT scan is always a wrong answer if an MRI can be done.

> Visual and auditory "evoked potentials" are always wrong answers.

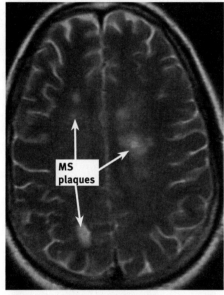

Figure 11.6: MRI with MS plaques. White matter plaques on an MRI is both the "best initial" and "most accurate" diagnostic test.

Source: Harman Chawla, MD

CSF Analysis

CSF analysis for oligoclonal bands of IgG is neither as sensitive nor as specific as an MRI. The main reason to assess CSF is to exclude other diseases in equivocal cases or to look for oligoclonal bands in the small percentage in whom the MRI is nondiagnostic. CSF in MS shows:

> A CSF WBC count higher than 50 to 100 or the presence of neutrophils should make you rethink the diagnosis. Maybe it is not MS.

- Mild elevation in protein
- Mild elevation in lymphocyte count (less than 50 to 100)

▶ **TIP**

For the boards, the question "What does this test show?" is not as important as "When is this test the right answer?"

TREATMENT

Acute exacerbations/deterioration: Treat with boluses of high doses of steroids.

Prevention of progression: One of the most important questions about MS is "How do you prevent progression?" Since there is no cure and no unique physical finding, the question is basically "**Do you know that steroids don't prevent progression?**"

Drugs that prevent progression:

- Glatiramer
- Beta interferon (causes flulike symptoms)
- Mitoxantrone (cardiotoxic)
- Natalizumab (causes progressive multifocal leukoencephalopathy)
- Fingolimod (oral)

Spasticity:

- Baclofen
- Tizanidine (central alpha agonist)
- Dantrolene

Fatigue:

- Amantadine
- Modafinil and methylphenidate (amphetamine-like stimulants)

> MS is one of the most frequent reasons physician-assisted suicide is requested.

> Don't forget to treat depression in MS.

PARKINSONISM

ETIOLOGY

Most cases have no clear etiology beyond aging. Damage to the brain that destroys the substantia nigra results in parkinsonism. Examples are:

- Trauma such as **boxing**
- Hypoxia and **stroke**
- **Encephalitis**
- Neuroleptic (antipsychotic) medications
- Carbon monoxide poisoning

PRESENTATION/"WHAT IS THE MOST LIKELY DIAGNOSIS?"

Since there is no blood or radiologic test that diagnoses parkinsonism, the presentation is the diagnosis. Mild disease presents with a tremor. As the disease advances, everything becomes slow. Look for:

- Rigidity
- Bradykinesia

- Tremor at rest, improved with movement
- Gait disturbance with shuffling and the need to turn very slowly "en bloc"
- Micrographia (small writing)
- Hypomimia (decreased facial expression)

Orthostasis in Parkinsonism

The same overall slowness (bradykinesia) also occurs in the autonomic nervous system. When a healthy person gets up from lying flat, there should be a transient tachycardia and constriction of blood vessels. Those with parkinsonism have "cogwheeling" of their autonomic nervous system as well. The normal tachycardia and vasoconstriction is absent or diminished, creating orthostatic hypotension.

Dementia in Parkinsonism

Parkinsonism is a movement and gait disorder. Mentation should remain intact when the diagnosis is first made. If there is prominent or early development of dementia, you should reevaluate your diagnosis. If the CT/MRI is normal, you should answer "Lewy body dementia." Treat with parkinsonian and dementia medications.

Psychosis and Mood Disorders in Parkinsonism

Psychosis with hallucinations and delusions is a part of the disease process and is often worsened by drug treatment. Up to 50% of patients are depressed.

TREATMENT

The answer to the treatment question is based on the severity of the disease presentation. Mild disease largely means just a tremor; such patients can still take care of themselves at home.

Mild Parkinsonism

Younger patients (below 60) with tremor as their main presentation are treated with **anticholinergic medications** such as benztropine, trihexyphenidyl, or procyclidine. Adverse effects can be severe such as:

- Dry mouth
- Constipation
- Urinary retention
- Glaucoma
- Confusion

Dopamine agonists such as ropinirole or pramipexole can also be used in mild disease. They do not have the adverse effects of the anticholinergic medications.

Older patients (above 60) get constipation and urine retention with anticholinergic medications. For older persons with tremor and rigidity, **amantadine** extracts dopamine from the substantia nigra.

Severe Parkinsonism

These patients will be described as "unable to take care of themselves" or as having "marked bradykinesia." The best initial therapy is either **levodopa/carbidopa** or a **direct-acting dopamine agonist** such as pramipexole or ropinerole, which can be used before, or with, levodopa/carbidopa. Dopamine agonists will have less efficacy (potency), but they will also have fewer adverse effects.

"On/Off" Phenomenon

The requirement for dopamine in the body is not constant. Unlike diabetes, however, you cannot monitor dopamine levels with a finger stick and just inject a little more. On/off phenomenon is from the variation in need for dopamine. When a patient needs less, he or she develops nausea, vomiting, hypotension, and cardiac abnormalities. When the requirement for dopamine goes up, the patient ends up being deficient. This is the "off" phenomenon. The patient appears frozen or locked in.

> On/off phenomenon is the swing between dyskinesia/restlessness ("on") and severe bradykinesia ("off").

Dopamine Augmenting Medications

These medications extend the half-life of dopamine to decrease the likelihood of on/off phenomenon.

- COMT inhibitors: **Tolcapone** and **entacapone** both block the metabolism of dopamine. They are added to levodopa/carbidopa.
- MAO inhibitors: **Selegiline** and **rasagiline** both inhibit the breakdown of dopamine and decrease the likelihood of on/off events.

> Deep brain stimulation is effective in drug-resistant Parkinson's.

Surgery and Deep Brain Stimulation

When all medical therapy has been tried and the patient still has severe parkinsonism, **surgically implanted electrodes** for deep-brain stimulation can alleviate symptoms of parkinsonism.

Antipsychotic Medications

Psychosis with hallucinations can be part of the disease process in parkinsonism. In addition, treatment with dopamine replacement (levodopa/carbidopa) and ancillary medications may result in symptoms of psychosis for the patient. In these patients, it is not possible to simply stop the medication. This would result in severe bradykinesia and immobility. These patients must continue their dopamine medications and take antipsychotic medications such as olanzapine, quetiapine, or clozapine. Quetiapine is least likely to cause tardive dyskinesia and movement problems.

> Beware of neutropenia with clozapine.

> Quetiapine has the smallest risk in Parkinson's.

TREMOR

Parkinsonism is a tremor at rest that improves with movement (intention). Cerebellar disorders give tremor only on reaching for things. When an otherwise healthy patient has a tremor with both rest and intention, this is an essential tremor.

Essential tremor is worsened by beta agonists and caffeine and is improved with alcohol. The case may describe a person with a "shaky hand that improves after a few drinks." **Essential tremor** is best treated with beta blockers such as **propranolol**.

Alternate therapies are:

- Primidone
- Benzodiazepines
- Gabapentin
- Topiramate

RESTLESS LEG SYNDROME

Restless leg syndrome (RLS) often comes to attention when the partners of affected people finds themselves bruised from being kicked at night in bed. RLS is precisely what the name says: an uncomfortable feeling in the lower extremities at night that improves with movement. RLS is best treated with the direct-acting dopamine agonist **ropinirole or pramipexole**. Rule out iron deficiency with a serum ferritin.

HEAD TRAUMA

All patients with head trauma severe enough to result in loss of consciousness or altered mental status should undergo a CT scan without contrast. Without head CT, there is no way to determine conclusively if the patient has a subdural or epidural hematoma. Both subdural and epidural hematomas have a "lucid interval," a period of normalcy between the initial loss of consciousness and the accumulation of blood later.

There are no focal neurological abnormalities in a person with concussion. The head CT is normal and there is no therapy. Patients with subdural and epidural hematoma can have focal neurological abnormalities. If they are large, both are treated with hyperventilation, mannitol, and surgical decompression. **Steroids are not useful for intracranial bleeding.**

Rapid decompression of intracranial hemorrhage is with:

- Mild hyperventilation
- Mannitol
- Surgical decompression
- Intracranial pressure monitoring
- Head of bed up

Hyperventilation

The rationale for hyperventilation with increased intracranial pressure is that there will be a **decrease in PCO$_2$, which constricts the blood vessels of the cerebral circulation**. This will cause a rapid decease in intracranial pressure. Hyperventilation is controversial because the same vasoconstriction may possibly decrease cerebral perfusion. The bottom-line answer is: hyperventilation with a mild decrease in pCO$_2$ (30 to 35 mm Hg) is considered useful in intracranial hemorrhage while awaiting surgical evacuation.

Head Trauma				
	Concussion	**Contusion**	**Subdural**	**Epidural**
LOC (loss of consciousness)	Yes	Yes	Yes	Yes
Focal findings	None	Rarely yes	Yes or no	Yes or no
CT result	Normal	Ecchymoses	Crescent	Lens-shaped bleed
Treatment	None	None	Drain	Drain

Ineffective Therapy

Steroids and loop diuretics are ineffective therapies.

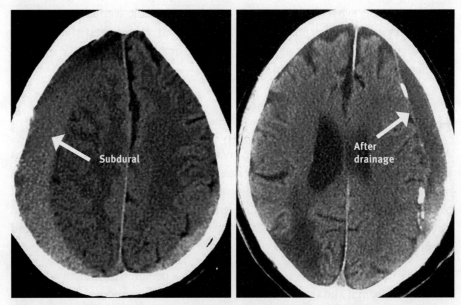

Figure 11.7: Head CT with subdural hematoma and post-surgical drainage. Blood is lighter than CSF. Subdural bleeding is from veins at lower pressure. (not the same patient)

Source: Rasik Parmar, MD, Nirav Thakkar, MD, and Nihar Shah, MD

WOMEN'S HEALTH

12

BREAST DISORDERS

Fibrocystic Condition

ETIOLOGY

Fibrocystic condition is a painful but histologically benign disorder of the breast. Although it seems to be related to estrogen and is worsened by even minor trauma, the true cause is unknown. The alternate name "cyclic mastalgia" sums up the disease in two words.

> Estrogen seems to be causative because this condition occurs only in premenopausal women or postmenopausal women on hormone replacement.

▶ TIP

Prepare to answer a "most likely diagnosis" question for fibrocystic condition since etiology and treatment are unclear.

PRESENTATION

Look for a woman between 30 and 50 who has **breast pain that is clearly described as cyclical**. The pain is worst in the time leading up to menstruation and improves when the menstrual period begins. Also look for:

- Rapid fluctuations in size of a breast mass
- Breast described as "lumpy and bumpy"

DIAGNOSTIC TESTS

Mammography is the best initial diagnostic test. The abnormal density of the breasts with fibrocystic condition can obscure the mammogram. Ultrasound is used with the mammogram and is of most value in differentiating cystic from solid lesions. Ultrasound has greater accuracy in those under age 30. The most accurate test is a biopsy.

Fine needle aspiration is for cystic lesions. Core needle or excisional biopsy is for persistent, solid lesions.

TREATMENT

There is no cure for fibrocystic condition. Therapy is vague. When asked for the "best initial therapy," your answer is:

1. Breast support with brassiere day and night can help avoid trauma.
2. Postmenopausal women should stop hormone replacement.
3. Danazol, a synthetic androgen, is the only FDA-approved treatment.
4. Less clear therapies include oil of evening primrose, vitamin E, and dietary modifications like avoiding fat, caffeine, and chocolate.

> Danazol gives androgenic adverse effects including:
> - Acne
> - Hirsutism

▶ TIP

If Danazol is one of the choices, then all dietary modifications are wrong answers.

VAGINAL BLEEDING DISORDERS

Abnormal Premenopausal Bleeding

DEFINITION

Abnormal bleeding is:

- **Menorrhagia:** excessive bleeding at regular menstrual intervals
- **Dysfunctional uterine bleeding:** occurs at irregular intervals

ETIOLOGY

Menorrhagia is most often caused by **fibroids** (uterine leiomyoma). Other causes are:

- Endometrial polyps (usually are benign)
- Intrauterine devices (IUD)
- Adenomyosis (endometrial glands within the uterine wall; the uterus markedly enlarges)

> Ectropion is when the columnar epithelium of the endocervix is exposed to the exocervix.

Dysfunctional uterine bleeding must first be evaluated by a pregnancy test. This is followed with a speculum examination. If these are negative, then other causes are:

- Endometrial hyperplasia
- Oral contraceptives (especially combination pills and progesterone-only pills)
- Polycystic ovary syndrome
- Thyroid dysfunction
- Infections (PID, cervicitis, endometritis)
- Cervical disorders (polyps, cancer, ectropion, endometriosis)
- Endometrial cancer

> Genital tract cancer at any level (cervix, vagina, endometrium, fallopian tubes) causes bleeding.

Diagnostic Tests

- **Pregnancy test**
- **Thyroid function tests**
- **Ultrasound:** adnexal masses, fibroids
- **Endovaginal or saline infusion ultrasound:** endometrial polyps, subserous myomas
- **Hysteroscopy:** polyps, endometrial cancer

Treatment

Treatment is based on the underlying cause. Polyps and cancer are removed surgically. Dysfunctional uterine bleeding not related to cancer, fibroids, or anatomic abnormalities is treated hormonally with:

- Progestins (medroxyprogesterone, norethindrone)
- High-dose estrogen oral contraceptives for short duration to "reset" the menstrual cycle
- Danazol
- GnRH agonists (leuprolide)

If hormonal treatment does not work, a hormone-containing IUD (levonorgestrel) or endometrial ablation is used. Hysterectomy is the answer only when all the other therapies have failed.

Fibroids (Leiomyomas)

Treatment of fibroids is based on the location, severity of symptoms, and desire to have children in the future.

- **Hysteroscopic myomectomy** allows removal of submucosal fibroids and preserves the ability to have children.
- **Abdominal myomectomy or laparoscopic removal** is used if the lesion is subserosal or intramural.
- **Uterine artery embolization** allows selective infarction of the blood supply to the fibroid without surgery.
- **Hysterectomy** is used for larger lesions. When childbearing is no longer desired.

> The route of removal of a fibroid is based on location. Hysteroscope the inside ones, and laparoscope the outside ones.

Postmenopausal Bleeding

Etiology/Presentation

Postmenopausal bleeding is usually painless and is more often from:

- Vaginal atrophy, friction ulcers, or trauma
- Endometrial polyps or cancer

- Cervical cancer
- Estrogen as hormone replacement therapy

DIAGNOSTIC TESTS

If physical examination does not reveal a clear cause of bleeding, the "next best step in management" is transvaginal ultrasound or endometrial biopsy. If the endometrium is less than 5 mm thick, the answer is:

- Endocervical curettage and biopsy
- Dilation & curettage (D&C) with hysteroscopy

TREATMENT

Endometrial biopsy or D&C may be curative. Hyperplasia is treated with progestins (medroxyprogesterone). If endometrial cancer is found, hysterectomy and surgical staging is needed.

Endometrial Cancer

Endometrial cancer presents with abnormal vaginal bleeding in a postmenopausal woman. Pain may occur from obstruction of the cervix with pus or blood. Pap smear is the most common wrong answer as a diagnostic test. Transvaginal ultrasound will show thickening of the endometrial lining. The most accurate diagnostic test is endometrial sampling. Treatment is with hysterectomy.

Polycystic Ovary Syndrome

DEFINITION/ETIOLOGY

Polycystic ovary syndrome (PCOS) is an idiopathic disorder with an **elevated luteinizing hormone (LH)** level leading to theca cell hyperplasia and the overproduction of estrogen and the androgen androstenedione.

PRESENTATION

PCOS presents with:

- **Obesity**
- **Menstrual abnormalities** (amenorrhea in 50%, dysfunctional uterine bleeding in 30%)
- **Diabetes** with hyperinsulinemia and insulin resistance
- **Virilization (rare):** hirsutism, acne, baldness, and deepening of the voice

DIAGNOSTIC TESTS

Ovarian ultrasound is the best initial test. There will be elevated levels of testosterone, androstenedione, and DHEA. Hyperlipidemia is common.

TREATMENT

1. **Metformin** and/or **pioglitazone** control diabetes and may induce ovulation if childbearing is desired.
2. **Medroxyprogesterone** or **oral contraceptives** help achieve regular shedding of the endometrium.
3. Hirsutism is treated with estrogen/progestin oral contraceptives. If there is an insufficient response, use spironolactone, flutamide, and finasteride.
4. **Weight** loss can lead to a decrease in testosterone levels and decreased insulin resistance.

> PCOS
> - LH > FSH
> - high androgens
> - metformin works!

MENSTRUAL DISORDERS

Premenstrual Syndrome

Premenstrual syndrome (PMS) is an idiopathic symptom complex with no objective physical or laboratory abnormalities. The symptoms are recurrent, developing 7 to 14 days before menses and resolving when it occurs. The symptoms are:

- Abdominal **bloating** and **breast pain**
- Extreme **fatigue**, irritability, depression, lethargy, and inability to concentrate
- Libido change

TREATMENT

The best initial therapy for moderate to severe PMS is selective **serotonin reuptake inhibitors** (SSRIs) such as fluoxetine, sertraline, or citalopram. In those not responding to SSRIs, ovarian function should be suppressed with:

- GnRH agonists
- Medroxyprogesterone
- Danazol

Mild symptoms may improve with **exercise** and **dietary modification** alone such as reducing salt, caffeine, and alcohol intake or increasing calcium intake.

Oral contraceptives and spironolactone may be effective. If SSRIs and these agents are both in the answers, the clear choice is an SSRI.

> Tricyclic antidepressants and lithium are **not** effective in PMS.

Dysmenorrhea

DEFINITION/PRESENTATION

Primary dysmenorrhea is defined as **painful menstruation** without identifiable pelvic pathology.

> Dysmenorrhea is "exertional angina" of the uterus.

There is low, midline cramping quite distinctly associated with ovulatory cycles. Women who suffer from dysmenorrhea are most likely to start within 1 to 2 years after menarche.

The pain may be accompanied by:

- Nausea
- Diarrhea
- Headache
- Flushing

The physical examination may reveal tenderness, but is otherwise normal.

TREATMENT

NSAIDs are the **best initial therapy**. Those not responding to NSAIDs are treated with:

- Oral contraceptives
- Medroxyprogesterone
- Levonorgestrel IUD

If the question describes dysmenorrhea and all of these therapies have been tried without success, the answer is laparoscopy.

Secondary Dysmenorrhea

Secondary dysmenorrhea is defined as pelvic pain with a clearly identified pelvic pathology. Secondary dysmenorrhea starts later in life (20s and 30s). Causes are:

- Endometriosis
- Submucosal myomas (fibroid)
- Cervical stenosis
- Pelvic inflammatory disease
- Adenomyosis

If a patient with dysmenorrhea is not responding to NSAIDs, oral contraceptives, or medroxyprogesterone, you should perform laparoscopy to identify one of the diseases as the cause of the pain.

Endometriosis

DEFINITION

Endometriosis is the abnormal growth of endometrial tissue outside the uterus. It is not clear why this happens. Endometrial tissue most commonly grows in the pelvis, or on the ovaries, fallopian tubes, or colon, but it can appear in almost any organ.

> Endometriosis is the most common cause of secondary dysmenorrhea.

PRESENTATION

Endometriosis presents with cyclical pelvic pain in timing with menstruation that is associated with:

- Infertility
- Dyspareunia
- Rectal pain and bleeding
- Dysfunctional uterine bleeding
- Chronic fatigue

DIAGNOSTIC TESTS

The best initial test is an ultrasound that shows fluid-filled masses. MRI is more accurate, but no imaging study can replace laparoscopy as the most accurate diagnostic test.

TREATMENT

The best initial therapy is with **NSAIDs** and **oral contraceptives**. These agents are unlikely to be able to control symptoms completely. The next best step in management is hormonal manipulation with:

- GnRH agonists (leuprolide, goserelin, nafarelin) to suppress ovulation
- Danazol
- Medroxyprogesterone
- Aromatase inhibitors

If medical therapy is inadequate to stop pain, **laparoscopy can be used to remove endometrial tissue** implants from where they are attached to pelvic structures.

Menopause

DEFINITION

Menopause is defined as 12 months of amenorrhea following the last menstrual period reflecting absence of ovarian estrogen production.

PRESENTATION

Menopause is associated with:

- **Hot flashes:** These occur in 80% of women. They are a feeling of intense heat over the trunk and face. The skin reddens and sweats.
- Vaginal atrophy
- Irritability

DIAGNOSTIC TESTS/TREATMENT

Although the FSH and LH levels are elevated, there is no routine test indicated for menopausal women. If the hot flashes (vasomotor symptoms) are uncomfortable, the "best initial therapy" is:

- Oral conjugated estrogen (combined with medroxyprogesterone to prevent endometrial hyperplasia)
- SSRIs

Vaginal atrophy is treated with estrogen cream or vaginal rings with estrogen.

CERVICAL CANCER

Screening

Indications for Pap smear:

- Start at the age of **21**.
- Do a Pap smear every 3 years for women ages 21–29. Interval can be extended to every 5 years for women ages 30–65 when Pap is combined with HPV testing.
- **Stop** screening at the age of **65**.

Changes in Pap Smear Screening Guidelines

The indication to start screening has nothing to do with onset of sexual activity. Your answer should always be what the guidelines are on the day of your examination. If these recommendations change again before your exam, answer based on what is current on the day of your exam. The examiners review the questions after the test to make sure that all the questions are current. They will discard inaccurate questions rather than include them in your grade. This is why you don't get your grade on the same day as the test. An exact percentage of questions correct is never published because it varies based on how many test questions are discarded.

> ▶ **TIP**
>
> **Never answer based on old recommendations because you think the exam cannot change fast enough.**

Management of Abnormal Pap Smears

Abnormal Pap smears range from very minor abnormalities with little significance such as atypical squamous cells of unknown significance (ASCUS) to low-grade squamous intraepithelial lesion (LSIL) to high-grade squamous intraepithelial lesion (HSIL). Each of these grades of abnormality comes with a progressively increasing frequency of developing invasive cervical cancer.

Pap smear every 3 years ages 21–65 or Pap smear + HPV testing 5 years ages 30–65

Human Papillomavirus

Testing for human papillomavirus (HPV): The presence of certain types of HPV DNA increases the risk of developing invasive cervical cancer. If high-risk HPV DNA types are present, more aggressive testing is indicated.

HPV vaccination: The indications for the HPV vaccine are:

1. Routine age 11 or 12 visit for girls
2. Catch-up vaccination for young women between the ages of 13 and 26
3. **Acceptable for boys**; no recommendation either for or against the vaccine

Answering "What Is the Next Step in Management?" Questions

If the Pap smear shows ASCUS, the "next step in management" is:

- **Repeat the Pap smear** in one year if the **HPV test is negative for high-risk DNA types**.
- **Perform colposcopy** if the **HPV test is positive for high-risk DNA types**.

If ASCUS is found a second time on Pap smear, the answer is:

- Colposcopic biopsy

If the Pap smear shows either **LSIL or HSIL**, the "next step in management" is:

- Colposcopic biopsy

Colposcopy Management

If the biopsy shows cervical intraepithelial neoplasia (CIN) I, the "next step in management" is:

- Repeat the Pap smear at 6 and 12 months.

If the biopsy shows CIN II or III, the "next step in management" is:

- Ablation or excision of the cervix

Methods of Ablation and Excision

There are many methods of removing CIN II and III that are similar in efficacy:

- Cauterization
- Cryosurgery
- Laser
- Loop excision with electrosurgery
- Conization (cutting off the transformation zone of the cervix)

> Between 80% and 85% of LSIL show CIN I on biopsy.

▶ **TIP**

You will not be asked to choose between methods of ablation and excision.

Invasive Cervical Cancer

PRESENTATION

Many cases of cervical cancer are detected by screening prior to the development of symptoms. When undetected by screening, cervical cancer presents with abnormal uterine bleeding and vaginal discharge. There may also be:

- Cervical ulceration
- Postcoital bleeding
- Purulent discharge
- Bladder and rectal involvement

DIAGNOSTIC TESTS/TREATMENT

The most accurate test is a **biopsy**. CT and MRI are used to determine the extent of disease. Carcinoma in situ can be treated with conization. Hysterectomy is the answer for all other stages. Radiation and chemotherapy are routinely used in conjunction with surgery.

> After hysterectomy, Pap smears are no longer indicated if the indication for the hysterectomy was for benign reasons and there has been no previous history of CIN II or III.

GYNECOLOGIC INFECTIONS

Vaginosis and Vaginitis

ETIOLOGY

Vaginosis has three main causes:

- Bacterial (*Gardnerella vaginalis*)
- *Trichomonas*
- *Candida*

Lactobacillus is the predominant normal organism of the vagina. *Lactobacillus* maintains the vagina at a pH of 4.5 or less. The acidic nature of the vagina is needed to suppress the growth of abnormal organisms such as *Trichomonas* and to prevent the overgrowth of normal commensal flora such as *Gardnerella*. **Only fungal vaginosis (vulvovaginal candidiasis) will grow at the normal low pH.**

Risk factors for vaginosis are:

- Cigarette smoking
- Recent **antibiotic use** decreasing normal flora
- Multiple or new **sexual partners**
- Obesity
- **Diabetes** predisposes to candidiasis
- *Trichomonas* is the only one that is sexually transmitted.

> Bacterial vaginosis is associated with preterm labor.

PRESENTATION

Vaginosis presents with an uncomfortable sensation that can be described as itching, sore, painful, vaginal irritation especially with penile insertion.

Unique Features of Each Cause of Vaginosis			
Organism	**Presentation**	**Diagnosis**	**Treatment**
Candida	"Cottage cheese," non-odorous discharge	pH normal <4.5 KOH prep with fungal hyphae	Topical antifungals Clotrimazole, econazole, terconazole, miconazole, nystatin Oral fluconazole
Trichomoniasis	Frothy greenish discharge	Wet mount with motile organisms with flagellae	Metronidazole or tinidazole orally only
Bacterial vaginosis	"Fishy odor" with KOH	"Clue cells" on wet mount	Metronidazole or clindamycin, either topical or oral

DIAGNOSTIC TESTS/TREATMENT

The best initial test for vaginosis is:

- Wet mount shows motile trichomonads.
- Wet mount also shows "clue cells," which are vaginal epithelial cells covered with bacteria.
- KOH for fungi

Metronidazole orally is useful for both bacterial vaginosis and trichomoniasis. Local metronidazole gel is **not** effective for trichomoniasis. There is **no human teratogenicity associated with the use of metronidazole** by any route of administration. Tinidazole is an alternative to metronidazole. It is acceptable to give a prescription to the patient to treat her partner.

> Metronidazole is **safe in pregnancy**, including the first trimester.

▶TIP

Vaginal culture and Gram stain are never correct answers for vaginosis.

Adverse effects of metronidazole
- Metallic taste
- Transient neutropenia
- **Disulfiram-like effect** with alcohol
- Peripheral **neuropathy**

> Routine "test of cure" is not needed when a patient is asymptomatic after treatment.

Which of the following requires treatment of the sexual partner?

a. Vulvovaginal candidiasis
b. Bacterial vaginosis
c. Trichomoniasis
d. Herpes simplex
e. Condylomata acuminata

Answer: The correct answer is (c). *Trichomonas* is *never part of normal vaginal flora*. It is exclusively acquired sexually. Although herpes and condylomata are acquired sexually, there is no benefit in treating the sexual partner because they cannot be eradicated. Without treating the partner, however, trichomoniasis will recur because of reinfection.

Pelvic Inflammatory Disease

Acute pelvic inflammatory disease (PID) presents with lower abdominal pain and tenderness that is associated with:

- Fever
- Leukocytosis
- **Cervical motion tenderness (CMT)**
- Cervical discharge
- Elevated ESR and C-reactive protein

The best initial test for any woman with lower abdominal pain/tenderness is a pregnancy test.

DIAGNOSTIC TESTS

After an ectopic pregnancy is excluded with a negative pregnancy test, the "next best step" is:

- Cervical swab for gonorrhea and chlamydia
- Nucleic acid amplification tests for both organisms
- Wet mount to look for increased white cells

The "most accurate test" for PID is a laparoscopy. Laparoscopy is done only if:

- Symptoms persisted despite repeated treatment.
- The diagnosis was unclear.
- There is evidence of a tubo-ovarian abscess

TREATMENT

- Penicillin-allergic patients are treated with clindamycin and gentamicin.
- Prompt treatment is essential to try to prevent tubal scarring and later, infertility.
- Metronidazole can be added to treatment for extra anaerobic coverage.
- **PID** and tubal scarring **increase the risk of an ectopic pregnancy**.

Treatment of PID	
Gonorrhea	**Chlamydia**
Cefoxitin or cefotetan or ceftriaxone	Doxycycline

> CMT is associated with **ectopic pregnancy** and **PID**.

> Sonography and CT show nothing in acute PID. Imaging excludes tubo-ovarian abscess.

> Fluoroquinolones are wrong in PID because of gonorrhea resistance.

> Treating the partner is essential in PID to prevent reinfection.

ONCOLOGY

13

ONCOLOGY

Breast Cancer

Screening and Prevention

Mammography is currently recommended to begin at age 50, repeated every 1 to 2 years. Aside from prophylactic mastectomy, the most effective method of preventing breast cancer is with tamoxifen (for premenopausal women) or raloxifene (for pre- and postmenopausal women) in those with two or more first-degree relatives affected (beginning at age 40) and in patients with ductal carcinoma in situ (DCIS).

> It is not clear how to use BRCA testing.

PRESENTATION/DIAGNOSTIC TESTS

Patients often present with a painless, firm lump in the breast; however, additional physical exam findings may include skin changes, lymph node enlargement, and lymphedema. The best initial test is a needle biopsy (although the "most accurate test" is an incisional or excisional biopsy). Mammography is done for every person with breast cancer, even those with an obvious lesion. Ten percent of patients have a lesion in the contralateral breast. Ten percent of patients have more than one focus in the breast. Estrogen and progesterone receptors should be tested on the biopsy as a predictive factor for response to endocrine therapy.

> Mammography is done to exclude multifocal disease even if you feel an obvious lesion.

Sentinel Lymph Node Biopsy

The "sentinel" lymph node is the first node that receives drainage from the breast cancer. Intraoperatively, a dye is injected into the operative field at the location of the lesion. The first node that the drainage goes to is the "sentinel" node. **If this node does not have cancer, no axillary lymph node dissection is necessary.**

> The "sentinel node" can spare hundreds of thousands of women an unnecessary axillary dissection.

TREATMENT

All five of these modalities can lower mortality.

1. **Lumpectomy and radiation** to the breast is equal to modified radical mastectomy (while causing less morbidity).
2. **Adjuvant chemotherapy** is given to every patient with a lesion larger than 1 cm or lymph node involvement.
3. **Tamoxifen or raloxifene** is given to every patient with positive estrogen or progesterone receptors (ER/PR).
4. **Aromatase inhibitors** are used in postmenopausal women either instead of tamoxifen or after tamoxifen.
5. The humanized monoclonal antibody **trastuzumab** targets the tyrosine kinase/epidermal growth factor receptor Her 2/neu, resulting in decreased recurrence and mortality.

> ER/PR therapy is either with tamoxifen/raloxifene followed by aromatase inhibitors or with aromatase inhibitors alone.

Toxicity of Therapy

- **Selective estrogen receptor modulator** (SERM) **medications:** Tamoxifen or raloxifene are both antagonistic on breast cancer (antiestrogenic on breast tissue); tamoxifen has an estrogen-like effect on the uterus (leading to increased rates of **endometrial cancer**), while raloxifene has antiestrogenic effects on the uterus. They both inhibit breast cancer and **protect from osteoporosis**.
- **Aromatase inhibitors:** The boards will not engage in the controversy of whether aromatase inhibitors should be used first instead of SERMs. Aromatase inhibitors clearly **cause increased osteoporosis** because they are antagonistic on the bone as well.

Ovarian Cancer

There are numerous associated risk factors for ovarian cancer; however, BRCA1 and BRCA2 positivity and hereditary nonpolyposis colorectal cancer syndrome are implicated in as many as 10% of all ovarian cancers. There is **no routine screening test** recommended. Look for:

- Woman over age 50
- Increasing abdominal girth from ascites and decreasing weight

The best **initial test is either a sonogram or a CT scan**. The most accurate test is a **biopsy**. Treatment is with surgical debridement and removal of the ovaries and pelvic contents.

The unique feature of ovarian cancer is that it is the only cancer in which **debulking** of the tumor in the pelvis and abdomen results in a major increase in survival even after the cancer has spread locally. This means surgical removal of all identifiable cancer is the answer even if the pelvic organs are covered with cancer, and the metastases are glued to the walls of the pelvis.

Debulking ovarian cancer = life

The more cancer the gynecologic oncologist removes, the longer the patient will live. There is no other cancer in which **removing multiple local metastatic lesions** will improve outcome. For each additional 10% of cancer volume removed, there is a 5% increase in the long-term survival. The object is to debulk the cancer down to metastatic nodules that are smaller than 1 cm in size. When used, **chemotherapy** is platinum-based.

Prostate Cancer
Screening

There is no routine screening that is to be universally offered for prostate cancer. The prostate-specific antigen **(PSA) has not been proven** to decrease mortality.

PRESENTATION/"WHAT IS THE MOST LIKELY DIAGNOSIS?"

Patients with prostate cancer may be asymptomatic or may present with symptoms of urinary tract obstruction such as dysuria, hesitancy, frequency, delay in initiating voiding, and post-void dribbling. There is burning only if the obstruction causes a urinary tract infection; in the absence of a urinary tract infection, there is no burning.

Digital rectal exam is not a proven strategy to reduce mortality from prostate cancer because the examiner may not detect the cancer (either due to the location within the prostate or due to the size of the lesion) and because once a nodule is detected, the disease may have already metastasized. If a lesion is suspected on digital examination, a transrectal ultrasound is performed to evaluate further.

DIAGNOSTIC TESTS

The most accurate test is prostate biopsy.

If there is a palpable mass, the patient should undergo a transrectal ultrasound followed by a biopsy. The purpose of the transrectal ultrasound is to add increased sensitivity to the digital examination. Without the guidance of the ultrasound, cancer can be definitively excluded only with the use of multiple blind biopsies. If the PSA is elevated, the prostate should be biopsied.

> PSA does **not** help screen for prostate cancer.

Prognosis

Given the intense variability in aggressiveness of prostate cancer even at the same level of localization, the most important prognostic factor is the **Gleason score**. Gleason scoring correlates with the likelihood that a patient's prostate cancer will metastasize. Hence, Gleason scoring will drive the likelihood of offering a person radical prostatectomy. If the patient has localized disease with a high Gleason score, the answer is radical prostatectomy. This is to be done before the disease can spread outside the prostate.

TREATMENT

In patients with disease localized to the prostate who are expected to live for several years, the best initial therapy is radical prostatectomy. **Radiation** therapy is slightly less effective at producing long-term remission. **Surgery** has a greater risk of erectile dysfunction and urinary incontinence.

There is no curative chemotherapy for prostate cancer; current regimens only prolong life. If surgery or radiation is in the choices, either one is always a better answer than chemotherapy.

Androgen Deprivation (Hormone Therapy)

The combination of the testosterone receptor blocker **flutamide** with a GnRH agonist is as effective as surgical castration in decreasing testosterone levels. **GnRH agonists** are goserelin and leuprolide. Complete androgen blockade with a combination of these medications will shrink the size of metastatic lesions and improve survival.

Pancreatic Cancer

Risk Factors

This is an excellent area for a "Which of the following is the strongest risk for pancreatic cancer?" type of question. The answer is clear: **tobacco smoking**. As much as 25% of all pancreatic cancer could be eliminated by the elimination of smoking. Pancreatic cancer may be familial or inherited in another 5% to 10% of cases. Obesity and physical inactivity present only a small risk.

Factors Clearly Not a Risk for Pancreatic Cancer

None of the following would be an answer to the "increases the risk of pancreatic cancer" question:

- Coffee and alcohol consumption
- Aspirin and NSAID use
- Diet
- *Helicobacter pylori*

▶ **TIP**

It is just as important to know the most common wrong answers as to know the right answer.

PRESENTATION/"WHAT IS THE MOST LIKELY DIAGNOSIS?"

Pancreatic cancer presents at a stage that is potentially resectable in only 15% to 20% of patients. Pancreatic cancer presents with:

- Nonspecific abdominal pain (80% to 85%)
- Weight loss
- Jaundice

> Only half of the jaundice in pancreatic cancer is painless.

Pancreatic head lesions present more often with **painless jaundice** and weight loss. Lesions in the body and tail present more often with pain and **weight loss**. Less common manifestations are steatorrhea, ascites, and a palpable, painless gallbladder.

DIAGNOSTIC TESTS

The testing of pancreatic cancer has become far more complex because of a marked expansion in the number of options. The "best initial test" when presented a patient with obstructive jaundice is either an **ultrasound** or a **CT scan**. CT scan is more accurate, and you should not expect to be asked to choose between these two methods. If the scan shows a clear mass, CT is the answer to the "next best step" question to look for distant metastases. A **CT-guided needle biopsy** is the most accurate test.

If CT does not show a mass in the pancreas, the "next best step" is an endoscopic retrograde cholangiopancreatography (**ERCP**) or endoscopic ultrasound (EUS). EUS is the most accurate of all the imaging studies, but is not always available. If the **EUS or ERCP** shows a mass, then the mass should be biopsied through that modality. ERCP also offers the benefit of the ability to place a biliary stent.

> The most accurate imaging study for pancreatic cancer is the endoscopic ultrasound.

Diagnostic Tests to Determine Resectability

This is a unique section solely for pancreatic cancer. After ultrasound, CT, ERCP, or EUS determine the presence of pancreatic cancer, a **biopsy** is performed. However, in order to determine if the patient is resectable, helical CT angiography, laparoscopy, or laparotomy is needed to determine the extent of spread. Pancreatic cancer often encases local vessels, making it unresectable; that is why a CT angiogram is performed.

The presence of distant metastases or involvement of the celiac axis, portal vein, or superior mesenteric artery makes the primary lesion unresectable.

▶ **TIP**

The questions in pancreatic cancer will center on assessing a patient for the possibility of resection.

TREATMENT

Surgery is the only potentially curative treatment. Metastatic disease treated with 5-FU and gemcitabine-centered regimens has been shown to prolong survival slightly. Though it is occasionally used, there is no evidence that radiation offers any survival benefit.

Testicular Cancer

PRESENTATION

Look for a young man with an incidentally found **painless mass** in the scrotum. About a third of patients have pain in the lower abdomen, perianal area, or scrotum.

DIAGNOSTIC TESTS

The best initial test is an **ultrasound**. Cystic lesions are rarely malignant. Solid lesions are removed by inguinal orchiectomy. **Do not cut the scrotum.** All patients need a CT or MRI of the abdomen to look for metastases. Those with negative scans will need a retroperitoneal lymph node dissection because the CT scan has a high rate of false negative scans.

Tumor Markers

Nonseminomatous cancers (embryonal cell tumors, choriocarcinomas, yolk sac tumors, and teratomas) are associated with elevation of:

1. Alpha-fetoprotein (**AFP**)
2. Human chorionic gonadotropin (**HCG**) (unique to nonseminomas)
3. LDH

TREATMENT

Seminomas: "Active surveillance" (**radiation to para-aortic nodes after orchiectomy**) alone is the best initial management. Active surveillance **prevents 95% of recurrences of seminomas** originally limited to the testicle. With advanced disease (disease spread outside the testicle), chemotherapy with etoposide and cisplatin is used.

Nonseminomas: Nonseminomas tend to have a poorer prognosis than seminomas and, therefore, require more aggressive treatment. For cancer limited to the testicle, patients may elect to have active surveillance or a retroperitoneal lymph node dissection. About **25% of cases will recur in the lymph nodes**, but as long as it is detected early, cure rates are equal. Patients with metastatic disease and those with elevated tumor markers postoperatively should receive a chemotherapy containing etoposide and cisplatin. Tumor markers (AFP and HCG) are used to follow the response to therapy.

Gynecomastia is found in 5% of men with testicular cancer.

Cryptorchidism is a risk of testicular cancer. This risk persists despite surgical correction earlier in life, as well as in the normally descended testis.

Scrotal violation (biopsy, surgery) increases rates of local recurrence.

AFP and HCG are elevated even in local disease.

Tumor markers and chest CT are used to detect recurrences.

Seminomas vs. Nonseminomas		
	Seminoma	**Nonseminoma**
Extent of spread	Local (80% limited to testicle)	More often outside testicle
Diagnostic tests	HCG may be elevated	AFP and HCG elevated in 85%
Primary management of local disease	Active surveillance	Active surveillance
Prevention of recurrence	Very radiosensitive	Retroperitoneal lymph node dissection used more
Treatment of recurrence	Chemotherapy with cisplatin-based regimen	Chemotherapy with cisplatin, bleomycin, and etoposide

PULMONOLOGY

14

DIAGNOSTIC TESTING IN LUNG DISEASE

Pulmonary Function Testing

Indications

Pulmonary function testing (PFT) is indicated for virtually any cause of chronic lung disease, dyspnea, cough, or wheezing. In addition, PFTs are useful for:

- Establishing the diagnosis of asthma in equivocal cases
- COPD, for both the diagnosis and assessing the severity of disease
- Determining the degree of the reactive airways component of COPD
- Preoperative assessment before thoracic or abdominal surgery
- Distinguishing restrictive from obstructive disease

> PFTs are the answer to establish the cause and severity of any suspected chronic lung disease.

▶ **TIP**

PFTs are not the answer when a patient is:

- Acutely ill, such as in the emergency department
- Uncooperative
- Confused

Spirometry

Spirometry is the portion of PFTs that establishes lung volumes and the degree of reversibility with bronchodilators. This can be assessed either formally or with a peak flow meter as a monitor of severity of airway obstruction. Reduction in value greater than 20% indicates moderate airway obstruction, while reduction greater than 50% suggests severe obstruction.

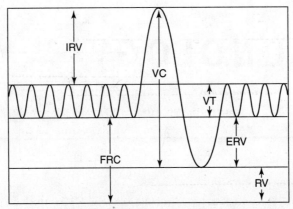

Figure 14.1: Normal spirography. This image shows the relative volumes of the different portions of normal spirography. IRV = Inspiratory Reserve Volume; VC = Vital Capacity; VT = Tidal Volume; RV = Residual Volume; ERV = Expiratory Reserve Volume.

Source: Conrad Fischer, MD

A healthy person should be able to exhale at least 80% of the FVC in one second (FEV1, the assessment of disease severity). The FEV1/FVC ratio (the diagnostic test) is normal if it is above 0.70. The residual volume is the portion of air that cannot be exhaled and does not participate in gas exchange. When the FEV1/FVC ratio is abnormally low, obstructive lung disease is present.

Forced Expiratory Flow 25%–75%

The forced expiratory flow (FEF) 25%–75% is the first part of the PFT to become abnormal in COPD. If a patient has a normal FEV1 or FEV1/FVC ratio, the FEF 25%–75% may still be abnormal, indicating the presence of early obstructive disease. The FEF 25%–75% is also known as the midmaximal flow rate.

Measurement of Residual Volume and Total Lung Capacity

Since the patient cannot exhale residual volume (RV), it is impossible to directly measure the RV from spirometry alone. You cannot measure from spirometry what you cannot move in and out of your lungs. Total lung capacity (TLC) and RV are **measured indirectly** via:

- Helium dilution
- Nitrogen washout
- Body plethysmography

Pre- and Post-bronchodilation FEV1

The most sensitive method of detecting airway reactivity (as seen in asthma) is the response to bronchodilation with a short-acting beta-2-agonist. The FEV1 and FVC are measured before and after albuterol. A positive (abnormal) test is an:

- Increase in FEV1 greater than 12%
- Increase in FVC greater than 200 mL

> Pre- and post-bronchodilation FEV1 is critical in determining how much a person with COPD will respond to bronchodilators and inhaled steroids.

Methacholine Stimulation Testing

Methacholine is artificial acetylcholine. Vagal stimulation and acetylcholine normally cause both bronchoconstriction and increased excretion of bronchial glands. Methacholine is considered positive (abnormal) if there is greater than 20% decrease in FEV1 after the inhalation of a minimal amount of methacholine. Methacholine stimulation testing is the answer when a person has intermittent dyspnea suggestive of asthma, but spirometry is normal or clear wheezing is not detected on physical examination.

> Methacholine is the most sensitive way of detecting asthma.

Diffusion Capacity of the Lung for Carbon Monoxide

The diffusion capacity of the lung for carbon monoxide **(DLCO) is used to detect damage to the lung parenchyma**. If the lung parenchyma and vasculature is damaged, gas diffusion cannot occur. The DLCO is used in:

1. • Interstitial or infiltrative lung disease
2. • COPD

In interstitial lung disease, the abnormally thickened interstitial membrane of the alveoli presents an obstruction to the passage of carbon monoxide. **Fibrosis** decreases the ability of gases to diffuse. In otherwise healthy lung parenchyma, carbon monoxide should easily pass the membrane. A decrease in DLCO means **the membrane is either missing or abnormally thick.** DLCO is also useful in assessing the type and severity of disease: If the lung parenchyma is destroyed from loss of elastin fibers, the DLCO will be impaired. If the obstructive disease is from chronic bronchitis, DLCO will be normal. Asthma has an increased DLCO.

> If the lung parenchyma is normal, carbon monoxide should pass into the blood easier than any other gas.

> More flow, more DLCO. Less flow, CO has nowhere to go, and DLCO is low.

DLCO must be corrected for the hematocrit. Anemia will artificially lower the DLCO and polycythemia will falsely raise it. Pulmonary hemorrhage will also spuriously increase the DLCO because blood in the lung will absorb the carbon monoxide, making it look as if more had been absorbed than really was.

> DLCO is strongly dependent on the amount of blood in the pulmonary capillaries.

Interpretation of DLCO Testing on Pulmonary Function Testing		
Normal DLCO	**Elevated DLCO**	**Decreased DLCO**
Chronic bronchitis	Asthma	Restrictive lung disease
Cystic fibrosis	Polycythemia	Interstitial fibrosis
	Obesity	Anemia
	Pulmonary hemorrhage	Emphysema
	Smoking	Sarcoidosis
	High altitude	Asbestosis
		Pulmonary hypertension
		Recurrent emboli

Peak Expiratory Flow Rate

The peak expiratory flow rate (PEFR or "peak flow") is a bedside test of respiratory function that has enormous benefit in the evaluation of asthma. The PEFR is closest to the FEV1 in terms of meaning. The PEFR is used to assess the severity of an asthma exacerbation. The "normal" value is not as important a term as what the patient's "usual" PEFR is. When you are presented a case in the emergency department, the PEFR is one of the most important means of determining whether the patient is improving or worsening in response to therapy.

Flow-Volume Loops

Flow-volume loops are a visual method of assessing obstruction or restriction to air flow in the lung. Spirometry simply assesses the volume of air and provides little information on the rate of flow. The flow-volume loop determines the volume of FVC, residual volume, tidal volume, rate of air movement, and location of obstruction.

Flow-volume loops can add sensitivity and specificity to spirometry. They are especially accurate in detecting the diminished pattern of expiratory flow characteristic of COPD.

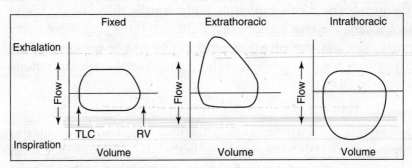

Figure 14.2: Flow-volume loops.

Source: Conrad Fischer, MD

When there is an obstruction to the flow of air in the major airways, the flow-volume loop appears flattened. The flattening occurs on inhalation when the obstruction is outside the thorax. The flattening is on exhalation when the obstruction is inside the thorax.

Assessing Oxygenation

Arterial Blood Gas

The arterial blood gas (ABG) is the most accurate method of assessing ventilation and acid-base status. An ABG does **not** have to be done to assess pH or oxygen saturation. The pulse oximeter is accurate to within 1 to 2 percentage points of an ABG, and pH can be accurately assessed on a venous blood gas (VBG) for the monitoring of metabolic disorders.

The venous pH is only 0.03 points lower than the arterial pH. The venous pCO_2 is only 4 points higher than the arterial pCO_2.

Where the ABG is indispensible is in the assessment of the alveolar-arterial (A-a) gradient. You can have two patients with identical pO_2 of 80 mm Hg. This would give them identical oxygen saturations on the oximeter of about 95%. However, if one had a respiratory rate of 24 and a pCO_2 of 20, and the other a respiratory rate of 12 and a pCO_2 of 40 mm Hg, the A-a gradient would be 45 in the first patient and 20 in the second. In other words, only the ABG can give a precise evaluation of ventilation and diffusion.

Alveolar-arterial Gradient

The A-a gradient is assessed as:

Alveolar oxygen level (A) = 150 mm Hg at sea level

Arterial oxygen level (a) = $pO_2 + pCO_2/0.8$

A-a = $150 - (pO_2 + pCO_2/0.8)$

> Calculating the A-a gradient is not as painful as it looks.

▶ **TIP**

You can also calculate "a" as: $pO_2 + pCO_2 \times 1.25$ (or add a quarter of the pCO_2 to itself).

> You cannot be a functional medical doctor without knowing how to calculate A-a gradient. Always calculate.

How the A-a Gradient Makes a Difference		
	Patient 1	**Patient 2**
pO_2/saturation	$pO_2$80/95%	$pO_2$80/95%
Respiratory rate	12/minute	24/minute
pCO_2	40 mm Hg	20 mm Hg
A-a gradient	20	45

> A simple difference in respiratory rate and pCO_2 has colossal implications for the health of the lungs.

Pulse Oximeter

The pulse oximeter is very precise for measuring saturation. It is accurate to within about 2% of the ABG; however, a number of factors can lead to an inaccurate pulse oximeter:

- **Carboxyhemoglobin:** Carbon monoxide can be present at a level of up to 50% to 70% and the pulse oximeter may read as a normal oxygen saturation above 90%. Carbon monoxide poisoning gives a falsely normal oxygen saturation.

> Cyanosis and dyspnea + normal pO_2 = methemoglobinemia

- **Methemoglobinemia:** Only half of methemoglobinemia registers on the oximeter. This gives a **falsely normal oxygen saturation** despite severe dyspnea and tissue hypoxia.

Other causes of inaccurate pulse oximetry are:

- Improper placement of the sensor
- Dark nail polish or skin pigment
- Hypothermia or anemia, which diminish flow

Normal Arterial and Venous Saturation

The normal **arterial saturation is 99%**; however, in patients with COPD, we would not consider the saturation pathologically low until it is below 90%. This has enormous significance for the use of home oxygen as treatment. Your answer is "home oxygen" as treatment when:

- pO_2 is less than 55 mm Hg or O_2 saturation is below 88%

Or, if there is evidence of right ventricular hypertrophy or an increased hematocrit:

- pO_2 less than 60 mm Hg or O_2 saturation below 90%

The normal venous saturation is 75%. Remember, although the venous saturation is 75%, the venous pO_2 is 40 mm Hg.

▶ **TIP**

Home oxygen is the answer to one of the critical COPD questions, "Which of the following will lower mortality?" but **only** if the pO_2 and oxygen saturation are low.

Oxygen Delivery

This section is not just irritating calculations. The ideas here underlie all critical care questions on targeted therapy.

Oxygen delivery is a function of:

- How much hemoglobin is being delivered?
- How well is it saturated?

The amount of hemoglobin delivered is a combination of the hemoglobin level **and** the cardiac output. If the hemoglobin level is normal, but there is no cardiac output, there is no oxygen delivery.

| Each gram of hemoglobin carries 1.34 mL of oxygen. |

Oxygen delivery = Hg level × 1.34 × cardiac output × saturation

This means:

- Anemia is perceived the same as hypoxia.
- Carbon monoxide poisoning is perceived the same as hypoxia.
- Methemoglobinemia is perceived the same as hypoxia.

Important Calculations

A normal hemoglobin level is 15 g per 100 mL of blood, so with 1.34 mL of oxygen per gram, there is 20 mL of oxygen delivered for each 100 mL of blood. Cardiac output is about 5 liters a minute.

20 mL O_2/100 mL blood × 5 liters cardiac output = 1,000 mL O_2 delivered

Oxygen leaves the heart and is delivered to tissue with 99% oxygen saturation. Blood leaves the tissues in the veins with about 75% saturation. The body consumes about 250 mL of oxygen per minute. The goal of targeted therapy for critically ill patients is to keep the oxygen saturation of the **central vein** above 70%. Fluids, vasopressors, and blood can be given to get the central venous oxygen saturation above 70%.

This is the same thing as saying "normal oxygen extraction is 25% to 30%." Watch for that question.

> If the central venous saturation is less than 70%, the body is extracting too much oxygen and working too hard.

PULMONARY NODULE

The fundamental question about the solitary pulmonary nodule is: When is biopsy the answer?

Despite the best predictive rules, some lesions that are removed will be benign, and that is the "cost" of making sure all the cancerous nodules are removed

When Is Biopsy the Answer?

Besides **tobacco smoking**, other characteristics associated with increased risk of malignancy are **size** of the lesion, **growth** of the lesion, and **older age**. Under age 40, malignancy is present in less than 5% of nodules. Above age 50 to 60, malignancy is present in more than 50% to 60%. When the size is smaller than 1 cm, less than 1% will have cancer. When the lesion is 2 cm or larger, the risk of cancer surpasses 50%.

Malignancy is more common in lesions that are enlarging, non-calcified, and have irregular "speculated" borders.

Management

Biopsy is the answer when the lesions are:

- Large (more than 2 cm)
- Enlarging (getting bigger on the repeat CT scan over 6 to 12 months)
- **Not** calcified
- With irregular speculated walls
- In older (above 50) smokers

Do **not biopsy** when the lesions are:

- **Small** (less than 1 cm)
- Calcified and smooth-walled
- In young (below 35 to 40) nonsmokers

Repeat the chest CT scan in 3 to 6 months. Compare current images to old images. Nodules stable for over 2 years are considered benign.

Equivocal or Unclear Presentations

When the lesion is between 1 and 2 cm in size in a person between 35 and 50 with no history of smoking, the answer can be either PET scanning or serial CT scans. CT remains the best initial test after detection of a nodule on a chest x-ray. The PET scan has 90% to 96% sensitivity and can be used to help exclude malignancy in lesions that are of intermediate risk (though it is much less effective for lesions smaller than 1 cm).

Sputum cytology has very limited, if any, utility. Although it is specific for the presence of malignancy, the false negative rate is too high to make it a useful modality.

▶ **TIP**

When you see sputum cytology as a choice for a diagnostic test, it is always a wrong answer. Transthoracic needle biopsy is used for the same type of equivocal lesions that are best evaluated by PET scan. Transthoracic needle biopsy has both a high false negative rate and the complication of pneumothorax.

> Calcification is the least precise of all the factors to distinguish benign from malignant lesions.

> Intermediate-sized nodules are best evaluated by PET scan. A negative PET scan has greater sensitivity than a negative needle biopsy.

Summary of Management of Solitary Pulmonary Nodule			
	Low probability	Intermediate probability	High probability
Characteristics	<1 cm Under age 35 Nonsmoker Calcified, with smooth edges	2–3 cm	>3 cm Over age 50 Smoker Uncalcified, with spicules
Management	Serial CT scans every 6 months	PET scan or needle biopsy	Excision

LUNG CANCER

PRESENTATION

There are **no pathognomonic features** to the presentation of lung cancer. There is no single symptom or physical finding unique to the most common cause of cancer death in "developed" countries. Patients present with the same cough, sputum, hemoptysis (25% to 50%), and shortness of breath that would accompany pneumonia, bronchitis, or COPD. The main difference is:

- History of smoking (personal or secondhand)
- **Weight loss**
- **Chronicity** and **recurrence** of symptoms
- **Chest pain** (20%)
- Hoarseness

> In "developing" countries, the most common cause of cancer death is hepatoma. In "developed" countries, the most common cause of cancer death is lung cancer.

> Any form of cancer can cause hypercalcemia. Squamous is the most common lung cancer to cause hypercalcemia.

Clinical Syndromes (Paraneoplastic Syndromes) Associated with Lung Cancer

- **Superior vena cava syndrome** presents with dilated neck and chest veins, facial "plethora," and widening of the mediastinum on chest x-ray.
- **Pancoast tumor** involves the superior sulcus in the chest. These patients present with upper extremity neuropathy and Horner syndrome.
- **Hypertrophic osteoarthropathy (clubbing)**
- **Clotting (Trousseau syndrome)**
- **Neuropathy**
- **Lambert-Eaton myasthenic syndrome** is muscular weakness that improves with repetitive use.

> Any form of lung disease can cause SIADH; small cell is the most common lung cancer to cause SIADH (and most other paraneoplastic syndromes).

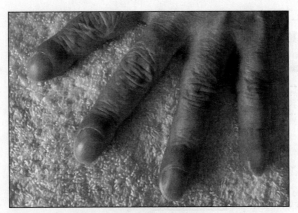

Figure 14.3: Clubbing of the finger. The precise cause of clubbing in respiratory illness is not known.

Source: Pablo Lam, MD

DIAGNOSTIC TESTS

Since the management of lung cancer is largely based on **surgery**, the diagnostic tests to determine the **extent of disease** is the center of the majority of questions.

Chest X-ray

The **best initial test is a chest x-ray**, which will show:

- Infiltrates that fail to resolve
- Nodules
- Pleural effusion
- Atelectasis

Chest CT

The "next best step in management" is a CT scan to add resolution and definition to the x-ray finding. **Sputum cytology is not accurate enough to be useful**. A negative cytology lacks sensitivity, and bronchoscopy for biopsy is done. A positive test to guide chemotherapy; radiation, surgery, and a biopsy must be done anyway.

PET Scan

PET scan is done to **stage the disease**, which dictates the treatment:

- **Establish the content of lung nodules** that are difficult to biopsy.
- Determine the **potential for curative resection**. If a patient seems to have a contralateral lesion that is cancerous, PET scan is an excellent tool to exclude cancer in what may simply be a reactively swollen node. In other words, if PET scan shows no cancer in a contralateral lesion, a previously

suspected unresectable metastatic cancer may now become a unilateral lesion that can be cured by surgery.

- Detection of distant metastases.

Lab Abnormalities in Lung Cancer

Lung cancer is associated with:

- Leukocytosis
- Anemia
- Thrombocytosis
- Cushing syndrome from ectopic ACTH production
- Hypercalcemia
- SIADH and resulting hyponatremia

Biopsy

Biopsy is the most accurate diagnostic test. The route of obtaining the biopsy is based on the location of the lesion and ease with which the lesion can be "reached."

Bronchoscopy: central lesions

Transthoracic needle biopsy: peripheral lesion

Mediastinoscopy: evaluation of central lymph nodes

Endobronchial ultrasound

TREATMENT

The only effective means of cure is surgical resection. The main question in lung cancer is: Can this patient's cancer be surgically removed?

Small Cell versus Non-Small Cell Lung Cancer

The reason lung cancers are described in two groups as either small cell lung cancer (SCLC) or non-small cell lung cancer (NSCLC) is because of the implications for treatment and prognosis. Small cell is almost never curable by surgery. Non-small cell may be curable by surgery.

> In 95% of cases, small cell is spread too far to be resectable at the time of diagnosis.

Contraindications to Surgery

The strongest contraindications to surgery are:

- **Metastatic disease**, in which it is fruitless to subject the patient to surgery without benefit
- **Severe lung disease**, in which removal of lung tissue will leave the patient without sufficient lung capacity to survive

Other reasons that make surgery an inappropriate treatment are widespread disease or cancer that is too close or attached to thoracic structures that cannot be resected, such as:

- Carina or trachea
- Heart or great vessels (vena cava, aorta)
- Bilateral disease
- Malignant pleural effusion
- Vertebral body
- Esophagus

Any one of these features is "T4" disease, which is by definition unresectable.

Nodes can be removed as long as they are on one side of the lung only. Hilar lymph nodes can be resected with the intent of curing the disease as long as the node is on the same side of the chest as the primary lesion.

> Ipsilateral mediastinal nodes are not as easy to remove as hilar nodes.

Preoperative Requirements
In order for surgery to be the answer, the patient should have:

- Preoperative FEV1 more than 2 liters (above 80%)
- Postoperative FEV1 greater than 40% of predicted
- DLCO more than 40% of predicted

Features that Are Not Critical in Treatment
Surprisingly, the size of the primary tumor is one of the least important features to drive curative resection. A small cancer attached to the carina, heart, or aorta is far more dangerous than a 5 cm cancer that is peripheral and not attached to important thoracic structures.

Other features that are **not** contraindications to surgery are involvement of the:

- Chest wall
- Diaphragmatic
- Pleura

Chemotherapy and Radiation
Chemotherapy is the treatment for SCLC. For those patients with limited SCLC, radiation is added to the treatment regimen. For NSCLC, adjuvant chemotherapy, and occasionally radiation, is used. Chemotherapy and radiation can be used as palliation.

> Platinum-based chemotherapy (either cisplatin or carboplatin) is best for lung cancer.

PLEURAL EFFUSION

Pleural effusion represents the accumulation of abnormal amounts of pleural fluid from virtually any form of lung or pleural disease. Any lung **malignancy** or **infection** can "weep" fluid into the pleural space. Although some infections frequently cause effusion (pneumococcus, tuberculosis) and some rarely cause effusion (viral, PCP), any form of infection can lead to an effusion. In addition to infection and cancer, any of the **connective tissue disorders** such as **systemic lupus erythmatosus, Wegener granulomatosis, Churg-Strauss** syndrome, or rheumatoid arthritis can cause an effusion. Finally, trauma to the chest, systemic causes of inflammation such as **uremia**, and most types of **cardiomyopathy** can cause excess fluid accumulation in the thoracic space.

> Causes of pleural effusion mimic the causes of pericarditis and pericardial effusion.

DIAGNOSTIC TESTS

The best initial test to detect a pleural effusion is the **chest x-ray**. It can sometimes be difficult to determine whether the opacity found on a chest x-ray is an effusion or an infiltrate in the lungs. The next step to confirm the presence of an effusion is:

- Decubitus chest x-ray
- Chest CT

On the decubitus films, the patients lies on her side and an x-ray is taken to see if the fluid forms a "layer" according to gravity. Chest CT does the same thing, and, although it is a more expensive test, the CT has the advantage of increased accuracy in detecting lung parenchymal disease or mass lesions that may have caused the effusion.

> Radiologic tests determine the presence of an effusion, but not the etiology.

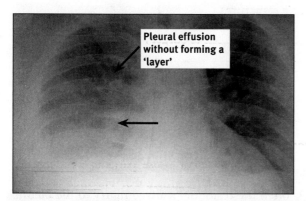

Figure 14.4: Pleural effusion testing. Chest x-ray is always the first test of an effusion.

Source: Mohammadomid Edrissian, MD

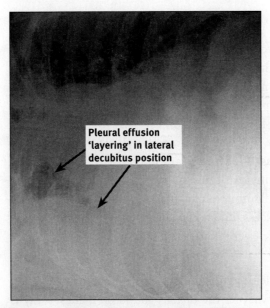

Figure 14.5: Pleural effusion testing. Movement of the fluid on an x-ray is still an excellent method of confirming that the x-ray abnormality is fluid and not a lung infiltrate.

Source: Mohammadomid Edrissian, MD

Thoracentesis and Pleural Fluid Analysis

The most accurate test of the cause of an effusion is a thoracentesis and analysis of pleural fluid. Routine evaluation includes:

- Protein
- Lactate dehydrogenase (LDH)
- pH
- Cell count
- Gram stain and culture

Thoracic Ultrasound

Ultrasound of the chest is not necessary to diagnose the presence of an effusion. Diagnostic thoracentesis is often done under sonographic guidance to obtain a sample.

Exudate vs. Transudate

Exudative pleural effusion is often the result of localized injury to the pleura. This injury leads to an elevated protein and LDH level. Exudates are most often from cancer and infection. Exudates are characterized by a protein level in the effusion above 50% of the serum level and an LDH in the fluid above 60% of the serum level.

Transudative pleural effusion is the result of hydrostatic forces squeezing fluid with a low protein and LDH level into the pleural space. CHF is the most important cause of a transudate.

Causes of Exudates and Transudates		
	Exudate	**Transudate**
Fluid protein	>50% of serum	<50% of serum
Fluid LDH	>2/3 of serum	<2/3 of serum
Causes	• Lung cancer • Empyema • Parapneumonic effusion (secondary to pneumonia) • Connective-tissue disease • Pancreatitis • Hypothyroidism • Pulmonary embolism	• CHF • Hypoalbuminemia • Atelectasis • Constrictive pericarditis • Cirrhosis (hepatic hydrothorax) • Nephritic syndrome

Empyema

An empyema refers to an **infected pleural effusion**. This is a very important diagnosis to make because of the implications for changing treatment. An empyema is a loculated pleural abscess and, because a chest tube is unable to drain all the fluid in the space, a thoractomy or VATS (video-assisted thorascopic surgery) must be performed to break down the loculations and drain the pus.

> Normal pleural fluid pH level is below 7.6.

Diagnosing an Empyema

The diagnosis is confirmed with:

- Pleural fluid **pH below 7.2** (or a low glucose)
- **Elevated WBC count** in the fluid above 1,000–2,000 neutrophils
- Positive Gram stain or culture growing an organism

Treatment of Empyema

The best initial treatment of an empyema is:

1. **Chest tube** drainage
2. Intravenous antibiotics

▶ **TIP**

Intrapleural antibiotics are not necessary.

Additional Diagnostic Tests for Effusions

- **Amylase level:** elevated with pancreatitis, rupture of the esophagus, lung or ovarian cancer
- **Triglycerides:** chylothorax
- **Adenosine deaminase level:** elevated in tuberculosis
- **Glucose level:** decreased with **rheumatoid arthritis**, lupus, malignancy, tuberculosis, parapneumonic effusion, esophageal rupture

Treatment of Recurrent Pleural Effusion

Drainage alone is often not curative for a pleural effusion, particularly if the cause is something essentially "incurable" such as a malignancy or cirrhosis. The treatment of recurrent effusion is either placement of an indwelling catheter or a pleurodesis, which is the attempt to fuse the visceral and parietal pleura to each other so that the potential "third space" of the pleura is eliminated.

Pleurodesis is accomplished by:

- Talcum powder instillation
- Doxycycline or bleomycin instillation

These substances are extremely irritating to the pleura. The inflammation that is produced results in the "fusion" of both sides of the pleura to each other.

Pleurectomy or Decortication

If the pleural effusion continues to recur despite pleurodesis, the most effective therapy is a decortication: the removal of the pleura from the lung by stripping it off. This has to be done in the operating room and requires thoracotomy. Both pleurodesis and decortication are specifically used only on those who cannot be controlled with medical therapy such as diuretics and antibiotics.

> Decortication is definitive treatment to eradicate recurrent pleural effusion.

ASTHMA

DEFINITION

Asthma is defined as a reactive airway with bronchospasm. This leads to either:

- **Increase in FEV1 of 12% or 200mL FVC** in response to inhaled beta agonist

or

- Decrease in FEV1 of 20% in response to methacholine stimulation

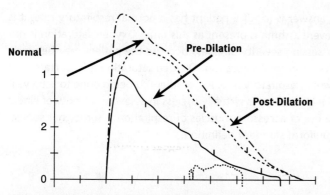

Figure 14.6: Pulmonary function testing. The shape of a flow-volume loop can make it easier to instantly diagnose a patient than looking at numbers on PFTs. You would not use PFTs to establish a diagnosis with an acutely ill patient.

Source: Mohammad Babury, MD

PRESENTATION

Ambulatory patients with mild and moderate asthma present with nocturnal symptoms and increasing frequency of use of metered dose inhalers (MDI). The severity of disease is based on:

- Frequency of nocturnal symptoms
- Frequency of use of MDIs
- Frequency of exacerbations (based on hospitalizations, requirements of systemic steroids, ICU admissions, and intubations)

Acute Asthma Exacerbation

Acutely ill patients come to the emergency department with severe episodes of shortness of breath **secondary to**:

- Respiratory **infection**
- **Nonadherence** to medications
- Environmental **allergens**
- **Emotions**

A patient comes to the emergency department with acute worsening of shortness of breath for the last day. Expiratory wheezing is heard on lung exam.

Which of the following is the best measure of severity of illness?

a. Oxygen saturation on oximeter
b. Oxygen saturation on arterial blood gas
c. Use of accessory muscles of respiration
d. Respiratory rate
e. Chest x-ray

Answer: The correct answer is (d). If a patient has a normal respiratory rate, it is highly unlikely that severe asthma is present as this time. Oxygen saturation is not the best method of assessing severity of illness because the patient may be working very hard to achieve a normal saturation. Oxygen saturation is important, but knowing how much work (respiratory rate, A-a gradient) is being done to achieve it is more important. The chest x-ray is virtually useless in assessing severity of illness acutely. Assessing the use of accessory muscles of respiration is somewhat subjective and lacking in a uniform standard definition.

Diagnostic Tests

The best initial test of respiratory function in asthma is the handheld peak flow meter. The most accurate test is the pre- and post-bronchodilation FEV1. Flow-volume loops before and after the use of bronchodilators is highly effective as well in assessing the diagnosis of asthma and its severity.

The DLCO is often increased in asthma.

Because the airway obstruction in asthma is reversible and transient, polycythemia is unusual.

▶ **TIP**

Radiologic tests (x-ray, CT, MRI) are never the correct answer to assess severity of asthma.

Assessing the Severity of Acute Asthma Exacerbation

The severity of illness in an acute asthma exacerbation is based on:

- Rapid respiratory rate (more than 30 per minute)
- Decreased peak expiratory flow
- Increased A-a gradient
- Inability to speak in complete sentences
- Normal CO_2 on an ABG with a rapid respiratory rate, an ominous sign that the patient is tiring out

Treatment

Chronic/Ambulatory Patients

The **best initial therapy** for anyone with reactive airway disease is an **inhaled beta agonist** as needed such as:

- Albuterol
- Levalbuterol
- Pirbuterol

Low saturation strongly indicates severe disease; however, severe disease can be present while still maintaining an oxygen saturation above 90%.

If the patient requires the inhaled beta agonist more than twice per week or more than twice at night per month, the following medications are **added** sequentially to the short-acting beta agonists:

1. **Inhaled steroids** (alternate therapies are cromolyn, nedocromil, or leukotriene modifiers)
2. **Long-acting beta agonists** such as salmeterol or formoterol (alternate therapies are leukotriene modifiers or theophylline)
3. **Omalizumab (anti-IgE)** antibodies for those with allergies. This anti-IgE antibody neutralizes the activation of mast cells.
4. **Oral steroids** are always the last choice for chronic use because of numerous adverse effects.

Role of Alternate Medications
It is very clear that inhaled beta agonists and inhaled steroids are the standard of care. It is very clear that oral steroids should be used. The best uses of alternate therapies are:

- **Cromolyn/nedocromil:** These agents are best for extrinsic allergies such as hay fever, animal dander sensitivity, and immediate IgE-mediated reactions.
- **Leukotriene modifiers/antagonists:** Best results are in those with atopic illness (eczema).
- **Antimuscarinic agents:** Ipratropium/tiotropium are best used in those with COPD. The precise role of these agents is not clear in asthma. They are very clearly beneficial in COPD.
- **Theophylline:** This is used as a third-line agent of limited value because of minimal efficacy and side effects such as arrhythmia and hypertension.

Treatment of Acute Asthma Exacerbations
The best initial therapy for an acute exacerbation of asthma in addition to oxygen is:

- Inhaled beta agonist (e.g., albuterol)
- Glucocorticoids
- Ipratropium
- Magnesium sulfate may add some efficacy if used in the emergency department.

There is **no maximum dose of short-acting beta agonists** (SABA). Glucocorticoids such as oral prednisone are equally efficacious as intravenous medications if absorption is normal. Steroids take 4 to 6 hours to work. Ipratropium does not have as rapid an effect as the SABAs, but it will help an acute asthma exacerbation.

> The exact role of antimuscarinic agents such as ipratropium and tiotropium is not precisely defined in asthma.

> The precise role of methylxanthines such as theophylline in the management of asthma is not clear.

> Theophylline and leukotriene modifiers have no benefit in the management of an acute asthma exacerbation.

Antibiotic Use in Asthma Exacerbation

Antibiotics are indicated only for a clear infection. There is no benefit in using antibiotics for every patient admitted for an exacerbation of asthma. Use antibiotics if there is:

- Fever

and

- Increased purulent sputum

and

- An abnormal chest x-ray with a new infiltrate

Endotracheal Intubation

Because emergency intubation is associated with more complications, such as aspiration pneumonia, esophageal intubation, and dental trauma, it should be done only for impending respiratory failure.

Intubation is performed for:

- Cyanosis
- Acute respiratory acidosis
- Depressed mental status from the acute asthma exacerbation

Allergic Bronchopulmonary Aspergillosis

DEFINITION/ETIOLOGY

Allergic bronchopulmonary aspergillosis (ABPA) is a hypersensitivity reaction of the airways seen in those with asthma and cystic fibrosis. This leads to impaction of mucus in the bronchi with eosinophil recruitment locally.

PRESENTATION

ABPA presents in asthmatics with:

- Recurrent and difficult-to-control episodes of bronchial obstruction
- Coughing up brownish mucous plugs
- Hemoptysis

DIAGNOSTIC TESTS

Look for:

- Eosinophilia
- Increased serum IgE levels
- Pulmonary infiltrates on chest x-ray, bronchiectasis on CT

The most accurate tests are:

- Skin testing for *Aspergillus*
- Precipitating antibodies for *Aspergillus*
- IgE and IgG antibodies for *Aspergillus*

TREATMENT

The best initial therapy to control the acute event is *oral* steroids, which can be combined with itraconazole.

▶ **TIP**

The most common wrong answer is to try using inhaled steroids.

CHRONIC OBSTRUCTIVE PULMONARY DISEASE

DEFINITION/ETIOLOGY

Often referred to as COPD, this condition is almost exclusively from tobacco smoking. It is defined as an irreversible decrease in FEV1/FVC ratio below 0.70. The patient will also have:

- Decreased FEV1
- Increased total lung capacity
- Increased residual volume

The DLCO may be either low (emphysema) or normal (chronic bronchitis) depending on the type of COPD.

> COPD increases TLC, but the air gained in the lung is not "usable" because it all becomes residual volume, which does not participate in gas exchange.

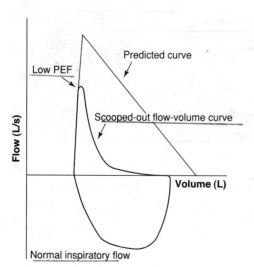

Figure 14.7: Pulmonary function testing. Flow-volume loops are a fast way of establishing the diagnosis by the visual impression. Notice the "C"-shaped exhalation in COPD.

Source: Mohammad Babury, MD, and Conrad Fischer, MD

PRESENTATION

Patients present with chronic, slowly progressive worsening of dyspnea, cough, or sputum production over months to years. Sputum production is variable, as is the presence of:

> COPD increases alveolar dead space.

- **Barrel chest**
- Clubbing
- Cyanosis

DIAGNOSTIC TESTS

The findings on pulmonary function testing previously described represent one of the strongest indications for office-based spirometric testing. Other abnormalities are:

- **Chest x-ray: flattened diaphragms**, narrow cardiac silhouette, retrosternal air trapping, bullae
- Polycythemia (elevated hematocrit)
- ABG: decreased pO_2, **chronic pCO_2 retention**. COPD routinely leads to chronic respiratory acidosis with **metabolic alkalosis as compensation**.

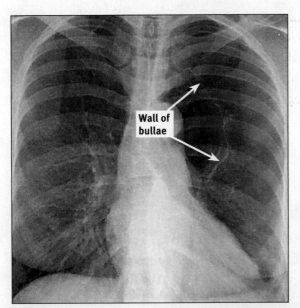

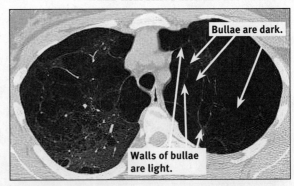

Figure 14.8–14.9: Chest x-ray and CT in COPD. Smoking destroys elastin fibers. The lungs lose their elastic recoil and bullae form.

Source: Mohammad Babury, MD, and Mahendra C. Patel, MD

TREATMENT

The management of COPD is very similar to the management of asthma. The best initial therapy is with inhaled bronchodilators. Start with albuterol and tiotropium. When symptoms are not controlled, inhaled steroids are added. Acute exacerbations of COPD are treated with the vigorous use of:

- Inhaled beta agonists (albuterol)
- Inhaled anticholinergics (ipratropium)
- Steroid bolus
- Antibiotics are often used, with hospitalized exacerbations.

> Combined inhalers (SABA + ipratropium) are superior to either as a single agent.

▶ TIP

Wrong answers are:

- Theophylline use in acute exacerbation of COPD
- Mucolytic agents such as N-acetylcysteine

Differences in COPD Management from Asthma Management

In COPD:

- **Anticholinergic medications are superior to albuterol or salmeterol.**
- Tiotropium is superior to ipratropium for chronic use.
- Short-acting bronchodilators are used for symptomatic benefit.
- Anticholinergic medications (such as tiotropium) are often used as first-line medication for symptomatic control, with long-acting beta-agonists added for further symptom control.
- Inhaled corticosteroids may be used in conjunction with long-acting beta-agonists.
- Leukotriene modifiers are useful in asthma, but not in COPD.
- **Intubation** should be **avoided unless there is severe, acute respiratory acidosis, in addition to CO_2 retention**.
- Smoking cessation lowers mortality.
- **Low-flow home oxygen** is one of the only methods to **lower mortality**.
- **CPAP and BiPAP are preferred** over intubation for establishing ventilation.

Criteria for Home Oxygen Use

Home oxygen is indicated for patients with PO2 below 55 mm Hg or saturation less than 88%, or for patients with PO2 below 60 mm Hg or saturation less than 90% in presence of medical complications of the disease.

Home oxygen and **smoking cessation** are the only two points of management associated with a **definite mortality benefit**. Pulmonary rehabilitation is also proven to improve functional status and quality of life.

Antibiotic Use in Acute Exacerbation of COPD

Antibiotic use is more liberal in COPD exacerbations. You will give antibiotics for:

- Increased sputum production in volume or change in character
- Worsening shortness of breath

This is despite the absence of fever or a new infiltrate on chest x-ray, because bacteria frequently colonize the airways in acute exacerbations of COPD.

The antibiotics to choose are: doxycycline, trimethoprim/sulfamethoxazole, azithromycin, cefdinir, cefpodoxime, cefprozil, and cefuroxime.

If the patient is older (65 or above), has severe disease defined as an FEV1 below 50%, or has more than three exacerbations a year, then treatment is a respiratory fluoroquinolone such as levofloxacin, moxifloxacin, or gemifloxacin.

BRONCHIECTASIS

DEFINITION/ETIOLOGY

Bronchiectasis is an abnormal widening of the bronchi that leads to a permanent anatomic change in the caliber of the airways. The most common causes are:

- Cystic fibrosis
- Respiratory infections such as allergic bronchopulmonary aspergillosis
- Foreign body aspiration
- Immune defects (hypogammaglobulinemia)
- Alpha 1-antitrypsin deficiency

PRESENTATION

Bronchiectasis presents with multiple, recurrent episodes of lung infections producing high volumes of sputum, fever, and cough. Less common manifestations are wheezing, chest pain, and dyspnea. Fever and chills are generally not present.

DIAGNOSTIC TESTS

The best initial test is a chest x-ray. The most accurate test is a high-resolution CT scan of the chest. Sputum culture is the only way to determine an infectious etiology.

> Immunoglobulin levels should be measured in bronchiectasis.

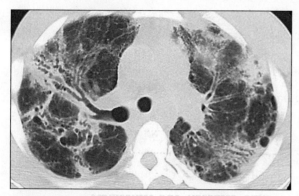

Figure 14.10: Chest CT showing bronchiectasis. Notice the widened, thickened bronchi.

Source: Craig Thurm, MD

TREATMENT

The best initial therapy is to treat the recurrent episodes of infection as they arise. The treatment of infections with *Pseudomonas* is a respiratory fluoroquinolone such as levofloxacin.

Maintenance therapy for all patients, regardless of the presence of an infection at the moment, is chest physiotherapy and postural drainage in an attempt to decrease the accumulation of mucus.

DIFFUSE PARENCHYMAL LUNG DISEASE

DEFINITION

Diffuse parenchymal lung disease, or DPLD, is often used interchangeably with the term "interstitial lung disease" (ILD). Diffuse parenchymal lung disease is a more precise term because the pathology may involve the entire lung, including the parenchyma, the alveolar space, the airways, and the interstitium.

▶**TIP**

The only **unique feature** of DPLD is the "exposure" in the history. Look for "most likely diagnosis" questions based on:

1. An **exposure to an inhaled or systemic toxin**

and

2. **Restrictive pattern** lung disease

ETIOLOGY

Acute DPLD

Rapid onset of symptoms over as little as a few days can be caused by:

- Acute interstitial pneumonia
- Vasculitis (Wegener, Churg-Strauss, microscopic polyangiitis)
- Eosinophilic pneumonia
- Hypersensitivity pneumonitis
- Alveolar hemorrhage syndromes

Slower Onset DPLD (Weeks to Months)

- Connective tissue disease (systemic lupus erythematosus or polymyositis)
- Idiopathic pulmonary fibrosis
- Sarcoidosis
- Radiation
- Pulmonary Langerhans cell histiocytosis

Toxin-induced Injury	
Antibiotics • Nitrofurantoin • Sulfasalazine • Minocycline	**Rheumatic Diseases** • Rheumatoid arthritis • Goodpasture • Wegener • Churg-Strauss • Scleroderma
Chemotherapy • Bleomycin • Mitomycin C • Busulfan • Melphalan • Cytosine arabinoside • Methotrexate • Nitrosoureas	**Toxins** • Radiation • Oxygen (>50% FiO_2) • Mercury • Amiodarone

Pneumoconioses	
Specific exposure	**Most likely diagnosis**
Computer manufacture	Berylliosis
Cotton	Byssinosis
Coal dust	Coal worker's pneumoconiosis
Fungi	Farmer's lung
Masons, glass	Silicosis

PRESENTATION

DPLD, despite its multifactorial nature, has tremendous similarity in its clinical presentation. Virtually every patient, no matter the etiology, presents with:

- Dry cough
- Crepitations/"Velcro" rales
- Dyspnea
- Hemoptysis
- Clubbing
- Loud P2 from cor pulmonale and pulmonary hypertension

Wheezing and cyanosis **are unusual** with interstitial lung diseases.

DIAGNOSTIC TESTS

The best initial test of DPLD is a chest x-ray. The causes of DPLD are indistinguishable from chest x-ray alone. They all show interstitial disease.

High-Resolution CT Scan

High-resolution CT scan (HRCT) is the "standard of care" as the "most accurate radiologic test" of DPLD. Although HRCT shows the same interstitial or "reticulonodular" pattern as a chest x-ray, it does so with much greater accuracy.

Severe interstitial disease is called "reticular" or "net-like."

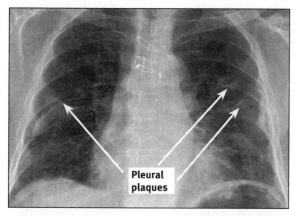
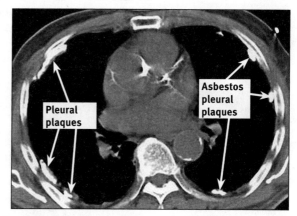

Figures 14.11–14.12: Chest x-ray and CT with pleural plaques. Asbestosis can give interstitial fibrosis, or focal lesions such as "plaques." These plaques are visible on both x-ray and CT scan.

Source: Mohammad Babury, MD, and Mahendra C. Patel, MD

Echocardiography

The echocardiogram will show:

- Pulmonary hypertension
- Right ventricular and right atrial hypertrophy
- Possible incompetence of the tricuspid and pulmonic valves

Unlike right bundle branch block, right ventricular hypertrophy has a normal width of QRS and only a single R wave.

EKG

EKG shows:

- Right ventricular hypertrophy (tall R waves in V1 and V2)
- Tall P waves in V1 and V2 (P pulmonale) indicative of right atrial hypertrophy
- Right axis deviation

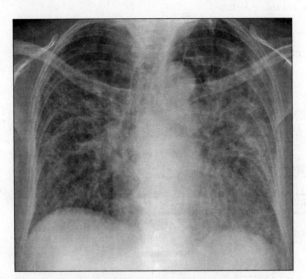

Figure 14.13: Pulmonary fibrosis on chest x-ray. The diffuse lung disease on x-ray cannot determine the etiology.

Source: Mohammad Babury, MD, and Mahendra C. Patel, MD

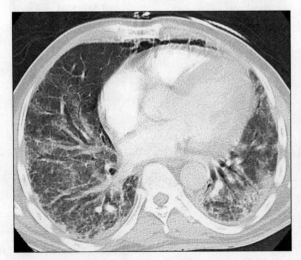 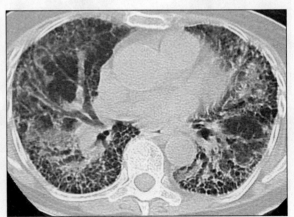

Figures 14.14–14.15: Pulmonary fibrosis on chest CT. High-resolution CT shows far more detail about lung fibrosis than a chest x-ray.

Source: Nirav Thakur, MD, and Nihar Shah, MD   *Source: Craig Thurm, MD*

Pulmonary Function Testing

PFT in DPLD shows a restrictive pattern with a decrease in DLCO. You should expect to see:

- Decreased FEV1
- Decreased FVC
- Normal FEV1/FVC ratio
- Decreased TLC, RV, and tidal volume

Everything will be diminished on PFTs in DPLD, but all the lung volumes will be decreased equally in all compartments.

Lung Biopsy

The "most accurate diagnostic test" is a lung biopsy. You are not doing a biopsy to establish the presence of restrictive lung disease of DPLD. The biopsy is used to:

- Exclude cancer and infection as a cause of DPLD
- Search for potentially treatable causes of disease, since the majority of causes of DPLD are not easily reversible by treatment

TREATMENT

The majority of causes of DPLD have **no specific therapy** that will reverse them. For the causes of occupational, environmental, and idiopathic pneumoconioses, there is no management other than removing the patient from exposure.

The point of doing the biopsy is to identify those cases with an active inflammatory component in whom glucocorticoids or other immunosuppressive agents may be beneficial. The **most treatable cases** are:

> Steroids work for sarcoid, berylliosis, biopsies with white cells, and some patients with pulmonary fibrosis.

- Infections
- Those with neutrophils, lymphocytes, or granulomas on biopsy
- Those with limited amount of fibrosis on biopsy

▶ TIP

Since the symptoms, physical findings, and diagnostic tests are nearly identical despite a huge array of causes, the most likely questions in DPLD center around the "most likely diagnosis" question.

> Start with the presentation (dry cough, restrictive pattern on PFTs), then look for a toxin in the history.

Sarcoidosis

DEFINITION

Sarcoidosis is a systemic illness of non-caseating granulomas that occur primarily in the lung, but can affect virtually any organ in the body.

PRESENTATION/"WHAT IS THE MOST LIKELY DIAGNOSIS?"

Look for a young, African American woman with **dyspnea, dry cough**, and skin lesions.

The most common extra-pulmonary sites of involvement are:

- **Skin:** Erythema nodosum, lupus pernio (of the face)
- **Neurologic:** Bilateral facial palsy, meningitis, central diabetes insipidus
- **Cardiac:** AV block, restrictive cardiomyopathy
- **Eye:** iritis, uveitis
- **Salivary gland**
- **Joint and muscle pain** (20%)
- **Liver, kidney, spleen, and bone** are "involved" with granulomas, but these are almost always clinically asymptomatic.

DIAGNOSTIC TESTS

The **best initial test is a chest x-ray**. More than 90% to 95% will have an abnormality on chest x-ray. Finding can be:

- Hilar nodes alone
- Hilar nodes and reticular opacities
- Reticular opacities with shrinking hilar nodes

The **most accurate test is a biopsy** of a lymph node. This is usually done through bronchoscopy and sometimes via mediastinoscopy.

- **Hypercalcemia:** Although an elevated urine calcium is present in 20% to 50% of patients, high blood calcium is found in only 10% to 20%.
- **ACE levels** are elevated in 60%.
- **PFTs** show a restrictive pattern with a decreased DLCO.
- Bronchoalveolar lavage shows increased CD4 cells.

Nonspecific findings of fatigue, malaise, and weight loss are common.

Half of sarcoidosis cases are found as an incidental finding on chest x-ray.

Hilar adenopathy is nearly universal in sarcoidosis.

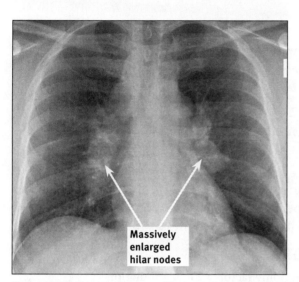

Figure 14.16: Chest x-ray in sarcoidosis. Notice massive whitish adenopathy in both hila.

Source: Mohammad Babury, MD, and Mahendra C. Patel, MD

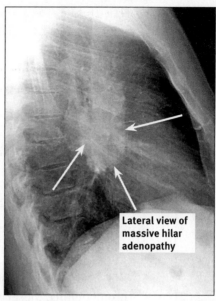

Figure 14.17: Lateral chest x-ray in sarcoidosis. Massive adenopathy appears as a "potato" in the center of the chest. Biopsy a piece of this for a certain diagnosis.

Source: Mohammad Babury, MD, and Mahendra C. Patel, MD

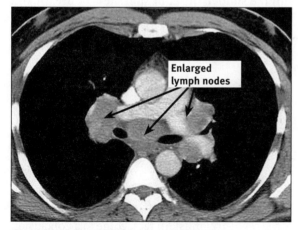

Figure 14.18: Chest CT with sarcoidosis. Chest CT shows more detail than an x-ray but is still not a substitute for a biopsy.

Source: Mohammad Babury, MD, and Mahendra C. Patel, MD

TREATMENT

The best initial therapy is prednisone (glucocorticoids); 90% of patients will either resolve spontaneously or resolve rapidly in response to steroids. For the small number of patients with progressive disease or who fail to improve with steroids, treatment is with:

> Failure of treatment with steroids is rare in sarcoidosis.

- Methotrexate
- Cyclophosphamide
- Azathioprine
- Cyclosporine
- TNF inhibitors

PULMONARY EMBOLUS

ETIOLOGY

Pulmonary embolus (PE) arises most often from the deep veins of the lower extremities (70%) and the pelvic veins (30%). The most common predispositions to the development of thromboembolic disease are:

- Immobility, surgery, and recent trauma
- Thrombophilia, most commonly factor V Leiden mutation
- Orthopedic surgical procedures, particularly knee and hip replacement
- Pregnancy

PRESENTATION

Pulmonary emboli present with the **sudden onset of shortness of breath** and **clear lungs** on auscultation. Other findings are based on the severity or size of the clot, such as:

- **Tachycardia and tachypnea**
- **Pleuritic chest pain**
- Pain in the legs
- Cough and hemoptysis
- Syncope and hypotension if severe

Pretest Probability

PE is unique in that the pretest likelihood of disease has enormous impact on the positive predictive value of the tests. You must, in fact, come to a conclusion about the likelihood of PE before you do any tests.

Healthy people do not clot on long plane rides. People who clot on planes most often have an underlying hypercoagulable state.

There is no single pathognomonic presentation of thromboembolic disease.

Clinical Criterion	Score
Clinical symptoms of DVT (leg swelling, pain with palpation)	3.0
Other diagnosis less likely than pulmonary embolism	3.0
Heart rate >100	1.5
Immobilization (3 days) or surgery in the previous 4 weeks	1.5
Previous DVT/PE	1.5
Hemoptysis	1.0
Malignancy	1.0
Clinical probability of PE (Wells criteria)	**Total Score**
High probability	>6.0
Moderate probability	2.0 to 6.0
Low probability	<2.0

Figure 14.19: Pulmonary emboli. Wells criteria for pretest probability of PE.

Source: Conrad Fischer, MD

DIAGNOSTIC TESTS

The "Best Initial Tests"

Chest x-ray:

- X-ray is usually obtained in setting of cardiopulmonary symptoms.
- The most common abnormality is atelectasis.
- Only 12% to 15% of chest x-rays are read as "normal."
- The most common wrong answer is a wedge-shaped infarction, also called a "Hampton hump."
- Pleural effusion is present in one-third of patients.

EKG:

- Most common finding: **sinus tachycardia**
- Most common abnormality: **nonspecific ST-T wave changes**
- **Most common wrong answer: S1, Q3, T3**

Arterial blood gas: Although an ABG often has hypoxia and an increased A-a gradient, the ABG can be normal in 10% to 15% of cases.

D-dimer: The D-dimer is extremely sensitive. A normal test reliably excludes the presence of PE or DVT. The D-dimer is nonspecific. This means that a positive test is insufficient to confirm the presence of a pulmonary embolus. This test should only be obtained in cases of low pretest probability of disease. A negative test in that circumstance can safely exclude PE as a cause of the symptoms.

> With a new machine and an expert reader, CTA is excellent in excluding PE.

The "Most Accurate Tests"

- CT angiogram (spiral CT)
- Ventilation perfusion (V/Q) test
- Lower extremity duplex: when positive, no other test is needed

CT Angiogram

The CT angiogram (CTA) is extremely specific for PE when it is positive. A positive CTA has a much greater positive predictive value than a high-probability V/Q scan.

- Radiation
- Contrast load in patients with renal disease or allergy

The emboli missed by the CTA are often small and potentially insignificant clinically. CTA is excellent at detecting large important clots and misses smaller, less dangerous clots. When reader expertise is strong and a new, high-sensitivity CT machine is used, the CTA has 95% sensitivity in excluding PE.

▶ **TIP**

When the baseline chest x-ray is abnormal, the V/Q scan is not accurate. The more abnormal the x-ray, the greater the need for CT angiogram.

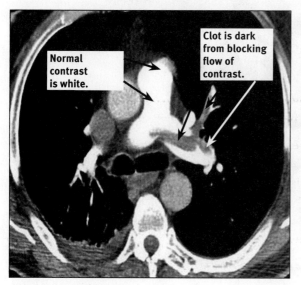
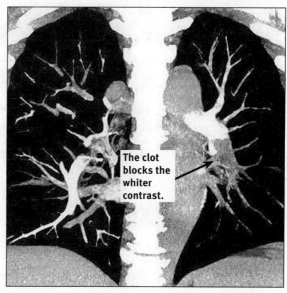

Figures 14.20–14.21: CT angiography. CT angiography is extremely specific for a clot. It is especially good for large clots.

Source: Echechukwu Elendu, MD

Source: Mohammad Babury, MD, and Mahendra C. Patel, MD

Ventilation/Perfusion Scan

- A normal V/Q scan is extremely sensitive. Normal V/Q essentially means there is no clot in the lungs. Even when there is no clot, the V/Q scan is rarely completely normal.
- **Low**-probability scan: PE is **still present** in 10% to 15%.
- **High**-probability scan: PE is **not present** in 10% to 15%.

Lower Extremity Duplex

This test is abnormal in 70% of those with PE. If it is positive, no further testing to detect the presence of a clot is necessary. If the duplex is abnormal, the patient needs heparin followed by 6 months of warfarin, so the CTA and V/Q will not change management.

> A negative lower extremity duplex is worthless in excluding a PE. It can originate from the pelvic veins or upper extremity.

Additional Lab Abnormalities with PE

The BNP and troponin levels may be elevated with PE. They are too nonspecific and insensitive to contribute to establishing or excluding a diagnosis of PE. When they are in the choices of "what to do next?" they are never the right answer.

Echocardiography is abnormal in 30% to 40% of patients with a PE. Abnormalities detected are:

- Abnormal RV size and function
- Tricuspid regurgitation

Echocardiography has limited sensitivity, but has none of the adverse effects of administering contrast material.

> Angiography is the single most accurate test for PE, but is rarely done.

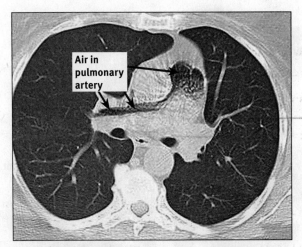

Figure 14.22: Air embolus on a CT. Look for air embolus when air is accidentally injected into the vessel.

Source: Mohammad Babury, MD, and Mahendra C. Patel, MD

TREATMENT

The best initial therapy is heparin or low molecular weight heparin followed by 6 months of warfarin with an INR of 2 to 3. Rivaroxaban alone is promising.

When are thrombolytics the answer?

- When the patient is hemodynamically unstable, defined as hypotensive, tachycardic, and severely hypoxic

When is a venous interruption filter the answer?

- When there is either a recurrent clot while the patient is already on heparin, or a contraindication to the use of heparin. Filter is also useful if the patient is already so unstable that any additional clot burden will overwhelm cardiac function: for example, a person with an embolus who is tachycardic and tachypneic with a normal blood pressure while on heparin. Although the patient is stable now, even a small additional clot will likely cause hypotension.

> Rivaroxaban orally is an alternative to heparin and warfarin treatment.

ACUTE RESPIRATORY DISTRESS SYNDROME

DEFINITION/ETIOLOGY

Acute respiratory distress syndrome (ARDS) is the most severe form of acute, idiopathic lung injury. The most common cause is **sepsis**, but there are numerous varieties of severe, overwhelming systemic illness resulting in a diffuse lung leak.

ARDS is defined as:

Acute lung failure + fluffy infiltrates on x-ray + normal wedge + pO_2/FiO_2 <200

Besides sepsis, ARDS is also caused by many kinds of infections such as **pneumonia** or **aspiration**. Lung and bone marrow **transplantation** are associated with ARDS even without the development of a specific infection.

Transfusion-related acute lung injury is when a patient develops acute shortness of breath after a transfusion from donor antibodies attacking recipient WBCs. The WBCs "clump" in the lungs like little pulmonary emboli. Therapy is supportive and it will resolve spontaneously over a few days.

ARDS is like pancreatitis in that any form of trauma or toxin can cause diffuse injury and inflammation of the organ.

PRESENTATION/DIAGNOSTIC TESTS

ARDS presents with sudden, severe lung injury with dyspnea, hypoxia, and a markedly elevated A-a gradient. By definition, ARDS is defined as having a pO_2/FiO_2 ratio below 200. The FiO_2 must be expressed as a decimal (e.g., room air is 0.21, **not** 21%).

For example:

Normal pO_2 is 100 mm Hg.

Normal FiO_2 is 0.20.

So, 100 divided by 0.2 = 500.

The chest x-ray will show diffuse bilateral infiltrates that look like pulmonary edema, but the pressures inside the heart and on the echocardiogram will be normal without any evidence (based on physical exam, lab results, or imaging) to suggest cardiac dysfunction as the cause. There will be bilateral fluffy infiltrates on the chest x-ray, and these patients usually require intubation.

TREATMENT

The most effective management is to use a smaller tidal volume of 6 mL/kg instead of the usual 12 mL/kg. This is referred to as low tidal volume ventilation (LTVV).

There is no specific therapy that will reverse ARDS. Steroids have not been shown to be universally effective.

Positive end-expiratory pressure (PEEP) is used to decrease the FiO_2 that is needed to maintain an oxygen saturation of more than 90%. PEEP keeps the alveoli open at the end of expiration, increasing the surface area for gas exchange that would decrease without treatment.

> ARDS is defined as having a normal wedge pressure.

> A normal pO_2/FiO_2 is about 500.

> The x-ray in ARDS looks like pulmonary edema, but all the pressures in the heart are normal.

Complications of Therapy with LTVV and PEEP

LTVV can cause:

- Respiratory acidosis from a decrease in minute ventilation; this is called "permissive hypercapnia"
- "Auto-PEEP," hypotension from increased intrathoracic pressure caused by decreasing the amount of time available for expiration

PEEP can cause:

- Barotrauma to the lungs, such as pneumothorax
- Hypotension by decreasing venous return to the left side of the heart

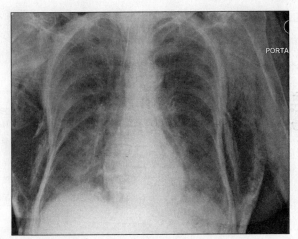

Figure 14.23: Barotrauma x-ray. Intubation and positive pressure ventilation can burst through the lungs into the surrounding soft tissue.

Source: Mohammad Babury, MD, and Mahendra C. Patel, MD

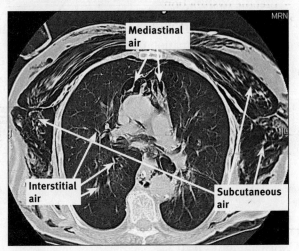

Figure 14.24: Barotrauma CT. Air can dissect into the skin, muscles, mediastinum, and all the soft tissues surrounding the chest.

Source: Mohammad Babury, MD, and Mahendra C. Patel, MD

SLEEP APNEA

DEFINITION/ETIOLOGY

Sleep apnea can be divided into either obstructive sleep apnea (OSA) or central sleep apnea (CSA). OSA is the more common of the two and is usually due to obesity and anatomic abnormalities of craniofacial structures.

> Smoking is an important risk for OSA.

Etiology of CSA

CSA is far less common and is from an idiopathic loss of central drive for respiration. CSA is associated with:

- Stroke
- Heart failure

- CNS disease
- Renal failure

PRESENTATION

Sleep apnea presents with daytime somnolence, snoring, and difficulties with attention. Patients have episodes of nocturnal choking and apnea witnessed by the bed partner. In addition, patients develop:

1. Hypertension
2. Headache
3. Lack of concentration
4. Erectile dysfunction
5. Pulmonary hypertension and right heart failure

> Central sleep apnea is nearly identical in presentation to OSA, but there is less snoring.

DIAGNOSTIC TESTS

The most accurate test is polysomnography, a "sleep study." Patients are observed during sleep in a lab for how many episodes of apnea/hypopnea they develop every hour. This is also known as the apnea-hypopnea index (AHI). Sleep apnea is defined as an AHI above 5. Severe OSA is defined as an AHI above 15 to 30 per hour.

Treatment of OSA

All patients with OSA should:

1. Lose weight.
2. Use oral appliances and devices to keep the airway open at night.
3. Avoid alcohol.

Once this plan is put in place, the next best step in the management of the patient is to use positive airway pressure devices such as CPAP and BiPAP.

If there is no resolution of symptoms with these methods, then surgery is needed to decompress the upper airway.

Continue Positive airway pressure (CPAP)

Treatment of CSA

CSA is managed in much the same way as OSA with CPAP and BiPAP. Weight loss is less likely to be effective and surgery is useless. Theophylline and acetazolamide have some modest benefit as medical therapy.

Ventilation:
Is defined as the product of the respiratory rate and
tidal volumen.

Respiratory Alkalosis results from Hyperventilation

In Mechanical ventilated patients with respiratory

Alkalosis in the setting of Appropiate tidal Volumen.

6ml x Kg = appropiety tidal volumen

the respiratory Rate should be lowered.

(Reduction in tidal Volume can trigger an increased

Ventilatory Rate) potential

RHEUMATOLOGY

15

RHEUMATOID ARTHRITIS

PRESENTATION/"WHAT IS THE MOST LIKELY DIAGNOSIS?"

The diagnosis of rheumatoid arthritis (RA) is based on the presence of a particular pattern of joint pain supported by a blood test.

These criteria lower the threshold for a diagnosis of RA:

- Synovitis—one joint alone is sufficient (though it is usually in multiple joints).

- More joints increase the certainty of diagnosis.

- Rheumatoid factor or anti-cyclic citrulinated peptide

- Increased C-reactive protein or ESR

- Longer than 6 weeks' duration

Expanding the diagnostic criteria allows earlier initiation of DMARDs.

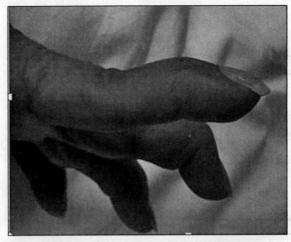

Figure 15.1: Rheumatoid arthritis with swan neck deformity.
Disease-modifying therapy is meant to prevent deformity such as this from ever occurring.

Source: Mayurkumar Gohel, MD

Additional Clinical Manifestations

Although they are not part of the definition of RA, this disorder also presents with:

Caplan syndrome is RA associated with pulmonary nodules or pneumoconiosis.

- Infection
- Fever, weight loss, myalgia
- Cardiac: pericarditis, atherosclerosis
- Dermatologic: rheumatoid nodules, vasculitis
- Ocular: scleritis, episcleritis, or keratitis
- Pulmonary: pulmonary fibrosis, pleuritis, bronchiolitis obliterans organizing pneumonia
- Neuro: mononeuritis multiplex
- Musculoskeletal: cervical spine instability (C1 and C2)
- Hematologic: Felty syndrome (neutropenia + splenomegaly), amyloidosis, thrombocytosis, leukocytosis, anemia

Felty syndrome is RA associated with:
- Neutropenia
- Splenomegaly

Nodules, morning stiffness, and being symmetrical are no longer required to establish a diagnosis.

Which of the following is the most common cause of death with rheumatoid arthritis?

a. Coronary artery disease
b. Lung infection or hemorrhage
c. Sepsis
d. Cervical spine cord compression
e. Hemorrhage

Answer: The correct answer is (a). Because of the immune defect, there is accelerated atherosclerosis leading to death by myocardial infarction. RA markedly worsens the effects of the usual risk factors for atherosclerosis such as hypertension, hyperlipidemia, diabetes, or tobacco smoking.

DIAGNOSTIC TESTS

Both rheumatoid factor (RF) and anti-cyclic citrullinated peptide (anti-CCP) should be obtained in all patients. RF is found in 75% to 85% of patients, but is nonspecific because it is present in numerous other rheumatologic disorders and chronic infections.

Radiologic tests looking for joint erosion are **no longer** an indispensable part of laboratory evaluation. X-ray abnormalities occur very late. Disease-modifying antirheumatic drugs (DMARDs) should be started before the x-ray becomes abnormal.

> Anti-CCP is specific to RA alone and is found in 70% to 80% of patients.

> X-ray is not necessary to diagnose RA.

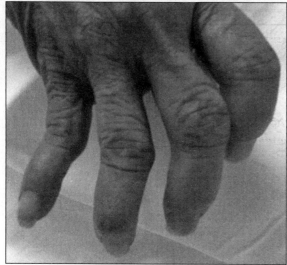

Figure 15.2: Rheumatoid arthritis with ulnar deviation. The presence of ulnar deviation is an automatic indication for DMARDs.

Source: Mayurkumar Gohel, MD

Additional Laboratory Abnormalities in RA

- ANA is often present, but is not useful.
- Anemia, thrombocytosis, or leukocytosis may be present.
- Joint fluid shows 10,000 to 20,000 WBCs/μl with increased neutrophils.
- ESR and CRP are elevated.

> Anti-CCP antibody levels correlate with aggressive disease activity; RF does not.

TREATMENT

The best initial therapy for the pain and stiffness of RA is **NSAIDs**; however, NSAIDs do not alter the course of the disease. **Methotrexate** has been and continues to be the mainstay of therapy. Methotrexate is an indispensible disease-modifying therapy. **Hydroxychloroquine and sulfasalazine are used in early, mild disease** that is not yet associated with erosive changes on x-ray. In patients with erosive disease, methotrexate and/or leflunomide should be used (generally in combination with hydroxychloroquine and/or sulfasalazine). If

> It is too late to wait for x-ray abnormalities to start treatment.

methotrexate does not fully control the disease, biological agents should be added, not substituted, for methotrexate or leflunomide as the initial DMARD. Generally, anti-tumor necrosis factor (anti-TNF) inhibiting agents, such as ebanercept, infliximab, golimumab, certolizumab, and adalimumab, are the first biologic agents used. There are numerous other biological DMARD agents such as:

- Abatacept (blocks T cell activation)
- Rituximab (anti-CD 20 agent that depletes B cells)
- Anakinra (interleukin-1 inhibitor)
- Tocilizumab (interleukin-6 inhibitor)

All of them are the answer to the question "What do you do when methotrexate **and** anti-TNF agents fail to fully control the disease?" or when the question describes a person intolerant of methotrexate.

▶ **TIP**

If anti-TNF medications do not control symptoms, use abatacept or rituximab as the next therapy instead of other anti-TNF medications.

Glucocorticoids are only used for:

1. Acute worsening/flare of RA
2. Short periods of time to allow the DMARDs to take effect ("bridge therapy")

▶ **TIP**

Gold is always a wrong answer. The other DMARDs and biological agents are more effective and do not cause nephrotic syndrome as occurs with gold salts.

Methotrexate

Methotrexate is unquestionably the answer as the **best initial DMARD**. Methotrexate should be started:

- Within 3 months of the diagnosis of rheumatoid arthritis

Methotrexate is associated with:

- Hepatic toxicity such as fibrosis
- Pulmonary fibrosis
- Cytopenias

> Leflunomide has the same efficacy/indications as methotrexate. Both are hepatotoxic.

Anti-TNF Agents (Etanercept, Adalimumab, Infliximab, Certolizumab)

These agents are added to methotrexate after several months of therapy. An adverse effect that needs to be monitored is the reactivation of tuberculosis. Patients are screened with a PPD prior to initiating therapy, and routinely during therapy. If the PPD is positive, give isoniazid. Anti-TNF agents can also cause drug-induced lupus. You do not have to wait for 9 months of isoniazid completion to start anti-TNF drugs.

Summary of RA Therapy

NSAIDs are used to control pain and stiffness, but do not modify the progression of disease. Glucocorticoids are used only to allow methotrexate several weeks to months to achieve a clinical response.

Anti-TNF **agents are the best initial biological agents to be added to methotrexate if the disease is not well-controlled.** There are many choices if methotrexate is either ineffective or not tolerated. Anti-TNF medications are always the first choice. Leflunomide is an alternative to methotrexate. Rituximab is an alternative biologic agent to anti-TNF medications.

ADULT STILL DISEASE

This is a complex of symptoms and signs without a confirmatory diagnostic test. Actually, the absence of rheumatoid factor and a negative ANA is part of the diagnostic criteria. Although the ferritin level is very high and the transaminases are elevated, these abnormalities are usually too nonspecific to be helpful. As with all rheumatologic diseases, there is joint pain and skin findings. Look for:

- Joint pain/arthritis
- **Fever** for at least a week that is **very high**
- Leukocytosis
- Salmon-colored, evanescent rash (commonly in the axilla and on the trunk)

> Ferritin is markedly elevated in adult Still disease.

Other features that will help answer the question are a sore throat, lymphadenopathy, and splenomegaly. Treat with NSAIDs. Use prednisone for those not responsive to NSAIDs. In those who have persistent disease (e.g., "the patient returns one week after stopping prednisone with return of joint pain and fever"), the answer is methotrexate or anti-TNF medications.

▶ **TIP**

The most likely question for adult Still disease is "What is the most likely diagnosis?" This is not so easy given the lack of a single specific feature. The key is the **collection** of findings.

> Look for the phrase "salmon-colored" with the rash.

Systemic Lupus Erythematosus

Presentation

Look for a patient with skin and joint problems and confirm with an elevated ANA. Systemic lupus erythematosus (SLE) has 11 "official" diagnostic criteria. A patient who exhibits four of these criteria is defined as having SLE.

Skin Manifestations

SLE has four dermatologic manifestations, which means you can carry a diagnosis of SLE exclusively from the dermatologic involvement. These are:

- Malar rash (distinguished from rosacea based on lack of involvement of nasolabial folds)
- Discoid rash (red, scaly plaques above the neck line, often in ear canals)
- Photosensitivity
- Oral ulcers (**painless** ulcers, typically on tongue or hard palate)

In addition, 30% of patients develop Raynaud phenomenon. Alopecia is even more common (70%). Raynaud phenomenon is treated with calcium channel blockers.

▶ **TIP**

Neither Raynaud nor alopecia is an official diagnostic criterion of SLE.

Arthritis (90%)

Joint involvement is defined as pain in two or more peripheral joints; the joints may or may not be tender or swollen.

Serositis

Serositis in SLE does not have just one symptom. Pleuritis can give chest pain that changes with respiration anywhere in the chest. Pericarditis can present with pain, effusion, or tamponade.

Neurological Involvement (15%)

Neurological involvement can be CNS, peripheral, or autonomic. The presentation is quite variable and may lead to:

- Seizures
- Stroke
- Psychosis (cognitive)
- Aseptic meningitis
- Peripheral neuropathy

Stroke in a young person (under 40) should provoke a test for ANA, ESR, anti-cardiolipins and vasculitis.

Renal (50%)

SLE has a broad range of presentation in terms of its renal involvement when it occurs. This can range from asymptomatic incidental findings to proteinuria, hematuria, membranous glomerulonephritis, or nephrotic syndrome. You cannot be certain of the precise level of involvement without a renal **biopsy.**

Hematologic

Patients with SLE most commonly have anemia of chronic disease (60%), not Coombs positive hemolytic anemia, which occurs in only 5% of patients. The WBC count is low exclusively from decreased lymphocytes, not neutropenia. Thrombocytopenia is from antibodies removing platelets from circulation in the same way as ITP.

> SLE can lower one, two, or all three cell lines.

Antiphospholipid Syndrome (40%)

Antiphospholipid (APL) syndrome can be due to either the lupus anticoagulant or the anticardiolipin antibody. There is little difference between them in terms of diagnosis or treatment. Lupus anticoagulant is more likely to present with an elevated aPTT and DVT or pulmonary embolus (PE). Anticardiolipin antibodies are more likely to be associated with spontaneous abortion. APL syndrome can cause a false positive VDRL, and is also associated with hemolytic anemia and levido reticularis. APL is treated with heparin followed by warfarin if DVT or PE occurs.

▶ **TIP**

When the case describes two first-trimester or a single second-trimester spontaneous abortion, look for anticardiolipin antibodies.

DIAGNOSTIC TESTS

The best initial test is an ANA, which is present in 95% to 100% of patients. The most specific tests are anti-double stranded (anti-DS) DNA and anti-Smith (anti-Sm). **Anti-DS DNA is present in 50% to 70%** and **anti-Sm** in 20% to 25%. Also present, though in less than 20% of patients, are antiribonucleoprotein, anti-Ro/SSA, and anti-La/SSB.

A 24-year-old woman with recently diagnosed SLE is admitted for atypical chest pain. She has pericarditis and had a pericardial window placed several months ago. Her EKG is equivocal. Which of the following would be most useful in determining the etiology of her chest pain?

a. Complement levels
b. ESR
c. Rheumatoid factor
d. Urinalysis
e. CBC
f. SS-A and SS-B antibodies

Answer: The correct answer is (a). Although rheumatoid factor (RF), anti-SS-A (Ro) and anti-SS-B (La) are present in 20% to 30%, they add little to the diagnosis. CBC, urinalysis, ESR, and complement levels should be obtained. The most important of these is the complement level because it can assess disease activity. During flares of lupus, complement levels drop and anti-DS DNA levels rise. This is very important because SLE can appear similar to many other diseases. This allows you to simply treat an acute manifestation such as a lupus flare by giving high-dose, short-course steroids instead of pursuing further investigation.

TREATMENT

Glucocorticoids are the **best initial therapy** for questions describing an acute flare of SLE symptoms. The best long-term disease-controlling therapy is hydroxychloroquine. For renal involvement, the best therapy is prednisone combined with either cyclophosphamide or mycophenolate.

Hydroxychloroquine has been the mainstay of therapy for SLE for 40 years, and is continued as a preventative measure even after resolution of symptoms. An annual eye exam is done because of the **retinal toxicity**.

Belimumab, azathioprine, cyclophosphamide, and mycophenolate are all effective for SLE and are the answer for these questions:

- A patient with SLE who continues to have frequent recurrences despite the use of hydroxychloroquine
- Severe symptoms that recur as soon as prednisone is discontinued
- SLE with renal involvement

Belimumab is the first SLE drug in 40 years.

> Some patients will get off steroids only by using azathioprine or cyclophosphamide.

> Belimumab restrains the effects of lymphocytes.

▶ **TIP**

Methotrexate is always a wrong answer for SLE.

Your patient with lupus becomes pregnant. Which of the following is the most accurate way to determine the risk of SLE in her child?

a. Titer of anti-DS DNA
b. Complement levels
c. Anti-SS-A (Ro)
d. Anti-Sm
e. Ultrasound

Answer: The correct answer is (c). Anti-SS-A or anti-Ro antibodies are associated with the development of neonatal lupus (congenital heart block, rash, and hematologic and hepatic abnormalities).

▶ **TIP**

The other frequently tested points on SLE and pregnancy are:

- A pregnant patient who **has anti-SS-A antibodies is at risk of neonatal lupus or AV heart block.**
- Steroids, hydroxychloroquine, and azathioprine should be continued during pregnancy; however, cyclophosphamide, mycophenolate, and methotrexate should be discontinued due to fetal abnormalities.
- Warfarin should be discontinued due to fetal abnormalities; aspirin and subcutaneous heparin should be substituted.

> SS–A = AV heart block in babies

A woman with a history of lupus comes in because of headache, fever, and neck stiffness. She has recently had worsening of her joint pain and was placed on high-dose NSAIDs and prednisone. Her CSF shows 185 white blood cells that are 92% lymphocytes. C3 and C4 levels are normal. Her anti-DS DNA titer is unchanged.

What is the best step in management of this patient?

a. Start ceftriaxone and vancomycin
b. Stop NSAIDs
c. Increase the dose of steroids
d. Add cyclophosphamide
e. Add hydroxychloroquine

Answer: The correct answer is (b). NSAIDs at high doses can cause an aseptic meningitis. The mechanism is unknown. Bacterial meningitis, which is treated empirically with ceftriaxone and vancomycin, is highly unlikely with a mild lymphocytic pleocytosis in the CSF. This is unlikely to be a lupus flare when she has just been placed on prednisone. In addition, complement levels will drop with a lupus flare and her complement levels are normal. Anti-DS DNA levels will rise with a lupus flare. Since this seems to be meningitis secondary to NSAIDs, cyclophosphamide and hydroxychloroquine will not help.

Drug-Induced Lupus

The major differences between drug-induced lupus and routine SLE is:

> Drug-induced lupus spares the brain and kidney.

- **Equal gender frequency:** Men get drug-induced lupus just as often as women
- **Absence of neurological and renal manifestations**
- Presence of **antihistone antibodies**; absence of all other antibodies
- Resolution with stopping offending agent (e.g., isoniazid, hydralazine, methyldopa, chlorpromazine)

SPINAL STENOSIS

PRESENTATION/"WHAT IS THE MOST LIKELY DIAGNOSIS?"

Look for a patient with back pain radiating to the buttocks and thighs. The pain is worse with walking and therefore can easily be confused with peripheral arterial disease. The key to the diagnosis is that the pain is worse when walking downhill or in any posture where there is a slight lean backward; resting brings rapid relief of pain. Cycling is pain free because the body is leaning forward.

Physical shows:

- Normal ankle/brachial arterial index
- Proximal muscle weakness in 60%
- Diminished reflexes in 25%
- Possible paresthesia

DIAGNOSTIC TESTS/TREATMENT

The most accurate diagnostic test is an MRI. X-ray and CT are always wrong answers.

The best initial therapy for severe pain is an epidural injection of corticosteroids. The most effective therapy is surgical decompression.

SYSTEMIC SCLEROSIS (SCLERODERMA)

Scleroderma presents with two forms:

1. Limited disease
2. Diffuse disease

Limited Disease (80%)

CREST syndrome (**C**alcinosis, **R**aynaud, **E**sophageal dysmotility, **S**clerodactyly, **T**elangiectasia)

Anti-centromere antibody is associated with CREST.

The skin changes of limited scleroderma do not progress more proximally than the elbows and comprise mainly sclerodactyly and facial involvement.

Patients with limited disease are more likely to develop **primary** pulmonary hypertension. It is primary because lungs are normal.

Primary pulmonary hypertension occurs in limited disease with normal lung parenchyma.

Esophageal dysmotility presents as GERD and is managed with proton pump inhibitors.

Diffuse Disease (20%)

Diffuse disease has all the same manifestations of CREST or limited disease as well as:

- **Pulmonary involvement:** Interstitial lung disease or secondary pulmonary hypertension may occur.
- **Renal involvement:** Hypertension, renal failure, or microangiopathic hemolytic anemia may be present.
- **Musculoskeletal involvement:** Myalgia and arthralgia that is nonerosive; tendon friction rubs may occur.
- **Cardiac involvement:** Fibrosis of the myocardium may occur (cardiomyopathy, pericarditis, arrhythmias).
- **Malabsorption:** Limited disease does not involve the GI tract past the esophagus; diffuse disease leads to malabsorption because of hypomotility of the GI tract.

> Only diffuse disease has renal, heart, and lung involvement.

> Remember: Telangiectasia can involve the GI tract as well as leading to bleeding.

DIAGNOSTIC TESTS

ESR may be elevated in a few patients, so whether it is up or down, it is never the right answer to any question about scleroderma. If asked "What is the most accurate test?" or "What is the most specific test?" the answer is **anti-SCL-70**, which is also known as **antitopoisomerase**. Anti-SCL-70 is present in only 30% of those with diffuse disease and 20% of those with limited disease; it is associated with an increased risk for ILD.

The **ANA is present in 80% to 95%**, so a negative test does have a fairly good negative predictive value. For CREST, test for anti-centromere antibodies.

> Gastric antral vascular ectasia (GAVE) are large vessels in the stomach.

> The diagnosis of scleroderma is not based on tests.

TREATMENT

- **Skin:** No treatment
- **Renal/hypertensive crisis:** ACE inhibitors (regardless of renal function)
- **Lung:**
  - The interstitial fibrosis is treated with cyclophosphamide.
  - Primary pulmonary hypertension is treated with bosentan, an endothelin inhibitor, and anticoagulation. Treprostinil, iloprost, and epoprostanil are prostacyclin analogs for primary pulmonary hypertension.
  - Anticoagulation with warfarin is indicated for most severe pulmonary hypertension
  - Sildenafil, tadalafil, and vardenafil all dilate pulmonary vasculature
- **Raynaud phenomenon:** Calcium channel blockers and occasionally sildenafil or alpha blockers

SJÖGREN SYNDROME

PRESENTATION/"WHAT IS THE MOST LIKELY DIAGNOSIS?"

Most autoimmune diseases occur more frequently in women, but Sjögren syndrome, with a 9:1 ratio, is almost exclusive to women. Because of loss of salivary and lacrimal glands, look for:

> Loss of saliva will lead to tooth loss.

- **Dry eyes** (xerophthalmia)
- **Dry mouth** (xerostomia)
- **Dry vagina** (dyspareunia)

A disease of exocrine gland function, Sjögren syndrome may exist as an isolated disorder; however, it most often occurs secondary to another auto-immune disorder (RA, SLE, systemic sclerosis). Although its presentations may be peripheral neuropathy, purpura, and muscle and joint pain, the most frequently asked questions concern the dryness previously described. The pancreas is only rarely affected. Sjögren syndrome can lead to lymphoma.

DIAGNOSTIC TESTS

The best initial test will be:

- Blood for **anti-Ro/SSA** and **anti-La/SSB**

And/or

- **Schirmer test:** filter paper touching the eye measuring lacrimal gland output (95% sensitive and specific)

The **most accurate test is a biopsy of the lip or the parotid salivary gland** (lymphocytic infiltration).

> ▶ **TIP**
>
> Additional diagnostic test abnormalities that will be in the choices include ANA and RF. Although found in Sjögren syndrome, they are neither the first nor the most accurate tests to perform.

> Sjögren syndrome is associated with a 44-fold increase in the risk of lymphoma.

A 32-year-old woman comes to the office for evaluation of dry, gritty eyes that "feel like sand got under my eyelids." She frequently sees the dentist, who cannot explain why a woman at her age is getting so many cavities. Her anti-Ro/SSA antibody is positive.

What is the most effective therapy for this patient?

a. Prednisone
b. Cyclophosphamide
c. Cevimeline
d. Azathioprine
e. Mycophenolate

Answer: The correct answer is (c). Cevimeline increases oral and ocular secretions. Although Sjögren syndrome is an autoimmune disorder, steroids and the usual immunosuppressive agents are, unfortunately, not effective.

TREATMENT

Hydroxychloroquine is used to control the underlying disease process in Sjögren syndrome. Symptomatic treatment is:

- **Pilocarpine** and **cevimeline** (these increase acetylcholine, which will increase secretions from the mouth, eyes, and vagina)
- **Artificial tears**
- Oral hygiene (this is critical, including fluoride treatments and frequent sips of water)

> Steroids will not help Sjögren syndrome.

RELAPSING POLYCHONDRITIS

This is a destructive inflammation of cartilaginous structures throughout the body. It is destructive in the sense that the cartilage not only is red, warm, and tender, but afterward becomes atrophic and deformed. Relapsing polychondritis is often associated with other autoimmune diseases such as SLE, RA, or vasculitis. Tracheal weakening may occur.

It is often associated with fever and migratory joint pains.

The most accurate test is a biopsy. Treatment is with prednisone. Dapsone and methotrexate are steroid sparing regimens.

> Destruction of the tracheal cartilage can damage the voice and lead to upper airway obstruction. Other manifestations may be ocular, cardiovascular/valvular, neurologic, and musculoskeletal.

BEHÇET SYNDROME

This is a syndrome of recurrent **lesions** of the **mouth** and **genitals** in persons of Asian or Middle Eastern ancestry. A unique skin lesion, known as pathergy, is a sterile abscess that occurs with minor trauma. Uveitis may be so severe as to cause **blindness**.

CNS lesions present in a similar fashion to multiple sclerosis in that virtually any manifestation is possible, such as seizures, sterile meningitis, encephalitis, or cranial nerve palsies.

Prednisone is the best initial therapy. Steroid sparing regimens are cyclophosphamide, colchicine, and thalidomide.

> There is no specific blood test for Behçet syndrome.

SERONEGATIVE SPONDYLOARTHROPATHIES

These disorders cause joint pain. They all present with the following findings in common:

- Often starts under the age of 40
- Involvement of the spine (spondylitis) and sacroiliitis
- Enthesopathy: inflammation of the point of attachment of ligaments and tendons at the joint capsule
- Uveitis
- No autoantibodies (seronegative)
- HLA B27 present in 50% to 95%
- Possible infectious trigger (nongonococcal genitourinary infections and infectious diarrhea)

Ankylosing Spondylitis

Ankylosing spondylitis begins as a chronic backache in young men in their 20s. The pain is worse in the morning and the stiffness lasts for more than an hour and radiates to the buttocks. The pain improves with activity.

Specific features (answering the "most likely diagnosis" question) are:

- Flattening of normal lumbar curvature
- Limitation of chest expansion
- Fusion of the spine over time
- Atrioventricular conduction defects in the heart
- Pulmonary fibrosis
- Arthritis of the hips (rare in RA)

Peripheral arthritis will occur in 50% of patients.

DIAGNOSTIC TESTS

The best initial test is an x-ray of the sacroiliac (SI) joint. The most accurate test is an MRI of the SI joint. In the first 2 years, SI joint abnormalities may be visible only on MRI. ESR is elevated in 85% of patients, but is not helpful enough to establish the diagnosis. It will be a wrong choice. CT scan is always a wrong answer in ankylosing spondylitis.

> ▶ **TIP**
>
> Do not choose HLA B27 testing as a specific diagnostic test. It is present in 8% of the general population.

> Only 5% of HLA-B27–positive patients develop ankylosing spondylitis.

> Bamboo spine is specific to ankylosing spondylitis.

TREATMENT

The best initial therapy is NSAIDs. The most effective therapy is anti-TNF medications such as etanercept, adalimumab, or infliximab.

▶ **TIP**

Steroids (prednisone) is the most common wrong answer as treatment.

Reactive Arthritis (Reiter Syndrome)

This is joint pain that occurs within 2 months of an infectious trigger (either gastrointestinal infection with *Shigella, Campylobacter, Yersinia,* or *Salmonella,* or a nongonoccocal genitourinary infection, such as with *Chlamydia*). The classic triad, present in only a third of patients, is:

- Joint pain
- Conjunctivitis
- Genital abnormalities such as urethritis or circinate balanitis

Treatment is with **NSAIDs**. If there is residual genital infection, it should be treated; however, by the time the arthritis develops, antibiotics will not resolve the joint pain. Use sulfasalazine in those not responding.

Psoriatic Arthritis

Arthritis occurs in 15% to 20% of those with psoriasis. It is more common in those with severe skin disease, which usually predates the arthritis. The two most specific physical findings for psoriatic arthritis are:

- Nail pitting
- Dactylitis ("sausage digits")

Psoriatic arthritis is similar to RA (symmetric polyarticular arthritis), but may have axial involvement and has an increased involvement of the DIP joints.

The best initial test is an x-ray of the joint showing such severe erosion of bone that it may come to a point and appear as a "pencil in a cup." Elevation of the ESR and uric acid level are present, but not useful. They are the wrong answer.

> Do not wait for x-ray abnormalities to treat psoriatic arthritis.

The **best initial therapy is NSAIDs**. The most effective therapy is **methotrexate**. Controlling the psoriasis with ultraviolet light may help control the disease. Anti-TNF agents are used if methotrexate is not effective.

Enteropathic Arthritis

This is joint pain as a manifestation of inflammatory bowel disease (IBD). Both ulcerative colitis and Crohn disease are associated with joint pain. The joint pain typically correlates with severity of GI, ocular, and dermatologic symptoms. Whipple disease is another intestinal infection associated with joint pain. Treatment is with NSAIDs initially to control pain. Anti-TNF medications are frequently used in IBD to control severe disease.

OSTEOARTHRITIS

Osteoarthritis (OA) is also known as degenerative joint disease. OA is a chronic, slowly progressive destruction of the joint space and articular cartilage without systemic symptoms. The etiology is not clear and damage to the joint space is so common as to be considered a normal part of the aging process.

ETIOLOGY

Obesity, competitive contact sports, trauma, female gender, and repetitive use of the joint predispose to OA, but it often occurs without these conditions.

PRESENTATION

Pain in the joint:

- Develops after inactivity
- Worsens with prolonged use; relieved with rest
- Lasts 20 to 30 minutes
- Lasts for less than 30 minutes in the morning
- Typically affects those over 50

Physical examination reveals:

- **Crepitation**
- Bony tenderness
- **Osteophytes** of the proximal interphalangeal joint (PIP) or Bouchard nodes, and distal interphalangeal joint (DIP) or Heberden nodes.

> OA rarely involves the wrists, elbows, shoulders, or ankles.

DIAGNOSTIC TESTS

All blood tests are normal (ESR, rheumatoid factor, C-reactive protein). Aspiration of the joint fluid shows less than 200 white blood cells with less than 50% neutrophils. The most accurate test is an x-ray, although the correlation between symptoms and x-ray findings is inconsistent.

X-ray shows:

- Joint space narrowing
- Osteophytes
- Dense subchondral bone

> Some patients have severe discomfort with mild x-ray changes or minor discomfort with extensive x-ray abnormalities.

▶ **TIP**

Although MRI is the answer to the question "What is the **most accurate diagnostic test?**" MRI is not routinely indicated. MRI is not the answer to "What would you do next?" When symptoms of OA are clear, giving analgesics and encouraging weight loss are what you should do first.

TREATMENT

NSAIDs are at least as effective as acetaminophen as the best initial treatment. NSAIDs are associated with gastrointestinal (bleeding) and renal adverse effects; acetaminophen can lead to hepatotoxicity.

A 73-year-old woman comes to the office with discomfort of her knee not responsive to acetaminophen or ibuprofen.

Which of the following will <u>not</u> improve her condition?

a. Chondroitin and glucosamine
b. Capsaicin cream
c. Intraarticular triamcinolone
d. Hyaluronic acid
e. Weight loss

Answer: The correct answer is (a). Chrondroitin and glucosamine are no more effective than placebo in relieving symptoms of OA. Hyaluronic acid relieves symptoms when it is injected into the joint by augmenting the viscoelastic properties of normal synovial fluid. Intraarticular injections of glucocorticoids can safely be given four times a year. Although they may cause some joint damage if overused, they lead to prompt resolution of pain. Capsaicin is an inhibitor of substance P.

> Although NSAIDs cause peptic ulcers, proton pump inhibitors should **not** be used routinely in every patient on an NSAID.

COX-2 Inhibitors

Only celecoxib remains on the market from this class of medications. Although never thought to be superior in terms of efficacy, these medications have a **decreased incidence of GI hemorrhage** because they do not inhibit the enzyme that generates prostaglandins that produce the mucous barrier in the stomach. The question most likely to be asked about celecoxib would be to test your knowledge about the **increased risk of cardiovascular events with the use of COX-2 inhibitors.**

> Celecoxib does not have better efficacy than the other NSAIDs.

CRYSTAL ARTHROPATHIES

Gout

ETIOLOGY

Gout is caused by the overproduction or underexcretion of uric acid. Acute attacks are precipitated by:

- Binge beer drinking
- Dehydration and acidosis
- Chemotherapy-induced cell death
- Rapid lowering of uric acid levels with allopurinol
- Trauma
- Surgery
- Medications such as diuretics and cyclosporine

PRESENTATION

Men account for 90% of those with gout. The most common presentation is the sudden onset of an extremely tender and painful metatarsophalangeal joint, known as podagra. The joint is warm and red and fever is common.

Other joints may be involved. Tophi are collections of monosodium urate crystals in the soft tissue around the ear, fingers, Achilles tendon, or extensor surfaces of the limbs.

> Gout is asymmetric and monoarticular.

> **Which of the following is most useful in determining a diagnosis of gout on the first attack of a painful joint in gout?**
>
> a. Serum uric acid level
> b. Urine uric acid level
> c. Joint fluid cell count and differential
> d. Joint fluid polarizing microscopy
> e. X-ray
> f. MRI
> g. Response to colchicine
>
> **Answer:** The correct answer is (d). Negatively birefringent needle-shaped crystals are the most specific test of an acute gouty attack. The cell count is generally above 10,000/µl but may be as high as 50,000. When markedly elevated, the synovial fluid cell count can be difficult to distinguish from infectious arthritis. The serum uric acid level, although elevated in 95% of cases over time, may be normal in 25% of acute attacks. Radiologic tests are normal with initial evaluation of gout. Colchicine can improve the pain of both gout and pseudogout. Using a response to treatment as a way of confirming a diagnosis is a poor way to establish any diagnosis.

DIAGNOSTIC TESTS

The most accurate way to establish a diagnosis with an acute gouty attack is with aspiration of the joint fluid. This is important to perform with the first attack of gout. Prior to establishing a diagnosis, an acute attack of gout can have numerous similarities to septic arthritis such as a markedly elevated cell count with increased neutrophils. Septic arthritis should have a cell count above 50,000/μl. Both disorders have a normal x-ray of the joint.

> Uric acid levels during an attack of gout may be normal.

Other abnormalities are:

- Elevated serum uric acid level
- Elevated ESR, C-reactive protein, and leukocytosis

TREATMENT

The best initial therapy for acute attacks is with NSAIDs. Indomethacin is not superior to other NSAIDs. Do not discontinue chronic therapy during attacks. Intra-articular steroids are superior to colchicine.

> Do not treat asymptomatic elevations in uric acid levels.

Treatment of Gout		
Circumstance	**Drug to use**	**Adverse effect**
Increased risk of GI bleeding	Celecoxib (COX-2 inhibitor)	Cardiovascular events
Renal insufficiency	Intraarticular corticosteroids or Systemic steroids	Exclude septic arthritis first Hyperglycemia
Preventing recurrent attacks	Colchicine	Bone marrow suppression

Preventing Recurrent Attacks

- Diet:
  - Limit the intake of alcohol, especially beer.
  - Limit the intake of red meat and seafood.
  - Increase liquids to increase urine output.
  - Lose weight.

- Uric acid lowering: Never start uric acid lowering agents during an acute attack of gout; treatment goal is uric acid below 6.0.
  - **Allopurinol:** best initial therapy especially if the renal excretion of uric acid is already high, patient is an overproducer of uric acid, renal insufficiency is present, or there is a history of nephrolithiasis or intolerance of uricosuric agents

> **Beware of drug hypersensitivity with allopurinol such as rash or Stevens-Johnson syndrome.**

> **When the blood level of uric acid is lowered sufficiently, uric acid crystals will dissolve.**

- **Febuxostat** is an inhibitor of xanthine oxidase that has similar efficacy to allopurinol in preventing acute gouty attacks. Febuxostat, being 50 times more expensive than allopurinol and generally not more efficacious, is the answer when the following are in the question:
  - Hypersensitivity to allopurinol
  - Renal insufficiency
  - Failure of allopurinol to control the level of uric acid
- **Colchicine is effective in preventing recurrent episodes of acute gout.** Colchicine is particularly indicated in the presence of renal insufficiency in which allopurinol or uricosuric agents are more dangerous or less effective. In addition to **bone marrow suppression**, colchicine leads to neuromuscular toxicity and **diarrhea**.
- Uricase agents rasburicase or pegloticase dissolve uric acid.

▶ **TIP**

Uricosuric agents must be used with a high daily urine output.

Uricosuric agents (probenecid, sulfinpyrazone): use as a third-line agent if renal excretion of uric acid is low on a 24-hour urine; contraindicated in renal insufficiency or with a history of nephrolithiasis

Pseudogout (Calcium Pyrophosphate Deposition Disease)

Pseudogout presents in a similar fashion to gout, but occurs in larger joints such as the knee. Certain conditions predispose to pseudogout. These include:

- Hyperparathyroidism
- Hypothyroidism
- Hemochromatosis
- Hypomagnesemia and hypophosphatemia

> **If NSAIDs can't be used, inject the joint with steroids.**

DIAGNOSTIC TESTS

The best initial and most accurate test is to aspirate the joint, looking for rhomboid-shaped crystals with positive birefringence on polarizing microscopy. As with gout, the cell count is typically elevated between 10,000 to 50,000 WBCs per μl.

> **X-rays are far more likely to be abnormal with pseudogout (chondrocalcinosis) compared with gout.**

TREATMENT

Treatment of pseudogout in an acute attack is the **same as that for gout**. The best initial therapy is an **NSAID**. If there is a contraindication to NSAIDs such as renal insufficiency, the best initial therapy is an **injection of intraarticular glucocorticoids**. Colchicine will be effective but should be avoided because of the risk of myelosuppression and gastrointestinal adverse effects such as diarrhea.

Prevention of recurrent attacks of pseudogout is to correct the underlying causes previously listed and to use colchicine.

> Allopurinol and febuxostat do not help pseudogout because it is not related to hyperuricemia.

SEPTIC ARTHRITIS

PRESENTATION

Infected joints present with the classic signs of infection such as redness, warmth, swelling, and tenderness. Two additional findings for joint infection are:

- Immobility, or pain on passive range of motion
- Palpable effusion

Which of the following confers the greatest risk of an infected joint?

a. Osteoarthritis
b. Prosthetic joint
c. Rheumatoid arthritis
d. Ankylosing spondylitis
e. Sexual promiscuity

Answer: The correct answer is (b). Prosthetic joints have the single greatest risk of becoming infected. Normal joints rarely become infected. The more deformed or damaged, the more likely there will be an infection. RA has a greater risk than OA, but a prosthetic joint is the most anatomically "abnormal" thing that can happen to a joint. Promiscuity confers a much greater risk of chlamydia than of gonorrhea, and only a small number of gonorrheal infections will disseminate to involve the joint.

Disseminated Gonorrhea

Because disseminated gonorrhea is a difficult diagnosis to establish from laboratory testing, it is important to know how the presentation is different in order to pursue additional testing. Look for:

- Migratory polyarthralgias
- Tenosynovitis: inflammation of the tendon sheaths, making movement of the fingers painful
- Rash: maculopapular lesions that evolve into sterile pustules

DIAGNOSTIC TESTS

The best initial test for septic arthritis is an arthrocentesis. The findings on joint fluid are essential in determining the diagnosis and guiding empiric therapy. With infectious diseases, results of culture are never available at the time initial treatment is started. The WBC count is usually > 50,000/μL.

▶ **TIP**

With infectious diseases, treatment is always empiric: based on the most likely organism to be found, while awaiting a confirmatory test.

Synovial Fluid Characteristics of Septic Arthritis			
Abnormality	**Crystal disease**	**Septic arthritis**	**Disseminated gonorrhea**
Cell count	2,000 to 50,000/µl	>50,000–100,000 (though it may be less in fungal or mycobacterial infections)	>30,000–100,000
Gram stain	Negative	50%–70% sensitive	25% sensitive
Fluid culture	Negative	90% sensitive	50% sensitive
Blood culture	Negative	25% sensitive	10% sensitive
Specific test	Polarizing microscopy	Joint fluid culture	Culture of fluid combined with culturing multiple distant sites

Diagnostic Tests for Disseminated Gonorrhea

Because the yield on joint fluid culture is so low (only 50%), it is essential to culture multiple distant sites such as:

- Pharynx
- Rectum
- Urethra
- Cervix

All of these have about a 10% to 20% sensitivity for growing gonorrhea, except for the cervix, which is positive in 20% to 30% of patients. Hence, the combination of culturing these multiple sites has a greater sensitivity (50% to 90%) than culturing the joint fluid itself.

> Terminal complement deficiency (C5 to C9) predisposes to recurrent *Neisseria* infection. You should always perform this test with recurrent gonorrhea infections.

> Do not rely on sexual history. The individual presentation is more important than risk factors.

▶ **TIP**

The presence of a rash, tenosynovitis, and migratory polyarthralgias is what will tell you to answer "culture multiple distant sites."

TREATMENT

The best initial treatment for septic arthritis is ceftriaxone and vancomycin. Ceftriaxone will cover gonorrhea and Gram-negative infections. Vancomycin will cover *Staphylococcus* and *Streptococcus*. Remember that this is only the empiric therapy before the results of culture are known.

Which of the following patients should receive their antibiotics directly into the joint fluid?

a. Prosthetic joints
b. Osteoarthritis
c. Gonorrhea
d. Methicillin-resistant Staphylococcus aureus
e. Rheumatoid arthritis
f. Injection drug users
g. SLE
h. None of the above

Answer: The correct answer is (h). No one needs injection of antibiotics directly into the joint fluid. Antibiotics of any kind will freely pass into the joint fluid from the blood. Synovial lining does not represent a significant barrier to the passage of antibiotics into the synovial fluid. This is because synovial lining has no basement membrane and the cellular connections are relatively loose compared to something like bone or the blood-brain barrier.

> All antibiotics should be altered once the specific organism and its sensitivities are identified.

Prosthetic Joint Infection

Infection of prosthetic joints represents two additional problems:

1. How to recognize the joint is infected
2. Two-stage treatment

In addition to the usual signs of an infected joint such as warmth, redness, and swelling, "loosening" of the joint or a radiolucent area in the bone around the implantation of the prosthetic joint suggests the prosthesis is infected.

Infections during the first year are generally causing by contamination of the prosthesis or wound site. Infections occurring after 1 year are generally spread hematogenously to the prosthesis.

Prosthetic joint infection is extremely difficult to eradicate. The metal joint obviously has no blood supply and is very hard to sterilize. You need to remove the joint. Treat for six weeks with intravenous antibiotics, then implant a new joint. Although it is possible to successfully treat with the metal in place, it is much less successful.

> Prosthetic joints need to be removed in order to ensure clearance of the infection.

VASCULITIS

Wegener Granulomatosis (Small Vessel Vasculitis)

PRESENTATION

Wegener presents predominantly with **upper and lower respiratory tract** involvement. It is a systemic vasculitis, so in addition to the nonspecific symptoms of fever and weight loss, the following organ systems may be involved:

> Look for sinusitis and otitis media in a person with unresolving respiratory symptoms and cavities on chest x-ray with renal involvement.

- Renal (80% to 90%; glomerulonephritis)
- Eyes
- Skin (petechiae and purpura)
- CNS (mononeuritis multiplex and stroke)
- Musculoskeletal (arthralgia)
- GI (bleeds)
- Hematologic (venous thromboembolism)

▶ **TIP**

Answer Wegener as "the most likely diagnosis" when a case is presented that looks like a respiratory infection but fails to resolve with antibiotics.

DIAGNOSTIC TESTS/TREATMENT

The best initial test in c-ANCA, also known as anti-proteinase-3. The most accurate test is a biopsy of the lung. Lung biopsy is superior in accuracy to sinus biopsy.

Anemia, white count abnormalities, and an elevated ESR are not specific or sensitive enough to be useful. The urinalysis will show protein, red cells, or red cell casts. However, urinalysis results alone are not specific enough to establish the diagnosis of Wegener granulomatosis.

Treatment is high-dose glucocorticoids (prednisone) and cyclophosphamide for 3 to 6 months, followed by 1 year of steroids plus azathioprine or methotrexate.

Polyarteritis Nodosa (Medium Vessel Vasculitis)

PRESENTATION

Polyarteritis nodosa (PAN) presents with damage of virtually every organ except the lung. The most common manifestations are:

| PAN = everything involved except lung |

- Fatigue, weight loss, and fever
- Renal insufficiency (from ischemia, not glomerulonephritis)
- Abdominal pain, especially with eating (mesenteric ischemia)
- Skin with petechiae, purpura, and livedo reticularis
- Peripheral neuropathy from vascular insufficiency of the vaso nervorum, which supplies the nerves (mononeuritis multiplex)
- Stroke in a young person (under 40)
- Testicular pain

DIAGNOSTIC TESTS/TREATMENT

The best initial tests are ANCA and hepatitis B surface antigen. Neither is specific.

The most accurate test is a biopsy of an involved organ such as skin, nerve, or muscle.

Angiography of the renal, mesenteric, or hepatic arteries can spare a patient a renal biopsy. Angiography in PAN shows "beading" of the involved vessel.

Anemia, leukocytosis, elevated ESR and C-reactive protein, and positive RF are sometimes present, but are not very helpful. They are not the answer to either the "best initial test" or the "most accurate test" question. ANCA is almost always negative.

Treatment is high-dose prednisone (glucocorticoids) plus cyclophosphamide (in severe cases).

> Always test PAN for hepatitis B surface antigen (approximately 50% of cases are associated with hepatitis B infection).

Churg-Strauss Syndrome (Small Vessel Vasculitis)

Churg-Strauss is a vasculitis similar to microscopic polyangiitis and Wegener granulomatosis. The main difference is that Churg-Strauss syndrome presents with:

- Asthma
- Eosinophilia

The most accurate test is a biopsy. In 40% of patients, p-ANCA (antimyeloperoxidase antibodies) are positive. Treatment is with prednisone and cyclophosphamide.

Microscopic Polyangiitis (Small Vessel Vasculitis)

PRESENTATION

Microscopic polyangiitis (MPA) is one of several pulmonary/renal syndromes. There is considerable similarity with PAN and Wegener. All of them can give skin, renal, and neurological involvement. However, unlike PAN, MPA very frequently and severely involves the lung. Unlike Wegener, MPA does not involve the upper respiratory organs such as the nose and ear.

> MPA is a lung/kidney syndrome that is much more common than Goodpasture syndrome.

▶ **TIP**

Any vasculitis can cause fever, weight loss, and fatigue.

DIAGNOSTIC TESTS/TREATMENT

The best initial test is p-ANCA, which is positive in 60% to 85% of patients. The most accurate test is a biopsy.

ESR and C-reactive protein are too nonspecific to be useful. Urinalysis will show proteinuria, hematuria, and red cell casts as it can in any form of glomerulonephritis.

Treatment is glucocorticoids and cyclophosphamide.

▶ **TIP**
Look for severe alveolar hemorrhage as the clue to the diagnosis.

Henoch-Schönlein Purpura (Small Vessel Vasculitis)

Henoch-Schönlein purpura (HSP) is a systemic vasculitis caused by IgA attacking small arteries. HSP presents with:

> HSP is similar to IgA nephropathy except that multiple organs are involved.

- Gastrointestinal: pain, bleeding, and diarrhea
- Joint: arthralgias
- Skin: leukocytoclastic, non-blanching purpuric lesions of the legs and buttocks
- Renal: hematuria, proteinuria, and when far advanced, nephrotic syndrome

There is no blood test for HSP. IgA levels are not routinely indicated or helpful. The most accurate test is a biopsy. Biopsy may not be necessary if there is a clear presentation with the previously described organs all involved.

Most cases of HSP will resolve spontaneously. Prednisone is not generally helpful or used, but glucocorticoids are used when:

- Resolution does not occur.
- Renal involvement and proteinuria are worsening.

Mononeuritis Multiplex

Mononeuritis multiplex is defined as a peripheral neuropathy of at least two peripheral nerves large enough to have names—for example, the ulnar and the peroneal, or the radial and the femoral. This disorder occurs in the majority of vasculitic disorders. This is different from peripheral neuropathy, which affects much smaller "twigs" or branches of the peripheral nerves. Mononeuritis multiplex affects both the sensory and motor components of the nerve. Vasculitis causes this because it damages the vaso nervorum, the vascular supply for these nerves. These large peripheral nerves are starved by the damage to their blood supply. Treatment is based on controlling the underlying disease.

Cryoglobulinemia

PRESENTATION

Cryoglobulins are an IgM occurring in association with hepatitis C. Patients present with vasculitis affecting:

- Kidney
- Skin
- Joints
- Peripheral neuropathy

As the name implies, symptoms are worse in the cold and in body parts that are gravity-dependent and more easily exposed to the cold such as:

- Nose
- Ears
- Fingers

DIAGNOSTIC TESTS/TREATMENT

Serum IgM cryoglobulin level is the most accurate test. Treat the underlying hepatitis C with interferon and ribavirin. For cryoglobulinemia, not for hepatitis C, use glucocorticoids such as prednisone and cyclophosphamide or rituximab. IgM-related diseases include cold agglutinin disease with *Mycoplasma* and cryoglobulinemia. Acute, severe cryoglobulinemia can be urgently improved with plasmapheresis.

> Do **not** treat asymptomatic cryoglobulinemia.

Summary of Vasculitic Disorders

All forms of vasculitis are essentially idiopathic inflammatory disorders of blood vessels. The vessels involved can be small as in PAN, or large as in Takayasu arteritis. All forms of vasculitis give fever, weight loss, malaise, and elevated ESR and C-reactive protein. They can all affect the kidney, skin, and joints. The most accurate test for all of them is a biopsy. The exception to this is Takayasu arteritis: You do not want to biopsy a large artery.

Comparison of Various Forms of Vasculitis: What Is the Difference?

Disease	Polyarteritis nodosa	Wegener granulomatosis	Microscopic polyangiitis	Churg-Strauss syndrome	Henoch-Schönlein purpura	Cryoglobulinemia
Presentation	• No lung involvement • History of hepatitis B	• Upper and lower respiratory involvement	• Alveolar hemorrhage • No upper respiratory involvement • Rapid renal failure	• Asthma, rhinitis, sinusitis	• No lung involvement • Limited to GI, joint, skin, and renal involvement	• History of hepatitis C
Diagnostic tests	Angiography	c-ANCA (anti-proteinase-3)	p-ANCA (anti-myeloperoxidase)	Eosinophilia in all, p-ANCA in half	Clinical pattern	IgM cryoglobulin level in blood
Treatment	Prednisone and cyclophosphamide	Prednisone and cyclophosphamide	Prednisone and cyclophosphamide	Prednisone and cyclophosphamide	Spontaneous resolution in most	Interferon and ribavirin for hepatitis C treatment

Takayasu Arteritis (Large Vessel Vasculitis)

This is a vasculitis that affects the aorta and its main branches such as the cerebral, renal, femoral, mesenteric, and coronary vessels. It presents with limb claudication and lightheadedness. When it is severe, the obstruction of flow makes the pulses nonpalpable, hence the name "pulseless disease."

Diagnostic Tests/Treatment

The most accurate test is angiography. Treatment is with glucocorticoids. Methotrexate, cyclophosphamide, and TNF-alpha inhibitors are used to help wean patients off of steroids. Severe disease can be bypassed surgically or treated with angioplasty.

> ▶ **TIP**
> Biopsy is never the answer with Takayasu arteritis.

> Look for a bruit over the subclavian arteries and a 10 mm Hg difference in blood pressure between the arms.

> All causes of vasculitis give fever, malaise, weight loss, and an elevated ESR and C-reactive protein.

FIBROMYALGIA

Fibromyalgia is a pain syndrome occurring mostly in women between the ages of 20 and 50. In addition to at least 3 months of aching pain and stiffness of 11 of 18 specific tender points, there is:

- Fatigue and sleep disturbance
- An association with irritable bowel syndrome (IBS), chronic fatigue syndrome, headaches, and interstitial cystitis

Blood tests are useful only to exclude other illnesses; as a matter of definition of the syndrome, they are all normal.

> Fibromyalgia is defined as pain in 11 of 18 identified trigger points for 3 months.

Treatment

Treatment of fibromyalgia is dissatisfying and a matter of trial and error. The best initial therapy is with cognitive/behavioral therapy and exercise. The best drug therapy is with milnacipran, pregabalin, tricyclic antidepressants, or duloxetine. NSAIDs, opiates, and steroids rarely work.

> ▶ **TIP**
> Steroids are always a wrong answer for treating fibromyalgia.

> Milnacipran is a combination serotonin/norepinephrine reuptake inhibitor that treats fibromyalgia.

POLYMYALGIA RHEUMATICA AND GIANT CELL ARTERITIS

Although polymyalgia rheumatica (PMR) and giant cell arteritis (GCA) may fall on the same spectrum of disease, their presentation and diagnostic tests are completely different.

Polymyalgia Rheumatica (Large Vessel Vasculitis)

PMR presents as:

> Look for pain/weakness in neck, hips, and shoulders in PMR.

- Proximal muscle pain and weakness (can't get up from a chair without using arms)
- Fatigue and malaise   *fever, Malaise, Fatigue*
- Age 50 or older
- Increased ESR and CRP — *Protein C Reactive*
- Normal CPK and normal aldolase
- Dramatic response to low-dose prednisone

Giant Cell Arteritis (Large Vessel Vasculitis)

Giant cell arteritis (GCA) is a systemic vasculitis, but predominantly presents with visual disturbance because of involvement of the temporal artery. GCA also presents with:

- Headache
- Jaw claudication

As with PMR, the best initial test is an ESR. The most accurate test is a biopsy and treatment is with prednisone (urgently to prevent vision loss). Biopsy within 4 weeks of initiation of steroids will not affect the results. Always start steroids first if you suspect GCA.

INFLAMMATORY MYOPATHIES (DERMATOMYOSITIS/ POLYMYOSITIS)

PRESENTATION

These disorders, also known as inflammatory myopathies, are idiopathic, autoimmune muscle weakness due to muscle destruction. They present with proximal muscle weakness and, less frequently, pain. There is no change in sensation, or coordination, and there is no cranial nerve or autonomic dysfunction. Look for the phrase "difficulty getting up from a chair without using the arms." There is also:

> Interstitial lung disease occurs in 10% to 30% of patients.

- Dysphagia
- Myocarditis

Although primarily a disorder of muscles, these conditions can result in interstitial lung disease and in malignancy.

▶ **TIP**

The most frequently tested point on presentation is the association of dermatomyositis with malignancy.

Skin Manifestations

- Gottron papules: scaly patches on the backs of the hands at the joints (pathognomic)
- Heliotrope rash: purplish discoloration around the eyes
- Shawl sign: erythematous area over the neck, upper chest, shoulders, and back
- Nailfold capillary abnormalities

DIAGNOSTIC TESTS

The "best initial test" is a CPK and aldolase level. The "most accurate test" is a muscle biopsy.

An elevated CPK is the main way to distinguish polymyalgia rheumatica from dermatomyositis. In PMR there is muscle pain and weakness, but no actual destruction of muscle. Hence, in PMR the CPK and aldolase are normal.

MRI and electromyography will both show abnormalities. They would not be done first, nor would they be considered as specific as a muscle biopsy. MRI is useful to guide the area of muscle to biopsy.

Other diagnostic tests that have limited benefit are the ESR, RF, and ANA. When they are normal they do not exclude the disease, and when they are positive they are too nonspecific to be very useful.

> MRI is useful only to tell you precisely where to biopsy.

Anti-Jo Antibodies

This is a unique test in inflammatory myositis. Anti-Jo antibodies indicate the increased likelihood of developing interstitial lung disease.

TREATMENT

Corticosteroids such as prednisone are the best initial therapy. Alternate therapies for those who are not controlled with prednisone or are steroid-dependent are:

- Azathioprine
- Methotrexate
- Intravenous immunoglobulin

APPENDIX: ABBREVIATIONS AND MNEMONICS

ABBREVIATIONS

A-a gradient: alveolar-arterial gradient

AA: amyloid from acute phase reactant amyloid A

AAA: abdominal aortic aneurysm

ABG: arterial blood gas

ABI: ankle/brachial index

ABIM: American Board of Internal Medicine

ABPA: allergic bronchopulmonary aspergillosis

ABVD: Adriamycin (doxorubicin), bleomycin, vinblastine, dacarbazine

ACE: angiotensin-converting enzyme

ACEI: angiotensin-converting enzyme inhibitor

ACS: acute coronary syndrome

ACTH: adrenocorticotropic hormone

AD: Alzheimer dementia

ADH: antidiuretic hormone

AED: antiepileptic drug

AFB: acid-fast bacillus

A-fib: atrial fibrillation

AFP: alpha-fetoprotein

AIDS: acquired immunodeficiency syndrome

AIN: allergic (acute) interstitial nephritis

AKI: acute kidney injury

AL: amyloid from light chains

ALL: acute lymphocytic leukemia

ALS: amyotrophic lateral sclerosis

ALT: alanine aminotransferase

AML: acute myeloid leukemia

ANA: antinuclear antibody

ANCA: anti-neutrophil cytoplasmic antibodies

Anti-CCP: anti-cyclic citrullinated peptide

Anti-DS DNA: anti-double stranded DNA

Anti-GBM: anti-glomerular basement membrane

Anti-TNF: anti-tumor necrosis factor

APL: antiphospholipid

APOE e4: apolipoprotein E

aPTT: activated partial thromboplastin time

AR: aortic regurgitation

ARB: angiotensin receptor blocker

ARDS: acute respiratory distress syndrome

ART: antiretroviral therapy

AS (disease): sickle cell trait

AS: aortic stenosis

ASCA: anti-saccharomyces cerevisiae antibody

ASCUS: atypical squamous cells of undetermined significance

ASD: atrial septal defect

ASLO: anti-streptolysin O

AST: aspartate aminotransferase

ATN: acute tubular necrosis

ATRA: all-trans-retinoic acid

AV: atrioventricular

AVM: arteriovenous malformation

BAL: bronchoalveolar lavage

BB: beta blocker

BCC: basal cell carcinoma

BCG: bacillus Calmette-Guérin

BiPAP: bilevel positive airway pressure

BMI: body mass index

BMT: bone marrow transplant

BNP: B-type natriuretic peptide

BP: blood pressure

BPV: benign positional vertigo

BUN: blood urea nitrogen

CABG: coronary artery bypass graft

CAD: coronary artery disease

C-ANCA: cytoplasmic anti-neutrophil cytoplasmic antibodies

CAP: community-acquired pneumonia

CBC: complete blood count

CBD: common bile duct

CCB: calcium channel blocker

CD (markers): cluster of differentiation

CDI: central diabetes insipidus

CEA: carcinoembryonic antigen

CGD: chronic granulomatous disease

CHF: congestive heart failure

CIN: cervical intraepithelial neoplasia

CJD: Creutzfeld-Jakob disease

CK-MB: creatine kinase-MB

CLL: chronic lymphocytic leukemia

CML: chronic myelogenous leukemia

CMT: cervical motion tenderness

CMV: cytomegalovirus

CNS: central nervous system

COMT (inhibitors): catechol-O-methyl transferase

COPD: chronic obstructive pulmonary disease

CPAP: continuous positive airway pressure

CPK: creatine phosphokinase

CPR: cardiopulmonary resuscitation

CRH: corticotropin-releasing hormone

CRP: C-reactive protein

CSA: central sleep apnea

CSF: cerebrospinal fluid

CT: computed tomography

CTA: CT angiogram

CVA: cerebrovascular accident

CVID: common variable immunodeficiency

D&C: dilation & curettage

DEXA: dual energy x-ray absorptiometry

DHEA: dehydroepiandrosterone

DI: diabetes insipidus

DIC: disseminated intravascular coagulation

DIP: distal interphalangeal joint

DKA: diabetic ketoacidosis

DLCO: diffusion capacity of the lung for carbon monoxide

DM: diabetes mellitus

DMARDs: disease modifying antirheumatic drugs

DNA: deoxyribonucleic acid

DPLD: diffuse parenchymal lung disease

DVT: deep vein thrombosis

EATL: enteropathy-associated T cell lymphoma

EBV: Epstein-Barr virus

ED: erectile dysfunction *or* emergency department

EEG: electroencephalogram

EF: ejection fraction

EGD: esophagogastroduodenoscopy

EIA: enzyme immunoassay

EKG: electrocardiography

ELISA: enzyme-linked immunosorbent assay

EM: erythema multiforme

EP: electrophysiology

ER: estrogen receptor

ERCP: endoscopic retrograde cholangiopancreatography

ERV: expiratory reserve volume

ESR: erythrocyte sedimentation rate

ESRD: end stage renal disease

ET: essential thrombocythemia *or* endotracheal

ETOH: ethanol

EUS: endoscopic ultrasound

FAP: familial adenomatous polyposis

FDA: Food and Drug Administration

FEF: forced expiratory flow

FeNA: fractional excretion of sodium

FFP: fresh frozen plasma

FSGS: focal segmental glomerulosclerosis

FSH: follicle-stimulating hormone

FTA-ABS: fluorescent treponemal antibody absorption

G6PD: glucose-6-phosphate dehydrogenase

GBS: Guillain-Barré syndrome

GCA: giant cell arteritis

GERD: gastroesophageal reflux disease

GFR: glomerular filtration rate

GGT *or* **GGTP**: gamma-glutamyl transpeptidase

GH: growth hormone

GI: gastrointestinal

GN: glomerulonephritis

GnRH: gonadotropin-releasing hormone

HAP: hospital-acquired pneumonia

HCG: human chorionic gonadotropin

HD: Hodgkin disease *or* Huntington disease

Her 2/neu: human epidermal growth factor receptor 2

HFE: gene associated with hemochromatosis

HIT: heparin-induced thrombocytopenia

HIV: human immunodeficiency virus

HOCM: hypertrophic obstructive cardiomyopathy

HP: *Helicobacter pylori*

HPF: high power field

HPV: human papillomavirus

HRCT: high-resolution CT

HSIL: high-grade squamous intraepithelial lesion

HSP: Henoch-Schönlein purpura

HSV: herpes simplex virus

IBD: inflammatory bowel disease

IBS: irritable bowel syndrome

IBS-A: irritable bowel syndrome, with alternating stool pattern

IBS-C: irritable bowel syndrome, constipation-predominant

IBS-D: irritable bowel syndrome, diarrhea-predominant

IBS-PI: postinfectious irritable bowel syndrome

ICU: intensive care unit

IgA: immunoglobulin A

IGF: insulinlike growth factor

IgG: immunoglobulin G

IgM: immunoglobulin M

IGRA: interferon gamma release assays

ILD: interstitial lung disease

IM: intramuscular

INR: international normalized ratio

IRIS: immune reconstitution inflammatory syndrome

ITP: idiopathic thrombocytopenic purpura

IUD: intrauterine device

IV: intravenous

IVIG: intravenous immunoglobulins

JVD: jugulovenous distension

KOH: potassium hydroxide

KS: Kaposi sarcoma

KUB: kidney, ureter, bladder

LA: left atrial

LAP: leukocyte alkaline phosphatase

LBD: Lewy body dementia

LDH: lactate dehydrogenase

LDL: low-density lipoprotein

LES: lower esophageal sphincter

LH: luteinizing hormone

LMW: low molecular weight

LOC: loss of consciousness

LP: lumbar puncture

LSIL: low-grade squamous intraepithelial lesion

LTVV: low tidal volume ventilation

LV: left ventricular

LVESD: left ventricular end systolic diameter

M (spike): monoclonal spike

MAC: mycobacterium avium complex

MAI: mycobacterium avium intracellular

MALT: mucosa-associated lymphoid tissue

MAOI: monoamine oxidase inhibitors

MAT: multifocal atrial tachycardia

MCA: middle cerebral artery

MCD: minimal change disease

MCHC: mean corpuscular hemoglobin concentration

MCV: mean corpuscular volume

MDI: metered dose inhaler

MDS: myelodysplastic syndrome

MENII: multiple endocrine neoplasia type II

MGUS: monoclonal gammopathy of undetermined significance

MHA-TP: microhemagglutination assay-Treponema palladium test

MI: myocardial infarction

MIBG: metaiodobenzylguanidine

MMA: methylmalonic acid

MOPP: mustargen, oncovin, procarbazine, prednisone

MPA: microscopic polyangiitis

MRA: magnetic resonance angiography

MRI: magnetic resonance imaging

MRSA: methicillin-resistant *Staphylococcus aureus*

MS: mitral stenosis *or* multiple sclerosis

MUGA: multigated acquisition

MVP: mitral valve prolapse

NASH: nonalcoholic steatohepatitis

NDI: nephrogenic diabetes insipidus

NHL: non-Hodgkin lymphoma

NIPPV: noninvasive positive pressure ventilation

NPH: neutral protamine hagedorn *or* normal pressure hydrocephalus

NPO: *nil per os* (nothing by mouth)

NSAIDs: nonsteroidal antiinflammatory drugs

NSCLC: non-small cell lung cancer

NSTEMI: non-ST segment elevation myocardial infarction

O&P: ova and parasite

OA: osteoarthritis

OI: opportunistic infection

OSA: obstructive sleep apnea

PA: pulmonary artery

PAD: peripheral arterial disease

PAN: polyarteritis nodosa

P-ANCA: perinuclear anti-neutrophil cytoplasmic antibodies

PAS: periodic acid-Schiff

PBC: primary biliary cirrhosis

PCI: percutaneous coronary intervention

PCOS: polycystic ovarian syndrome

PCP: pneumocystis pneumonia

PCR: polymerase chain reaction

PCT: porphyria cutanea tarda

PE: pulmonary embolus

PEA: pulseless electrical activity

PEEP: positive end-expiratory pressure

PEFR: peak expiratory flow rate

PET scan: positron emission tomography scan

PFO: patent foramen ovale

PFT: pulmonary function test(ing)

PID: pelvic inflammatory disease

PIP: proximal interphalangeal joint

PMI: point of maximal impulse

PML: progressive multifocal leukoencephalopathy

PMR: polymyalgia rheumatica

PMS: premenstrual syndrome

PNH: paroxysmal nocturnal hemoglobinuria

PPD: purified protein derivative

PPI: proton pump inhibitors

PR: progesterone receptor

PSA: prostate-specific antigen

PSGN: post-streptococcal glomerulonephritis

PSP: progressive supranuclear palsy

PT: prothrombin time

PTH: parathyroid hormone

PTU: propylthiouracil

PUD: peptic ulcer disease

P. vera: polycythemia vera

RA: rheumatoid arthritis *or* right atrium

RAIU: radioactive iodine uptake

RAST: radioallergosorbent

RBC: red blood cell

RDW: red cell distribution of width

RF: rheumatoid factor

RLS: restless leg syndrome

RMSF: Rocky Mountain spotted fever

RPGN: rapidly progressive glomerulonephritis

RPR: rapid plasma reagin

RTA: renal tubular acidosis

RUQ: right upper quadrant

RV: right ventricular *or* residual volume

SAAG: serum ascites albumin gradient

SABA: short-acting beta agonists

SAH: subarachnoid hemorrhage

SBP: spontaneous bacterial peritonitis

SC (disease): sickle-hemoglobin C disease

SCC: squamous cell carcinoma

SCD: subacute combined degeneration

SCID: severe combined immunodeficiency

SCLC: small cell lung cancer

SERM: selective estrogen receptor modulator

SI: sacroiliac

SIADH: syndrome of inappropriate antidiuretic hormone

SJS: Stevens-Johnson syndrome

SLE: systemic lupus erythematosus

SMA: smooth muscle antibodies

SPEP: serum protein electrophoresis

SRI: serotonin reuptake inhibitors

SS (disease): sickle cell anemia

SSRI: selective serotonin reuptake inhibitor

SSSS: staphylococcal scalded skin syndrome

SSTI: skin and soft tissue infections

STD: sexually transmitted disease

STEMI: ST segment elevation myocardial infarction

SVT: supraventricular tachycardia

TB: tuberculosis

TEE: transesophageal echocardiography

TEN: toxic epidermal necrolysis

TIF: transoral incisionless fundoplication

TIPS: transjugular intrahepatic portosystemic shunt

TLC: total lung capacity

TMG: toxic multinodular goiter

TMP-SMZ: trimethoprim-sulfamethoxazole

TRALI: transfusion-related acute lung injury

TRAP: tartrate resistant acid phosphatase

TRH: thyrotropin releasing hormone

TSH: thyroid-stimulating hormone

TSP: tropical spastic paraparesis

TSS: toxic shock syndrome

TTE: transthroacic echocardiography

TTP: thrombotic thrombocytopenic purpura

UA: urinalysis

UAG: urinary anion gap

UC: ulcerative colitis

USPSTF: United States Preventive Services Task Force

V/Q scan: ventilation/perfusion scan

VAD: vincristine, adriamycin, dexamethasone

VAP: ventilator-associated pneumonia

VATS: video-assisted thoracic surgery

VBG: venous blood gas

VC: vital capacity

VDRL: Venereal Disease Research Laboratory

VEGF: vascular endothelial growth factor

V-fib: ventricular fibrillation

VSD: ventricular septal defect

VT: tidal volume

V-tach: ventricular tachycardia

VWD: von Willebrand disease

VWF: von Willebrand factor

VZIG: varicella zoster immune globulin

VZV: varicella zoster virus

WBC: white blood count

WPW: Wolff-Parkinson-White syndrome

ZES: Zollinger-Ellison syndrome

MNEMONICS

ABCDE: Asymmetric; Borders are uneven; Color changes; Diameter changes; Evolution

CHADS$_2$: Congestive failure (defined as an EF <35%); Hypertension; Age >75; Diabetes mellitus; Stroke (2 points)

CHOP: Cyclophosphamide, Adriamycin, Vincristine (Oncovin), Prednisone

CREST syndrome: Calcinosis, Raynaud, Esophageal dysmotility, Sclerodactyly, Telangiectasia

CURB65: Confusion; Urea (BUN above 20); Respiratory rate >30 per minute; Blood pressure (Systolic <90, diastolic <60); age above 65

DIAPERS: Drugs; Infections; Atrophic vaginitis; Psychiatric or neurologic; Endocrine/metabolic; Restriction of mobility; Stool impaction

HACEK: *Haemophilus parainfluenzae, Aggregatibacter actinomycetemcomitans, Cardiobacterium hominis, Eikenella corrodens, Kingella kingae* (Gram-negative bacterial causes of culture-negative endocarditis)

INDEX